Prevention of Skin Cancer

Cancer Prevention – Cancer Causes

Volume 3

Prevention of Skin Cancer

Edited by

David Hill, Ph.D.
Centre for Behavioural Research in Cancer,
The Cancer Council Victoria, Melbourne, Victoria, Australia

J. Mark Elwood, M.D., D.Sc.
National Cancer Control Initiative,
Melbourne, Victoria, Australia

and

Dallas R. English, Ph.D.
Cancer Epidemiology Centre,
The Cancer Council Victoria, Melbourne, Victoria, Australia

KLUWER ACADEMIC PUBLISHERS
DORDRECHT / BOSTON / LONDON

A C.I.P. Catalogue record for this book is available from the Library of Congress.

ISBN 1-4020-1435-x

Published by Kluwer Academic Publishers,
P.O. Box 17, 3300 AA Dordrecht, The Netherlands.

Sold and distributed in North, Central and South America
by Kluwer Academic Publishers,
101 Philip Drive, Norwell, MA 02061, U.S.A.

In all other countries, sold and distributed
by Kluwer Academic Publishers,
P.O. Box 322, 3300 AH Dordrecht, The Netherlands.

Printed on acid-free paper

Printed in the Netherlands.

Contents

Contributors

We are grateful to our colleagues who contributed to this volume, whose participation makes it a unique contribution to the prevention of skin cancer.

Bruce K. Armstrong M.B., B.S., D.Phil.
Philippe Autier, M.D., M.P.H.
Chris D. Bajdik, Ph.D.
Peter Briss, M.D.
Rob Carter, Grad.Dip.Pop.Health, B.A.(Hons), M.A.S., Ph.D.
Frank R. de Gruijl, Ph.D.
Brian L. Diffey, D.Sc., Ph.D.,
Suzanne Dobbinson, M.Sc., Ph.D.
Richard P. Gallagher, F.A.C.E., M.A.
Peter Gies, Ph.D.
Karen Glanz, M.P.H., Ph.D.
Tim K. Lee, Ph.D
Ronald D.Ley, Ph.D.
Rachel Neale, Ph.D.
Vivienne E. Reeve, Ph.D.
Colin Roy, Ph.D.
Mona Saraiya, M.P.H., M.D.
Gianluca Severi, Ph.D.
Harry Slaper, Ph.D.
Petra Udelhofen, Ph.D. (deceased).
David Whiteman, B.Med.Sc., M.B., B.S.(Hons), Ph.D.

Editors:
David J. Hill, Ph.D.
J. Mark Elwood, M.D., D.Sc.
Dallas R. English, Ph.D.

Acknowledgements

We are deeply grateful to Anne Gibbs for her commitment to this project. She brought a high level of editorial skill and a remarkable ability to master the diverse technical contents of the material in this book to ensure the result was coherent, consistent and of a high quality.

Our thanks to Margaret Byron, whose production skills and computer expertise have contributed greatly to the quality of this volume.

We are grateful to Professor Robin Marks for his advice and input, especially in regard to Chapter 2.

The writing of this book was materially assisted by the opportunity for most of the authors to attend a workshop in Melbourne, Australia. Support for the workshop was provided by the National Cancer Control Initiative, the Australian Government Department of Health and Ageing, and The Cancer Council Victoria.

Preface

Our series Cancer Prevention - Cancer Control continues to address the causes and prevention of cancer. In this volume, Hill, Elwood, and English bring together a rich resource summarizing the state of science underpinning the primary prevention of skin cancer. While skin cancer causes an increasing burden, particularly in populations of European origin, our understanding of the role of sun exposure together with the genetic components of skin cancer continues to grow. Given the emphasis on evidence-based medicine and public health prevention efforts, it is noteworthy that, although we can all access the same evidence base, countries around the world have had remarkably different responses to the application of this knowledge to prevent skin cancer. The outstanding contribution of the Australian public health community to the scientific understanding of skin cancer etiology and the translation of this knowledge into national prevention efforts uniquely positions the editors to compile this volume focused on the primary prevention of skin cancer. In so doing they draw on an international team of authors to present a "state of the science" summary of skin cancer prevention and to identify those areas where uncertainty remains.

To achieve successful prevention of cancer we must translate our scientific knowledge base into effective prevention programs. This book offers the reader keen insights into the depth of our understanding of etiologic pathways for skin cancer. This etiologic science base is complemented by rigorous prevention science placing emphasis on the social context for effective and sustained prevention efforts. Examples set forth in this book are noteworthy for their success in reduction of skin cancer risk, but they will also serve as a model for other cancer prevention programs. This book, like the series in general, should help bring this evidence to the broader prevention community.

Graham A. Colditz, M.D., Dr. P.H.
Editor in Chief
Cancer Causes and Control

Chapter 1

The scope of the book

David J. Hill[1], Ph.D.; J. Mark Elwood[2], M.D., D.Sc.; Dallas R. English[3], Ph.D.
[1]Centre for Behavioural Research in Cancer, The Cancer Council Victoria, Melbourne, Australia; [2]National Cancer Control Initiative, Melbourne, Victoria, Australia; [3]Cancer Epidemiology Centre, The Cancer Council Victoria, Melbourne, Australia

Cancers of the skin are the most commonly occurring cancers in humans. Predominantly found in populations of European origin, the frequency of these cancers and the consequent impact on medical services, as well as their morbidity and mortality, mean that prevention is an important public health issue.

While there are a number of texts that deal comprehensively with clinical aspects of skin cancer, none appears to have brought together the full spectrum of issues relating to primary prevention. Prevention, early detection, and treatment inevitably interrelate in practice. Public information about skin cancer, even if focused on prevention, may also precipitate concern about skin lesions within the target population, leading individuals to present for medical assessment. However, this volume focuses solely on primary prevention.

In some countries the approach to prevention of skin cancer has been largely science-based and well organized, elsewhere it has been very variable. In this book, we present a critical assessment of the current state of the science relating to prevention of skin cancer, and identify the key issues in prevention and the factors that need to be considered when intervention programs are planned. We examine the preventability of skin cancers, the most effective techniques for preventive interventions, and what benefits can be expected from prevention programs.

1

D. Hill et al. (eds.), Prevention of Skin Cancer, 1-2.
© 2004 *Kluwer Academic Publishers. Printed in the Netherlands.*

In focusing on the prevention of skin cancer by the modification of the effects of ultraviolet radiation (UVR), the book provides the basis of sound public health theory and practice. We review the individual risk factors for the three main types of skin cancer. From an examination of the physics and climatology of solar UVR, we describe how UVR is measured and how it is affected by atmospheric factors. We present up to date summaries of the epidemiology and genetics of skin cancers, and critically assess the epidemiological evidence for the relationship between sun exposure and skin cancer. We review results of animal studies that provide a significant understanding of photocarcinogenesis. We identify cross-linkages between molecular, animal, and epidemiological studies on UV-induced skin cancers and discuss current risk models. With this background, we discuss the behavioral considerations in solar and artificial UVR exposure, the efficacy of behavioral interventions to reduce exposure, and the economic impact of preventive programs. The book includes current critical reviews of ozone depletion trends, the use and effects of solaria, and the use and efficacy of sunscreens. The authors are all active researchers who present the latest findings in their areas of study and also discuss the implications that arise from their work for programs to prevent skin cancer.

This book draws together a succinct summary of what is known about the causes of skin cancer, the effectiveness of interventions, and what they can achieve.

Chapter 2

Who gets skin cancer: individual risk factors

J. Mark Elwood, M.D., D.Sc.

National Cancer Control Initiative, Melbourne, Victoria, Australia

Key words: skin cancer, skin type, actinic keratoses, nevi, risk factors

INTRODUCTION

This chapter will describe some pathological and clinical aspects of skin cancer which will be useful in regard to the more detailed material presented later in the book. It will describe the different types of skin cancer and what is known of their cellular origins and precursor lesions. Factors that affect the risk of skin cancer in individuals are described, including skin color and skin type, family history, and a range of other investigated factors.

1. THE BIOLOGY OF SKIN CANCER

Cancers of the skin are the most commonly occurring cancers in humans, and are also common in many mammals including cattle, horses, dogs, and cats. The most common types of cancer occurring in the skin in humans (and the only ones to be addressed in this book) are squamous cell cancer, basal cell cancer, and melanoma.

The skin consists of an outer layer of epidermis, under which lies the basal layer. The epidermis consists of layers of epithelial cells, replaced by proliferation from the deeper layers by division of the basal cells. Cells from

3

D. Hill et al. (eds.), Prevention of Skin Cancer, 3-20.
© 2004 *Kluwer Academic Publishers. Printed in the Netherlands.*

the basal layer migrate towards the surface, as large cells containing keratin; as the cells migrate towards the surface they become flatter, and the nucleus becomes smaller, until the most superficial layers of epidermis are composed of flat cells without nuclei. The basal cells are separated from the dermis by a thin layer of protein material called the basal lamina. Below this is the dermis, connective tissue carrying blood vessels and nerves. The skin contains hair follicles, sebaceous glands, and eccrine and apocrine glands (sweat glands).

Basal cell and squamous cell cancers

These two tumors together, and perhaps including rarer types, are often grouped as "non-melanoma skin cancer" or NMSC. While ideally they should be treated as separate diseases, as there are major differences in their etiology, natural history, and treatment, they are grouped together in much of the literature, so the general term is useful when more specific information is not available.

Basal cell carcinomas (BCC) originate from cells in the basal layer of the epidermis, and some but not all authorities regard the cells of origin as non-keratinizing. They may also arise from cells in hair follicles or sebaceous glands. BCCs are a feature of a number of rare inherited conditions, including the nevoid basal cell carcinoma syndrome. BCCs invade locally, and complications can ensue from local spread. The tumor spreads through tissues following a path of least resistance, and higher recurrence rates have been noted for tumors involving the eyelid, nose and scalp. Metastatic spread, while extremely rare, does occur. BCCs are normally curable, with five and 10-year survival rates on large series of patients being nearly 100%. Several clinical and pathological sub-types are recognized which may vary in their biological aggressiveness, but differences in etiology between sub-types have not been described.

Squamous cell cancers (SCC) arise from the keratinocytes in the basal layer of the epidermis. The tumors grow slowly. In Australia in 1995 there were about 190,000 people treated for basal cell cancer, and 80,000 for squamous cell cancer [1]; there were about 330 deaths ascribed to these two diseases combined, suggesting an overall mortality of only 0.1%. However, if they have invaded into the dermis, they may recur after treatment, and they can metastasize, commonly to regional lymph nodes and to more distant sites. For squamous cell cancers the worst prognosis lesions tend to be on the lip, ear, and the scalp in men (Marks, R., personal communication) [2]. Metastatic spread is more likely if there is immunosuppression or corticosteroid therapy. A poor outcome with these tumors is often related to patient delay and an isolated or unconventional lifestyle.

Both BCC and SCC may recur, although the risk of recurrence is low. Also patients have a high risk of developing a further primary skin tumor, with follow-up studies showing rates of incidence of new primaries of 20 to 50% within five years. These are presumably due to the same etiological factors, predominantly sun exposure, which caused the first primary. Both BCC and SCC are usually treated surgically, by excision, curettage, or electrosurgery, or by Mohs micrographic surgery which is particularly useful for tumors in difficult sites such as the face. Radiotherapy can also be effective and is used mainly for older patients with extensive lesions. Cryosurgery and ablation by lasers has also been used [3,4]. Treatment by destructive means such as ablations or curettage in the absence of biopsy is not recommended as standard treatment, but does occur. Imiquimod applied topically is an immune modulator, inducing interferon alpha and interleukin 12. It has shown success in treatment of superficial BCC, actinic keratoses, and Bowen's disease (SCC in situ) [5,6].

The frequency of multiple lesions, new primaries and recurrences, added to the ease of treatment without necessarily having pathological confirmation, and the high frequency of the condition makes routine registration of these cancers something undertaken only by a few registries. Therefore obtaining accurate information on incidence is difficult, as discussed in Chapter 5.

Melanoma

Melanoma is a tumor of melanocytes, which are derived from the embryonic neural crest. Melanoma may arise in or close to a nevus or distinct from it, and usually begins with a radial or horizontal growth phase, where the lesion remains confined to the epidermis. Growth involving extension downward from the epidermis, the vertical growth phase, may result in a visible nodule on the skin surface. Melanomas with an adjacent intra-epidermal component are referred to as superficial spreading or lentiginous type melanomas, which include lentigo maligna, acral, and mucosal melanomas. Melanoma may develop without such an epidermal component, classified as nodular melanoma.

Melanoma is usually diagnosed before any spread beyond the primary site is clinically apparent, and such stage 1 melanoma has an overall 10-year survival rate of around 85%, in comparison to melanoma with nodal or distant metastasis which has a 10-year survival of 30% or less. Within stage 1 tumors, the outcome depends critically on the depth of the lesion, measured by Breslow's method, and ten year survival rates vary from well over 90% for tumors less than 0.76 mm deep to less than 50% for tumors thicker than 4mm [7]. Other prognostic variables are the presence of ulceration of the primary tumor; the anatomical site, with tumors on the limbs having a better prognosis; and gender, female patients having a better prognosis even when other factors are taken into consideration [8].

Treatment is by excision of the primary lesion. There has been considerable controversy about the effect of removing the draining lymph nodes. There have been many trials of adjuvant therapies with chemotherapy, non-specific immunotherapy, and levamisole, mostly with unclear results on survival. Imiquimod (see above) has shown some success in the treatment of lentigo maligna lesions [9].

Patients with melanoma are at increased risk of a subsequent primary. A Swedish registry based study showed relative risks of subsequent melanoma compared to the general population of 10 in males and 8.6 in females [10], and risks of 3.6 and 2.4 respectively for non-melanoma skin cancer. In Australia the absolute risk of a second primary was 4.5% within five years – higher in males, with evidence of some concordance by body site [11].

Other skin cancers

There are many much rarer types of skin cancer, and in addition cancers originating in other sites can spread or metastasize to the skin. Merkel cell carcinoma arises in cells of neuroendocrine origin in the basal layer, and has been associated with ultraviolet exposure and immunosuppression. Some of these other rare skin cancers have been associated with ultraviolet exposure, immunosuppression, or genetic syndromes, and Kaposi's sarcoma has become more common with the increase in HIV [12].

2.   RISK FACTORS FOR SKIN CANCER IN INDIVIDUALS

The cause of the great majority of skin cancers in pale skinned subjects is a combination of the effects of one predominant environmental physical factor, ultraviolet radiation, and characteristics that determine the response of the body to that radiation. The details of the relationship with ultraviolet radiation and the mechanism are different for SCC, BCC, and for melanoma, as discussed in Chapter 6. Unlike melanoma, the relationship for NMSC has many analogies in experimental animals, and the quantitative relationships of exposure to cancer occurrence have been established with great precision in experimental situations, as shown in Chapter 10. The other etiological factors for the major types of skin cancer frequently differ, and so will be described for melanoma and for non-melanoma skin cancer (NMSC) separately.

3.   PRECURSOR LESIONS AND DERMATOLOGICAL RISK FACTORS

3.1   SCC - actinic keratoses

Actinic or solar keratoses are recognized as precursor lesions for SCC [13], and SCC in situ is often called Bowen's disease. The progression rate of actinic keratoses has been estimated as around 1 per 1000 per year, and about 25% regress each year [14,15]. Actinic keratoses themselves are associated with cumulative sunlight exposure and the same skin characteristics as confer a high risk of skin cancers, and can be prevented by sunscreens. There is no known precursor lesion for BCC.

3.2   Melanoma – nevi

Nevi are benign focal proliferations of differentiated melanocytes, and have been studied in great detail since the major studies in the 1980s showed them to be a very strong predictor of melanoma. Studies using various counting methods and size classifications have consistently shown an increased risk of melanoma in association with an increased number of nevi. Categorization by size of nevus, or calculation of total nevus density rather than number, does not produce consistently different associations. Strong associations have been seen in complex studies which employ full body examinations by dermatologists, but also with very simple measures, such as a count of nevi over a certain size on a single site such as the arm or back, or even self report of total or site-limited nevus counts [16-18].

Atypical nevi show clinically recognized features that indicate histological dysplasia, although the correlation, as with common nevi, between clinical and pathological findings is variable [19]. Some studies suggest a stronger association of melanoma risk with number of atypical nevi than with the number of ordinary nevi, but as the categorizations and reference groups differ, it is difficult to compare studies. Studies which have assessed both, with mutual adjustment, have usually shown that both are independent risk factors for melanoma [20-22].

In general the factors associated with melanoma are also associated with nevi, suggesting that ultraviolet or solar radiation is a major cause of nevi [23]. Nevi develop from birth and increase in number to adolescence, with higher numbers in males. The much higher rate of development of nevi in Australian than in Scottish children [24] suggests that sun exposure has a dominant effect even very early in life, and that the number of nevi in adult life may be determined by early sun exposure. There is a higher prevalence of both common and of atypical nevi in children at lower latitude within Australia [25]. The numbers generally decrease with increasing age in adult populations, which could be due to a true decrease with increasing age in adults, or a birth cohort effect, with older people having fewer nevi because of their different lifetime experience of factors such as sun exposure.

In children, the highest nevus densities tend to be on the face, back, shoulders, and the lateral surface of the arms; the legs have a low density [26,27]. The site distribution of melanoma in childhood in Australia was similar to the distribution of nevi [28], but the site distribution of adult melanoma is different, particularly the high rate on the female leg. Nevi in different body sites must vary in their susceptibility to malignant change; this variation might depend on acquired resistance to ultraviolet radiation, or on other features [26,29].

Nevi are also a risk factor for BCC [30]. Studies of the prevention of nevi are discussed in Chapter 8.

3.3   Skin, hair and eye color, and "skin type"

Melanoma

Skin characteristics are important in determining the response to ultraviolet radiation. Cutaneous melanoma occurs much more commonly in light skinned ethnic groups, being least common in deeply pigmented groups, and of intermediate frequency in ethnic groups with intermediate skin tones, such as those characteristic of Eastern Asia. Within European origin populations, most studies show modest but consistent increases in risk of melanoma in association with light or red hair color, blue eye color, and high degrees of freckling [31]. While the first studies were mainly in British and northern European origin groups, these associations have also been seen in Italy [32] and Israel [33]. Most of these associations are moderate in strength, with relative risks of between 2 and 4 in lightly pigmented rather than darkly pigmented subjects. A strongly correlated factor is that people whose skin tends to burn easily and tan poorly have a greater risk of melanoma. "Skin type" is usually described as a four point scale from 1 "Always burn, never tan" to 4 "Rarely burn, tan easily" but definitions differ considerably [34,35].

NMSC

The pigmentation factors which give rise to high risk of melanoma also relate to a high risk of NMSC, with light hair, skin and eye color, and poor ability to tan being risk factors, usually with risks in the 2-4 range [36,37]. Albinism, where pigmentation is greatly reduced, increases NMSC risk.

4. FAMILY HISTORY AND GENETICS

Melanoma

A small proportion of melanomas occurs in individuals with a very strong family history of melanoma, and a family or personal history of dysplastic nevi. Investigations of such families have identified several relevant genes [38,39], as discussed in Chapter 7. This section will deal only with the empiric risk associated with a family history of melanoma. In a meta-analysis of eight case-control studies including about 3000 patients, the relative risk associated with having one affected first degree relative was 2.2, and this was consistent in studies from a wide range of latitudes [40]. This association is independent of the associations with eye and hair color, nevi, and freckling. There is no clear relationship between having a positive family history and the age at onset or body site of the melanoma in the index case [41]. In contrast, studies of extremely high-risk families show a younger age at onset. As with other common cancers, specific genetic linkages only apply to a minority of cases with a positive family history. A large study in Australia showed that 45% of positive family histories could not be confirmed on more detailed inquiry [42,43]. The method of verifying family histories may influence the strength of the associations seen [44].

Both melanoma and NMSC are increased in patients with xeroderma pigmentosum, a genetic condition with reduced ability to repair DNA damage. The relative risk of melanoma in subjects under age 20 is over 1000, and the site distribution of the melanomas is different from the general population [45]. This is discussed further in Chapter 7.

NMSC

Apart from xeroderma pigmentosum, several hereditary diseases predispose to NMSC primarily by increasing susceptibility to the effects of ultraviolet radiation, such as nevoid basal cell carcinoma syndrome. These are discussed in Chapter 7.

5.   OTHER RISK FACTORS

5.1   Hormonal factors

Melanoma

In many countries, melanoma incidence is higher in women than in men at ages 20-49, whereas above these ages incidence is higher in men. In a large study using record linkage techniques in Sweden [46] the risk of melanoma increased with increasing age at first birth, and decreased with increasing parity. Some, but not all, other studies have shown protective effects of high parity, or an increased risk with late age at first birth [46,47]. There has been no consistent relationship observed with age at menarche, or with a prior oophorectomy [48]. These inconsistent relationships may be still confounded by sun exposure, despite the methods used in some studies to adjust for sun exposure.

Particular attention has been paid to oral contraceptive use; a meta-analysis of studies up to 1996 showed no association with ever-use, and only a modest increase in risk with long term use, which could be due to confounding by sun exposure [48], or affected by increased surveillance of contraceptive users [49]. In pre-menopausal women in the US Nurses' Health Study, current use was associated with a relative risk of 2.0, and risk was further increased with many years of use, but was not elevated amongst past users [50]. But overall there is no clear association with oral contraceptive use. Similarly there is no clear association with the use of estrogen therapy, with some studies reporting increased risks, but others finding no association [48].

5.2   Diet and chemoprevention

Melanoma

In a cohort study in Norway, melanoma risk in women was increased with higher intakes of polyunsaturated fats and with cod liver oil supplementation, but decreased in association with coffee drinking; but no corresponding associations were found in men, confounding by sun exposure could not be taken into account [51], and no consistent association with dietary intake of polyunsaturated fat was found in several case-control studies. Apparent protective effects of vitamin E, beta-carotene, or zinc intake have been seen in some studies [52], although serum zinc levels have been reported to be increased in melanoma patients [53]. Vitamin D intake showed no associations [54].

Most studies have shown no associations with consumption of alcohol, coffee or tea. A modest positive association with body mass index has been found [55]; and risk was found to be associated with obesity and natural menopause in one study [56]. It is an interesting point whether the risk of melanoma should be computed per unit area of skin in regard to these associations.

NMSC

There have been studies reporting a reduced risk of NMSC with low fat diets or diets with enhanced micronutrients, but the results have been somewhat inconsistent. One study reports a protective effect of citrus peel consumption, but no association with citrus fruit or juice [57].

Non-melanoma skin cancer is one of the most extensively studied areas in chemoprevention, because early skin lesions are easily accessible for analysis. Much attention has focused on retinoids, derivatives of retinol (vitamin A), in which some experimental results suggest a protective effect. However, in larger studies, a double blind trial of oral beta-carotene in people with previous NMSC showed no effect on the prevention of tumor recurrence over five years [58], and a randomized trial of isotretinoin in patients with a previous BCC showed no preventive effects but substantial toxicity [59]. A randomized trial of selenium supplements in NMSC patients showed no reduction in subsequent NMSC incidence despite encouraging results from previous case control studies, although a reduction in total cancer incidence and in prostate cancer was observed [60].

5.3   Smoking

The major case control studies have not shown associations of melanoma with smoking, and a Dutch case control study showing an association between tobacco smoking and SCC showed no association with melanoma or with BCC [61]. An increase in SCC was seen with current smoking (relative risk 1.5) in a cohort study of nurses [62], and in two earlier studies; no excess of BCC was found [63].

5.4   Prescribed drugs

While no consistent associations have been reported, a reduction in risk of melanoma was seen in association with the use of non-steroidal anti-inflammatory drugs such as aspirin and ibuprofen, adjusted for sun exposure [64].

5.5   PUVA treatment

Psoralens given orally and combined with ultraviolet A radiation
(PUVA) is an effective treatment for psoriasis and other skin conditions
[65]. Follow-up studies in Europe and North America have shown a great
increase in SCC after PUVA treatment, with relative risks compared to the
general population of up to 10 [66,67]. However, no excess of SCC was
reported in nearly 1000 European patients treated with ultraviolet A and a
trioxsalen bath, rather than oral therapy, with an average follow-up time of
15 years [68]. Most studies show no increased risk of BCC, or an increase
only in patients with very high numbers of treatments [66].

Most early studies did not show any increased risk of melanoma, but in a
series of 1380 patients first treated with PUVA between 1975 and 1976,
follow up of more than 20 years has shown a relative incidence of melanoma
of 8.4, the excess beginning 15 years after first exposure and being greater
with longer follow up and with higher dosages of PUVA [69].

5.6   Infections, immunosuppression, and other cancers

In a large case-control study in Europe and Israel, a negative association
was found between melanoma and previous infectious disease [70].
However, other studies have shown no associations with infections.

NMSC is greatly increased in subjects with epidermodysplasia
verruciformis, which is associated with HPV (human papilloma virus)
infection, the tumors occurring in sun exposed skin [71]. HPV sequences
have been found in SCC and BCC specimens from both immunosuppressed
and normal patients [72-74]. A study of 12 patients with advanced
melanoma showed that seven were positive for HPV, and these patients had
a worse prognosis [75].

The risk of SCC, and to a lesser extent BCC, is greatly increased amongst
organ transplant patients with immunosuppression produced by drugs, and
the tumors occur primarily on exposed areas and are probably related to
ultraviolet exposure [2,76]. However, infectious agents such as HPV may
also be relevant. Patients with PUVA treatment had a further increased risk
of SCC if they had therapy with ciclosporin, an immunosuppressant [77].
Melanoma is increased in patients who have received renal transplantation.
In a study of 38 children with renal allograft transplantation, the total body
nevus count was increased, and the count was positively associated with
duration of immunosuppression [78]. Both melanoma and NMSC have been
shown to be increased in patients with sarcoidosis, a chronic disease of
unknown etiology characterized by exaggerated immunological responses
[79].

Follow up of patients with non-Hodgkin's lymphoma or chronic lymphocytic leukemia has shown significantly elevated risks of SCC (relative risks 5.5 and 8.6) and of melanoma (relative risks 2.4 and 3.1 respectively). Follow up of SCC patients showed a significantly elevated risk of lymphomas and leukemias [80]. Excesses of many other cancers after NMSC have been found [81,82].

5.7 Trauma

Squamous cell cancers can arise as a complication of skin trauma, for example from burns and scars or chronic infection, particularly seen in developing countries. SCC has been reported in scars from tuberculosis, leprosy, and injuries. The kangri cancer of the skin described in Kashmir affects the lower abdomen and thighs and is due to contact with clay pots containing burning charcoal; somewhat similar cancers have been reported in Japan and China [83].

5.8 Ionizing radiation, chemicals, and occupation

Excess risks of NMSC have been described in association with ionizing radiation since early in the 20th century, occurring amongst radiologists, uranium miners, and atomic bomb survivors. The risk of NMSC has been elevated in patients after treatment by x-ray therapy for enlargement of the thymus gland in infancy, tinea capitis of the scalp, and various other diseases. Overall, there appears to be a linear dose-response relationship, and there is consistency with induction of skin cancers by ionizing radiation in laboratory animals [84]. Prior radiation therapy increased the risk of BCC but not SCC [85].

Detailed investigations have been made of an apparent excess of melanomas at the Lawrence Livermore nuclear laboratory in the US. There was evidence of surveillance bias [86], but associations with exposures to chemicals, high explosives, photographic chemicals, and ionizing radiation were seen [87]. In contrast, there was no excess of melanoma at the Los Alamos nuclear laboratory with likely similar exposures [88].

Many earlier studies, particularly in Europe, have shown that NMSC, unlike melanoma, is increased in long-term outdoor workers. However, recent studies in Australia and Sweden do not show any excess in outdoor workers, perhaps due to self-selection in terms of skin susceptibility [89,90]. A meta-analysis of studies of farmers showed no excess of skin cancers, but a modest excess of lip cancer, relative risk 2.0 [91].

Non-melanoma skin cancer of the scrotum was described in 1775 in chimney sweeps in Britain, and is generally regarded as the first reported environmental cancer [92]. Since then, many chemicals have been associated with skin cancers, including polycyclic aromatic hydrocarbons, which occur in soot, coal tars, asphalt, and lubricating and cutting oils, giving increases in skin cancer amongst workers exposed to machine tools, and many other groups. Skin cancers along with squamous cell carcinomas of the lung occur in workers exposed to coal gas and tar, and amongst roofers and foundry workers [83].

Arsenic increases the risk of both squamous and basal cell tumors, often in association with hyperpigmentation and keratoses [93]. Arsenic exposure is encountered in the manufacturing of paints, insecticides, and herbicides, and smelting of mineral ores, and exposure can occur by drinking water or medicinal agents such as Fowler's solution, used in the past to treat many conditions including psoriasis and asthma. Arsenic in water supplies has been related to NMSC in Taiwan and Mexico [94], although a study of toenail arsenic concentrations of NMSC patients and controls in the US showed no association [95].

Studies of occupational factors in melanoma are difficult to interpret because few such studies have the ability to control for sun exposure, which may vary considerably between occupational groups. There have been several reports of increased risks of melanoma in connection with many industries, involving the petrochemical, rubber products, and electronics industries, and exposure to compounds such as vinyl chloride and polychlorinated biphenyls [87]. Many of these associations are confounded by the positive socioeconomic gradient of melanoma; high socioeconomic groups such as professional engineers may have higher rates of melanoma for this reason. No specific occupational exposure association has been consistently observed in studies that have the ability to control for the effects of socioeconomic status and of sun exposure.

CONCLUSIONS

Skin cancers are produced by a predominant environmental agent, sun exposure, the effects of which are modified by the biological characteristics of skin including its color and its ability to evoke protective mechanisms against the effects of sun exposure. The three main types of skin cancer – squamous cell carcinoma, basal cell carcinoma, and melanoma – all share these features although the details of the relationships with both sun exposure and host factors differ. A wide range of other factors has been assessed in regard to causes of skin cancer. The established causal factors are sun exposure, ultraviolet radiation from other sources, skin characteristics (including pigmentation), and reaction to sun, family history and genetics, immunosuppression, ionizing radiation, and chemicals including hydrocarbons in soot and arsenic. No clear relationships have been seen with smoking, diet, hormonal factors, or drugs.

SUMMARY POINTS

- There are three main types of skin cancer: squamous cell carcinoma, basal cell carcinoma, and melanoma. Basal and squamous cell carcinomas are extremely common but cause very few deaths. The prognosis in melanoma depends primarily on the thickness of the primary tumor.
- Most skin cancers are treated by surgical removal, with a wide range of other treatments for selected cases.
- Squamous cell cancers and melanoma are related to, respectively, actinic keratoses and nevi, which share the distributional characteristics of these tumors. Basal cell cancer has no recognized precursor lesion.
- All three types of skin cancer are more common in light skinned and lightly pigmented individuals, and those who burn easily and tan poorly on sun exposure.
- A positive family history confers a modest increased risk of melanoma, with a small proportion of patients having linkage to particular genetic alleles. Skin cancers are increased with several rare genetic abnormalities, including xeroderma pigmentosum.
- Hormonal factors, diet, and smoking have no clear relationship with skin cancers.
- Melanoma and squamous cell cancer are increased after treatments with psolarens combined with ultraviolet A radiation (PUVA).
- Skin cancers are increased in immunosuppressed patients, and there are indications of links to infectious agents such as human papilloma virus.
- Chronic trauma, ionizing radiation, and chemicals including hydrocarbons in soot and arsenic have been associated primarily with squamous or basal cell cancers.

IMPLICATIONS FOR PUBLIC HEALTH

The range of individual susceptibilities to skin cancers is very wide. These are diseases of lightly skinned individuals, and subjects with darker natural skin color are at much lower risk. Preventive programs targeted to the more susceptible population groups may be inappropriate or irrelevant for other groups.

The main modifiable causal factor is sun exposure, and a range of approaches, described later in this book, should minimize excessive exposure. Exposure to artificial ultraviolet sources should be controlled.

These diseases are increased in individuals with rare genetic conditions or unusual exposures, such as patients with xeroderma pigmentosum, or patients who have received artificial immunosuppressants. Such individuals may need specifically tailored surveillance and preventive programs.

REFERENCES

1. Staples M, Marks R, Giles G (1998) Trends in the incidence of non-melanocytic skin cancer (NMSC) treated in Australia 1985-1995: are primary prevention programs starting to have an effect? *Int J Cancer* **78**: 144-148.
2. Koh HK, Lew RA, Geller AC *et al.* (2002) Skin cancer: prevention and control. In: Greenwald P, Kramer BS, Weed DL, eds. *Cancer Prevention and Control*. New York: Marcel Dekker Inc., pp. 611-640.
3. American Academy of Dermatology Committee on Guidelines of Care, Drake LA, Ceilley RI *et al.* (1992) Guidelines of care for basal cell carcinoma. *J Am Acad Dermatol* **26**: 117-120.
4. American Academy of Dermatology Committee on Guidelines of Care (1993) Guidelines of care for cutaneous squamous cell carcinoma. *J Am Acad Dermatol* **28**: 628-631.
5. Marks R, Gebauer K, Shumack S *et al.* (2001) Imiquimod 5% cream in the treatment of superficial basal cell carcinoma: results of a multicenter 6-week dose-response trial. *J Am Acad Dermatol.* **44**: 807-813.
6. Stockfleth E, Meyer T, Benninghoff B *et al.* (2001) Successful treatment of actinic keratosis with imiquimod cream 5%: a report of six cases. *Br J Dermatol* **144**: 1050-1053.
7. Soong S, Weiss HL (1998) Predicting outcome in patients with localized melanoma. In: Balch CM, Houghton AN, Sober AJ, Soong S, eds. *Cutaneous Melanoma.* St. Louis, Missouri: Quality Medical Publishing Inc., pp. 51-79.
8. Balch CM, Buzaid AC, Atkins MB *et al.* (2000) A new American joint committee on cancer staging system for cutaneous melanoma. *Cancer* **88**: 1484-1491.
9. Ahmed I, Berth-Jones J (2000) Imiquimod: a novel treatment for lentigo maligna. *Br J Dermatol* **143**: 843-845.
10. Wassberg C, Thorn M, Yuen J *et al.* (1996) Second primary cancers in patients with cutaneous malignant melanoma: a population-based study in Sweden. *Br J Cancer* **73**: 255-259.
11. Giles G, Staples M, McCredie M *et al.* (1995) Multiple primary melanomas: an analysis of cancer registry data from Victoria and New South Wales. *Melanoma Res* **5**: 433-438.
12. Brash DE, Bale AE (2001) Cancer of the skin. In: De Vita VT, Jr., Hellman S, and Rosenberg SA, eds. *Cancer: principles and practice of oncology*. Philadelpia: Lippincott Williams and Wilkins, pp. 1971-1975.
13. Brash DE, Ponten J (1998) Skin precancer. *Cancer Surv* **32**: 69-113.
14. Marks R, Foley P, Goodman G *et al.* (1986) Spontaneous remission of solar keratoses: the case for conservative management. *Br J Dermatol* **115**: 649-655.

15. Dodson JM, DeSpain J, Hewett JE *et al.* (1991) Malignant potential of actinic keratoses and the controversy over treatment. A patient-oriented perspective. *Arch Dermatol* **127**: 1029-1031.
16. Skender-Kalnenas TM, English DR, Heenan PJ (1995) Benign melanocytic lesions: risk markers or precursors of cutaneous melanoma? *J Am Acad Dermatol* **33**: 780-785.
17. Armstrong BK, English DR (1988) The epidemiology of acquired melanocytic naevi and their relationship to malignant melanoma. In: Elwood JM ed. *Melanoma and Naevi, Pigment Cell, Vol.9.* Basle: Karger, pp. 27-47.
18. Barnhill RL, Mihm CM Jr (2002) Histopathology and precursor lesions. In: Balch CM, Houghton AN, Sober AJ, Soong S, eds. *Cutaneous Melanoma.* St. Louis, Missouri: Quality Medical Publishing Inc., pp. 103-133
19. Grob JJ, Andrac L, Romano MH *et al.* (1988) Dysplastic naevus in non-familial melanoma. A clinicopathological study of 101 cases. *Br J Dermatol* **118**: 745-752.
20. Carli P, Biggeri A, Nardini P *et al.* (1998) Sun exposure and large numbers of common and atypical melanocytic naevi: an analytical study in a southern European population. *Br J Dermatol* **138**: 422-425.
21. Garbe C, Buttner P, Weiss J *et al.* (1994) Risk factors for developing cutaneous melanoma and criteria for identifying persons at risk: multicentre case-control study of the Central Malignant Melanoma Registry of the German Dermatological Society. *J Invest Dermatol* **102**: 695-699.
22. Schneider JS, Moore DH, Sagebiel RW (1994) Risk factors for melanoma incidence in prospective follow-up. The importance of atypical (dysplastic) nevi. *Arch Dermatol* **130**: 1002-1007.
23. Green A, Swerdlow AJ (1989) Epidemiology of melanocytic nevi. *Epidemiol Rev* **11**: 204-221.
24. Harrison SL, MacKie RM, MacLennan R (2000) Development of melanocytic nevi in the first three years of life. *J Natl Cancer Inst* **92**: 1436-1438.
25. Kelly JW, Rivers JK, MacLennan R *et al.* (1994) Sunlight: A major factor associated with the development of melanocytic nevi in Australian schoolchildren. *J Am Acad Dermatol.* **30**: 40-48.
26. Autier P, Boniol M, Severi G *et al.* (2001) The body site distribution of melanocytic naevi in 6-7 year old European children. *Melanoma Res* **11**: 123-131.
27. Harrison SL, Buettner PG, MacLennan R (1999) Body-site distribution of melanocytic nevi in young Australian children. *Arch Dermatol* **135**: 47-52.
28. Whiteman DC, Valery P, McWhirter W *et al.* (1997) Risk factors for childhood melanoma in Queensland, Australia. *Int. J Cancer* **70**: 26-31.
29. Green A (1992) A theory of site distribution of melanomas: Queensland, Australia. *Cancer Causes Control* **3**: 513-516.
30. Lock-Andersen J, Drzewiecki KT, Wulf HC (1999) Naevi as a risk factor for basal cell carcinoma in Caucasians: a Danish case-control study. *Acta Derm Venereol* **79**: 314-319.
31. Bliss JM, Ford D, Swerdlow AJ *et al.* (1995) Risk of cutaneous melanoma associated with pigmentation characteristics and freckling: systematic overview of 10 case-control studies. *Int J Cancer* **62**: 367-376.
32. Naldi L, Lorenzo IG, Parazzini F *et al.* (2000) Pigmentary traits, modalities of sun reaction, history of sunburns, and melanocytic nevi as risk factors for cutaneous malignant melanoma in the Italian population: results of a collaborative case-control study. *Cancer* **88**: 2703-2710.
33. Tabenkin H, Tamir A, Sperber AD *et al.* (1999) A case-control study of malignant melanoma in Israeli kibbutzim. *Isr Med Assoc J* **1**: 154-157.

34. Stern RS, Momtaz K (1984) Skin typing for assessment of skin cancer risk and acute response to UV-B and oral methoxsalen photochemotherapy. *Arch Dermatol* **120**: 869-873.
35. Weinstock MA (1992) Assessment of sun sensitivity by questionnaire: validity of items and formulation of a prediction rule. *J Clin Epidemiol* **45**: 547-552.
36. Green A, Battistutta D (1990) Incidence and determinants of skin cancer in a high-risk Australian population. *Int J Cancer* **46**: 356-361.
37. van Dam RM, Huang Z, Rimm EB *et al.* (1999) Risk factors for basal cell carcinoma of the skin in men: results from the health professionals follow-up study. *Am J Epidemiol* **150**: 459-468.
38. Greene MH (1999) The genetics of hereditary melanoma and nevi. 1998 update. *Cancer* **86**: 2464-2477.
39. Hayward N (2000) New developments in melanoma genetics. *Curr Oncol Rep* **2**: 300-306.
40. Ford D, Bliss JM, Swerdlow AJ *et al.* (1995) Risk of cutaneous melanoma associated with a family history of the disease. *Int. J Cancer* **62**: 377-381.
41. Greene MH, Clark WH Jr., Tucker MA *et al.* (1985) High risk of malignant melanoma in melanoma-prone families with dysplastic nevi. *Ann Intern Med* **102**: 458-465.
42. Aitken JF, Youl P, Green A *et al.* (1996) Accuracy of case-reported family history of melanoma in Queensland, Australia. *Melanoma Res* **6**: 313-317.
43. Aitken JF, Green AC, MacLennan R *et al.* (1996) The Queensland Familial Melanoma Project: study design and characteristics of participants. *Melanoma Res* **6**: 155-165.
44. Weinstock MA, Brodsky GL (1998) Bias in the assessment of family history of melanoma and its association with dysplastic nevi in a case-control study. *J Clin Epidemiol* **51**: 1299-1303.
45. Kraemer KH, Lee MM, Andrews AD *et al.* (1994) The role of sunlight and DNA repair in melanoma and nonmelanoma skin cancer. The xeroderma pigmentosum paradigm. *Arch Dermatol* **130**: 1018-1021.
46. Lambe M, Thörn M, Sparén P *et al.* (1996) Malignant melanoma: reduced risk associated with early childbearing and multiparity. *Melanoma Res* **6**: 147-153.
47. Gallagher RP, Elwood JM, Hill GB *et al.* (1985) Reproductive factors, oral contraceptives and risk of malignant melanoma: Western Canada melanoma study. *Br J Cancer* **52**: 891-907.
48. Armstrong BK, English DR (1996) Cutaneous malignant melanoma. In: Schottenfeld D, Fraumeni, JF Jr, eds. *Cancer epidemiology and prevention.* New York: Oxford University Press, pp. 1282-1312.
49. Palmer JR, Rosenberg L, Strom BL *et al.* (1992) Oral contraceptive use and risk of cutaneous malignant melanoma. *Cancer Causes Control* **3**: 547-554.
50. Feskanich D, Hunter DJ, Willett WC *et al.* (1999) Oral contraceptive use and risk of melanoma in premenopausal women. *Br J Cancer* **81**: 918-923.
51. Veierod MB, Thelle DS, Laake P (1997) Diet and risk of cutaneous malignant melanoma: a prospective study of 50,757 Norwegian men and women. *Int. J Cancer* **71**: 600-604.
52. Kirkpatrick CS, White E, Lee JAH (1994) Case-control study of malignant melanoma in Washington State. 2. Diet, alcohol, and obesity. *Am J Epidemiol* **139**: 869-880.
53. Ros-Bullón MR, Sánchez-Pedreño P, Martínez-Liarte JH (1998) Serum zinc levels are increased in melanoma patients. *Melanoma Res* **8**: 273-277.
54. Weinstock MA, Stampfer MJ, Lew RA *et al.* (1992) Case-control study of melanoma and dietary vitamin D: implications for advocacy of sun protection and sunscreen use. *J Invest Dermatol* **98**: 809-811.

55. Thune I, Olsen A, Albrektsen G *et al.* (1993) Cutaneous malignant melanoma: association with height, weight and body-surface area. A prospective study in Norway. *Int J Cancer* **55**: 555-561.
56. Smith MA, Fine JA, Barnhill RL *et al.* (1998) Hormonal and reproductive influences and risk of melanoma in women. *Int J Epidemiol* **27**: 751-757.
57. Hakim IA, Harris RB, Ritenbaugh C (2000) Citrus peel use is associated with reduced risk of squamous cell carcinoma of the skin. *Nutr Cancer* **37**: 161-168.
58. Greenberg ER, Baron JA, Stukel TA *et al.* (1990) A clinical trial of beta carotene to prevent basal-cell and squamous-cell cancers of the skin. The Skin Cancer Prevention Study Group. *N Engl J Med* **323**: 789-795.
59. Tangrea JA, Edwards BK, Taylor PR *et al.* (1992) Long-term therapy with low-dose isotretinoin for prevention of basal cell carcinoma: a multicenter clinical trial. Isotretinoin-Basal Cell Carcinoma Study Group. *J Natl Cancer Inst* **84**: 328-332.
60. Clark LC, Combs GF, Jr., Turnbull BW *et al.* (1996) Effects of selenium supplementation for cancer prevention in patients with carcinoma of the skin. A randomized controlled trial. Nutritional Prevention of Cancer Study Group. *JAMA* **276**: 1957-1963.
61. De Hertog SA, Wensveen CA, Bastiaens MT *et al.* (2001) Relation between smoking and skin cancer. *J Clin Oncol* **19**: 231-238.
62. Grodstein F, Speizer FE, Hunter DJ (1995) A prospective study of incident squamous cell carcinoma of the skin in the Nurses' Health Study. *J Natl Cancer Inst* **87**: 1061-1066.
63. Hunter DJ, Colditz GA, Stampfer MJ *et al.* (1990) Risk factors for basal cell carcinoma in a prospective cohort of women. *Ann Epidemiol* **1**: 13-23.
64. Harris RE, Beebe-Donk J, Namboodiri KK (2001) Inverse association of non-steroidal anti-inflammatory drugs and malignant melanoma among women. *Oncol Rep* **8**: 655-657.
65. Halpern SM, Anstey AV, Dawe RS *et al.* (2000) Guidelines for topical PUVA: a report of a workshop of the British photodermatology group. *Br J Dermatol* **142**: 22-31.
66. Stern RS, Liebman EJ, Väkevä L *et al.* (1998) Oral psoralen and ultraviolet-A light (PUVA) treatment of psoriasis and persistent risk of nonmelanoma skin cancer. *J Natl Cancer Inst* **90**: 1278-1284.
67. Lindelof B, Sigurgeirsson B, Tegner E *et al.* (1999) PUVA and cancer risk: the Swedish follow-up study. *Br J Dermatol* **141**: 108-112.
68. Hannuksela-Svahn A, Sigurgeirsson B, Pukkala E *et al.* (1999) Trioxsalen bath PUVA did not increase the risk of squamous cell skin carcinoma and cutaneous malignant melanoma in a joint analysis of 944 Swedish and Finnish patients with psoriasis. *Br J Dermatol* **141**: 497-501.
69. Stern RS (2001) The risk of melanoma in association with long-term exposure to PUVA. *J Am Acad. Dermatol* **44**: 755-761.
70. Kolmel KF, Pfahlberg A, Mastrangelo G *et al.* (1999) Infections and melanoma risk: results of a multicentre EORTC case-control study. *Melanoma Res* **9**: 511-519.
71. Jablonska S (1991) Epidermodysplasia verruciformis. In: Friedman RJ, Rigel DS, Kopf AW, Harris MN, Baker D, eds. *Cancer of the skin.* Philadelphia: WB Saunders Co., pp. 101-113.
72. Shamanin V, zur Hausen H, Lavergne D *et al.* (1996) Human papillomavirus infections in nonmelanoma skin cancers from renal transplant recipients and nonimmunosuppressed patients. *J Natl Cancer Inst* **88**: 802-811.
73. Burk RD, Kadish AS (1996) Treasure hunt for human papillomavirus in nonmelanoma skin cancers. *J Natl Cancer Inst* **88**: 781-782.
74. Kiviat NB (1999) Papillomaviruses in non-melanoma skin cancer: epidemiological aspects. *Semin Cancer Biol* **9**: 397-403.

75. Dreau D, Culberson C, Wyatt S *et al.* (2000) Human papilloma virus in melanoma biopsy specimens and its relation to melanoma progression. *Ann Surg* **231**: 664-671.
76. Jensen P, Hansen S, Moller B *et al.* (1999) Skin cancer in kidney and heart transplant recipients and different long-term immunosuppressive therapy regimens. *J Am Acad Dermatol.* **40**: 177-186.
77. Marcil I, Stern RS (2000) Risk of developing a subsequent nonmelanoma skin cancer in patients with a history of nonmelanoma skin cancer: a critical review of the literature and meta-analysis. *Arch Dermatol* **136**: 1524-1530.
78. Smith CH, McGregor JM, Barker JNWN *et al.* (1993) Excess melanocytic nevi in children with renal allografts. *J Am Acad Dermatol.* **28**: 51-55.
79. Askling J, Grunewald J, Eklund A *et al.* (1999) Increased risk for cancer following sarcoidosis. *Am J Respir Crit Care Med* **160**: 1668-1672.
80. Adami J, Frisch M, Yuen J *et al.* (1995) Evidence of an association between non-Hodgkin's lymphoma and skin cancer. *BMJ* **310**: 1491-1495.
81. Frisch M, Melbye M (1995) New primary cancers after squamous cell skin cancer. *Am J Epidemiol* **141**: 916-922.
82. Kahn HS, Tatham LM, Patel AV *et al.* (1998) Increased cancer mortality following a history of nonmelanoma skin cancer. *JAMA* **280**: 910-912.
83. Scotto J, Fears TR, Kraemer KH *et al.* (1996) Nonmelanoma skin cancer. In: Schottenfeld D, Fraumeni JF Jr, eds. *Cancer epidemiology and prevention.* New York: Oxford University Press, pp. 1313-1330.
84. Shore RE (2001) Radiation-induced skin cancer in humans. *Med Pediatr Oncol* **36**: 549-554.
85. Karagas MR, McDonald JA, Greenberg ER *et al.* (1996) Risk of basal cell and squamous cell skin cancers after ionizing radiation therapy. *J Natl Cancer Inst* **88**: 1848-1853.
86. Hiatt RA, Krieger N, Sagebiel RW *et al.* (1993) Surveillance bias and the excess risk of malignant melanoma among employees of the Lawrence Livermore National Laboratory. *Epidemiology* **4**: 43-47.
87. Austin DF, Reynolds P (1997) Investigation of an excess of melanoma among employees of the Lawrence Livermore National Laboratory. *Am J Epidemiol* **145**: 524-531.
88. Acquavella JF, Wilkinson GS, Tietjen GL *et al.* (1983) A melanoma case-control study at the Los Alamos National Laboratory. *Health Phys* **45**: 587-592.
89. Green A, Battistutta D, Hart V *et al.* (1996) Skin cancer in a subtropical Australian population: incidence and lack of association with occupation. *Am J Epidemiol* **144**: 1034-1040.
90. Hakansson N, Floderus B, Gustavsson P *et al.* (2001) Occupational sunlight exposure and cancer incidence among Swedish construction workers. *Epidemiology* **12**: 552-557.
91. Khuder SA (1999) Etiologic clues to lip cancer from epidemiologic studies on farmers. *Scand J Work Environ Health* **25**: 125-130.
92. Pott P (1775) *Chirurgical observations relative to the cataract, the polypus of the nose, the cancer of the scrotum, the different kinds of ruptures, and the mortification of the hands and feet.* London: Hawse Clark and Collins.
93. Shannon RL, Strayer DS (1989) Arsenic induced skin toxicity. *Hum Toxicol* **8**: 99-104.
94. Hsueh S, Cheng GS, Wu MM *et al.* (1995) Multiple risk factors associated with arsenic-induced skin cancer: Effects of chronic liver disease and malnutritional status. *Br J Cancer* **71**: 109-114.
95. Karagas MR, Stukel TA, Morris JS *et al.* (2001) Skin cancer risk in relation to toenail arsenic concentrations in a US population-based case-control study. *Am J Epidemiol* **153**: 559-565.

Chapter 3

Solar and ultraviolet radiation

Peter Gies[1], Ph.D.; Colin Roy[1], Ph.D.; Petra Udelhofen[2], Ph.D. (deceased)
[1]*Australian Radiation Protection and Nuclear Safety Agency ,Victoria, Australia;*
[2]*formerly of Institute for Terrestrial and Planetary Atmospheres, State University of New York, USA*

Key words: UV Index, biological effectiveness, solar UVR climatology, artificial UVR

INTRODUCTION

Solar UVR is the most important source of ultraviolet radiation (UVR) to which the world's population is exposed. The long-term effects of these UVR exposures are dealt with in later chapters but a brief description of the biological effects of UVR is given here and an overview of the measurement of UVR is also provided. The chapter provides a detailed exploration of the range of factors that affect solar UVR at the earth's surface and includes a summary of solar UVR levels around the world. The role of personal behavior when outdoors, perhaps the most important factor determining an individual's exposure to solar UVR, is then examined as being the main potential avenue to modify and reduce these exposures. The chapter concludes with an overview of artificial sources of UVR and their associated hazards.

D. Hill et al. (eds.), Prevention of Skin Cancer, 21-54.
© *2004 Kluwer Academic Publishers. Printed in the Netherlands.*

1.   THE BIOLOGICAL EFFECTS OF UVR

Ultraviolet radiation (UVR) is part of the solar electromagnetic radiation spectrum, which includes visible radiation (wavelength range 400-770 nm) and infrared radiation (wavelengths greater than 770 nm). The UVR region covers the wavelength range 100-400 nm and consists of three sub regions, UVA (315-400 nm), UVB (280-315 nm) and UVC (100-280 nm) as defined by the International Committee of Illumination (CIE).

Only UVR in the range 200-400 nm can have a direct interaction with living organisms, since at wavelengths shorter than 200 nm the UVR is strongly absorbed by oxygen in the air. The penetration depth of UVR into human tissue is between 0.1 and 1 mm, so the organs at risk are the skin and the eyes. UVR has shorter wavelengths and thus more energetic photons than visible light and hence is capable of producing more damage when absorbed in biological tissue.

1.1   UVR and the skin

The effectiveness of the different UVR wavelengths in producing biological damage varies markedly. Exposure to UVB and UVC can result in erythema or reddening of the skin (sunburn). A similar effect can also be obtained with UVA but the dose required is much greater. Generally, the shorter the UVR wavelength, the greater the biological effectiveness of the radiation. A given quantity of UVB can be up to 1000 times as effective as the same quantity of UVA in producing erythema. In 1987 McKinlay and Diffey reviewed published data on the effectiveness of UVR in producing erythema in human skin and proposed a standard erythemal response curve, which was subsequently adopted by the CIE [1]. This curve, shown in Figure 3.1, exhibits a marked variation in effectiveness with wavelength, decreasing by orders of magnitude between 300 nm and 320 nm and continuing to decrease across the UVA to 400 nm.

UVR irradiance is described in terms of power (watts) per unit area (square meter) and is denoted $W.m^{-2}$. The time integral of the irradiance gives the energy per unit area. For example, 1 watt is 1 joule per second - therefore $1\ W.m^{-2}$ incident for 1 second is a dose of $1\ J.m^{-2}$ and incident for 1 minute is a dose of $60\ J.m^{-2}$.

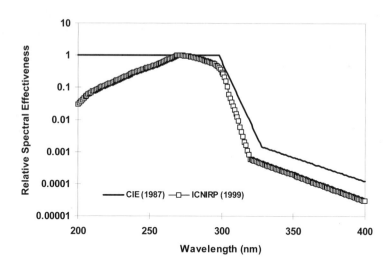

Figure 3.1 The erythemal effectiveness of UVR versus wavelength of the CIE [1] compared with the relative spectral effectiveness of the ICNIRP [5] exposure guidelines.

Apart from UVR lasers, which can emit a single UVR wavelength, sources of UVR generally emit at multiple wavelengths in the UVR and the combined effect of the different wavelengths on a biological system must be assessed. It is therefore necessary to measure the amount of energy present at each wavelength, multiply by the relative biological effectiveness of that wavelength and add all the contributions, as in Equation 3.1. When the biological effectiveness is measured in terms of erythema, the resultant total is called the erythemally effective UVR irradiance, denoted as UVR_{eff}. The inclusion of the CIE [1] spectral effectiveness function in the calculation ensures that proper weighting is given to the biologically effective wavelengths below 315 nm.

For determination of the erythemally effective irradiance of a broadband source weighted against the CIE [1] spectral effectiveness curve, the following weighting formula is used:
Where:

$$UVR_{eff} = \sum_{\lambda_1}^{\lambda_2} E_\lambda \cdot S_\lambda \cdot \Delta_\lambda \qquad (1)$$

$UVR_{eff} =$	biologically effective irradiance in $W.m^{-2}$
$E_\lambda =$	spectral irradiance in $W.m^{-2}.nm^{-1}$
$S_\lambda =$	relative spectral effectiveness (action spectra),
λ_1, λ_2	are the lower and upper wavelength limits
$\Delta_\lambda =$	bandwidth in nanometers of the calculated or measurement intervals

Equation 3.1

Previously the MED (minimum erythema dose) was used to quantify UVR, where the MED was the amount of UVR sufficient to cause a barely perceptible erythema or reddening in individuals with a sensitive or fair, unadapted skin. The MED (in terms of UVR_{eff}) from a number of studies was in the range 200 to 300 $J.m^{-2}$ and depended upon the susceptibility of the test subject.

Recently a new term, the SED (standard erythema dose) [2] has been defined. The SED represents a CIE weighted UVR_{eff} dose of 100 $J.m^{-2}$. It is not related to any individual's MED. However, the SED can be used to describe the erythemal effectiveness of various UVR sources and as such is a useful measure of biologically effective UVR.

1.2   UVR and the eye

The lens of the eye is a strong absorber of wavelengths shorter than 400 nm. UVB and UVC are absorbed by the cornea and conjunctiva and in sufficient doses will cause photokeratitis and conjunctivitis. These painful effects are often referred to as "welder's flash" in industry. The action spectrum and threshold dose for this condition have been widely investigated. The peak of the photokeratitis action spectrum occurs at approximately 270 nm with a threshold dose of approximately 40 $J.m^{-2}$ for both primate and human eyes. As with erythema induction, the spectral effectiveness of UVR on the eye shows a similar rapid decrease in effect of several orders of magnitude between 300 and 320 nm, with the shorter wavelength UVB being far more effective at causing damage than UVA. The response of the retina to UVA and visible radiation is similar but very little UVR reaches the retina.

The International Radiation Protection Association/International Non-Ionizing Radiation Committee (IRPA/INIRC) produced guidelines [3] on exposure to UVR in 1985, which were revised [4] in 1989 and republished by the International Commission on Non-Ionizing Radiation Protection (ICNIRP) in 1999 [5]. The guidelines list exposure limits for UVR that provide protection for both the skin and the eyes from acute effects of exposure. The ICNIRP [5] guidelines are useful in quantifying the hazards associated with sources of UVR, in particular artificial sources. For example, it is possible to calculate the effective irradiance (UVR_{eff}) of a broadband source by using Equation 3.1 with the ICNIRP [5] spectral effectiveness curve for S_{λ}. (The ICNIRP spectral effectiveness curve differs slightly from the CIE curve (Figure 3.1) because the effect on eyes and skin differs slightly.) The maximum allowed exposures dose of ICNIRP is 30 $J.m^{-2}$ and the time to exceed this, called the maximum allowed exposure time T_{max}, can be calculated using Equation 3.2.

$$T_{max} \ (seconds) = \frac{30 \quad (J.m^{-2})}{UVR_{eff} \ (W.m^{-2})} \quad (2)$$

Equation 3.2

The more powerful the source of UVR, the higher UVR_{eff} and thus the shorter will be the allowed exposure time. Exposure for a duration of less than T_{max} should not result in adverse short-term health effects. Spectral weighting as in Equation 3.1 and exposure times will be applied later in this chapter to a number of examples, including solar UVR and artificial sources.

2.   MEASUREMENT OF UVR

This section is a general introduction to the measurement of UVR. Measurement of UVR from both solar and artificial sources can be accomplished using a variety of instrumental and measurement techniques, many of which are quite complex and beyond the scope of this chapter. The major difficulty with measuring UVR is the need to block out stray radiation, such as visible. If measurement of UVB is required, then the detector should respond only to UVB and not to UVA or visible radiation. The sun's spectrum at the earth's surface is predominately visible and infrared, with UVR comprising just 8% of the total and UVB accounting for only 1 to 3 % of UVR. Most detectors are quite sensitive to visible (unless specifically engineered to respond only to UVR), so the visible and infrared wavelengths must be blocked or the measurement will be in error.

2.1   Spectral measurement systems

The most fundamental and accurate way of determining the characteristics of a UVR source is to measure its emission at each wavelength and thereby obtain its spectral distribution. Such spectral measurements require a spectroradiometer, which measures in sequence the intensity at individual wavelengths, by using a dispersive element such as a prism or diffraction grating mounted inside the unit. Radiation is admitted into this monochromator by specially designed input optics, either a diffuser or an integrating sphere, is dispersed and selected by the monochromator and relayed to a detector, either a photomultiplier, photodiode, or photographic film. Many factors such as bandwidth and resolution, wavelength response, stray light, linearity, and calibration (both wavelength and irradiance) must be carefully characterized [6-8].

Once the spectral output of a UVR source has been measured, the results can be used to calculate various quantities of interest. The spectral output, usually a spectral irradiance, can be integrated across the different wavebands such as the UVC, UVB and UVA to determine the irradiance, expressed in $W.m^{-2}$. Alternatively, the spectral output can be weighted with a function such as the CIE [1] erythemal response, the ICNIRP [5] response curve or with a DNA damage response to determine the total effect due to the sum of all the UVR wavelengths, as in Equation 3.1. Having the basic spectral measurement means that different weightings can be applied at any time. For highly accurate work, double monochromators (essentially two monochromators, one after the other) reduce the amount of extraneous radiation (stray light) selected by the system. This is critically important when the spectral irradiance of the source varies rapidly with wavelength, as it does in the solar spectrum at wavelengths below 300 nm.

2.2   Broadband measurement

As spectral UVR measurement equipment is generally very expensive, an alternative approach is to use a radiometric detector. There are two main types of radiometers: thermal detectors, which generally have a flat response with wavelength, and wavelength dependent radiometric detectors. These detectors have the advantage over spectral measurement systems in that they allow continuous measurement of UVR. There are a number of features that are desirable for any UVR detector, such as stability (both with time and temperature), constant low level dark current, suitable spectral response and uniformity of response across the detector [8]. Very few UVR detectors satisfy all the conditions, but nevertheless they can provide useful measurements as long as the investigators are aware of and make allowances for the instrumental shortcomings.

Thermal detectors, such as thermopiles, absorb the incoming radiation resulting in a temperature increase, which when carefully measured is related to the intensity of radiation. These detectors have a response across a very wide spectral range and are stable but less sensitive than other UVR detectors.

Many radiometric detectors have been developed to measure specific wavebands (UVA or UVB) or the biological effectiveness of the solar UVR. They utilize optical filters to select the wavelength range and a vacuum photodiode or photovoltaic cell to respond to the UVR. The filters attempt to select only the wavelength range of interest, such as UVB or UVA, but it is difficult to tailor the filter characteristics exactly to such narrow wavebands.

These radiometric detectors can be used for measurement of solar UVR but also have application in the measurement of artificial UVR sources. However, to accurately measure an artificial source it is necessary to know both the spectral responsivity of the detector as well as the spectral distribution of the source.

Alternatively, by interposing a selected filter, the responsivity of the radiometer can be modified to approximate the erythemal response of human skin. The matching of the erythemal detector response with that of the human erythemal response has been achieved with varying degree of success and these detectors are widely used for the measurement of solar UVR.

2.3   Films and biological detectors

A number of UVR-sensitive films or mediums have been used to measure UVR. The most widely used of these is polysulphone (PS) film, which was first introduced by Davis *et al.* [9] in 1976. Upon exposure to UVR the absorbance of the film in the UVR part of the spectrum changes. The film is calibrated under known conditions. Following UVR exposure, measurements of the film absorbance pre and post UVR exposure allows the determination of cumulative exposure dose. The spectral response of the PS film depends upon the film thickness, with films between 30 and 45 microns thickness showing a spectral response that is similar although not identical to the human erythemal response. PS film has been used as a dosimeter in numerous human solar UVR exposure studies, but it can also be used to measure exposure to artificial sources of UVR. However, its dose response needs to be calibrated for the particular source it is to be used with. Other films that have been used successfully are phenothiazine, 8-MOP and diazo film. There has been considerable interest in biological detectors using spores or biofilm [10,11] to measure UVR. The advantage of these detectors is that they are small, inexpensive in most cases, and can be used in personal exposure studies, where the use of bulky radiometric detectors would be either difficult or impossible, although recent miniaturization of radiometric detectors has largely eliminated this advantage.

3.   SOLAR UVR

3.1   The solar spectrum

A comparison between the extraterrestrial solar spectrum and one measured at the earth's surface is shown in Figure 3.2. The effects due to absorption in the atmosphere can be clearly seen. While sunspot activity can increase the extraterrestrial intensity, this effect is more marked at wavelengths less than 290 nm, which are completely absorbed as they pass through the atmosphere and are not present in the solar spectrum at the earth's surface. The intensity of the extraterrestrial spectrum generally has a yearly variation of less than 10%, but the intensity of solar radiation at the earth's surface is subject to large variations due to numerous factors, discussed later in this chapter. From Figure 3.2, the proportion of energy at wavelengths below 400 nm in solar UVR at the earth's surface is very minor and is generally less than 7% with the UVB contributing just 0.04% (Table 3.1).

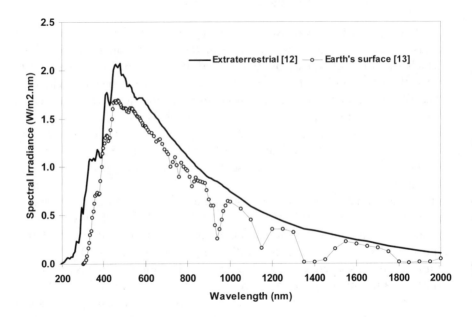

Figure 3.2 Comparison of the extraterrestrial solar spectrum [12] with the measured spectrum at the earth's surface [13].

Table 3.1 Distribution energy of the extraterrestrial solar spectrum [12] and the solar spectrum measured at the earth's surface [13].

Wavelength region	Extraterrestrial		Earth's surface	
	Irradiance (W.m^{-2})	Percentage of total	Irradiance (W.m^{-2})	Percentage of total
UVC	7.6	0.56	–	0
UVB	18.3	1.4	2.0	0.04
UVA	92.1	6.8	60	6.5
Visible	606	44.8	313	55
Infrared	629	46.5	355	38

Ozone, although being only a minor constituent of the earth's atmosphere, nevertheless plays a vital role in the absorption of incoming solar UVR, in particular, the lower wavelengths of the UVB. The absorption by ozone in most of the UVA region is virtually zero but below about 340 nm it increases rapidly with decreasing wavelength. The effect of this can be seen in Figure 3.3 and Table 3.1 as the difference between the extraterrestrial and surface solar spectra. Stratospheric ozone is responsible for preventing much of the UVR below 290 nm from reaching to the earth's surface (molecular oxygen also plays a role). Concern about the effects of increased solar UVB as the result of stratospheric ozone depletion is not new but the discovery of the springtime Antarctic ozone hole by Farman *et al.* [14] in 1985 increased the general awareness and has heightened concern. The worry is that long-term ozone depletion will add significantly to the UVB levels (and hence UVR$_{eff}$) the population is exposed to, which in turn may ultimately result in increased skin cancer and melanoma rates. At mid-latitudes, where most of the world's population lives, ozone depletion is currently estimated at 3% per decade by UNEP [15]. However, it is unlikely that long-term ozone depletion effects on the measured UVR will be verified for some years by the existing UV measurement networks [16]. The effects of ozone depletion are covered in more detail in Chapter 4.

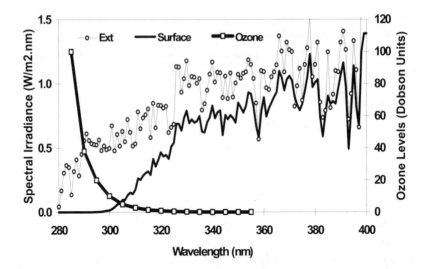

Figure 3.3 A comparison of the extraterrestrial spectrum with that measured at the earth's surface (Melbourne, Australia, January 1990) for the UVR wavelength range 280 to 400 nm. Also shown are the absorption coefficients of ozone (right axis), which increase sharply at wavelengths below 340 nm and are responsible for reducing the hazardous UVR below 300 nm.

3.2   UV Index

The introduction of the Global Solar UV Index [17,18] by the World Health Organisation (WHO), the World Meteorological Office (WMO), the United Nations Environment Programme (UNEP) and the International Commission on Non-Ionizing Radiation Protection (ICNIRP) was aimed at standardizing the global reporting of solar UVR. The UV Index provides the public with a numerical indication of the maximum potential solar UVR hazard during the day: the higher the number, the higher the predicted solar UVR hazard. The use of such a standardized quantity also allows comparison of the potential UVR hazard between widely separated geographical locations; this can be particularly important for tourists. It is anticipated that the UV Index will play a key role in future educational campaigns [19] to change people's behavior and reduce their solar UVR exposures.

When presented as a forecast, the UV Index is calculated using computer models which require the input of various atmospheric parameters including ozone, potential cloud cover and to a lesser extent water vapour and aerosols. Computations of clear sky solar UVR can give an accurate estimate of the maximum UVR. The prediction of cloud cover is difficult and results in more uncertainties for non-clear sky conditions.

Originally, the UV Index was defined and reported in forecasts as the daily maximum value. It is now a continuous measure so it can be used for real-time displays, although daily forecasting still uses the maximum value. The UV Index is not an instantaneous value but the average over either 10 or 30 minutes. Since measurements of UV Index are made under all weather conditions, they are generally lower than the predicted maximum for clear sky conditions. The UV Index is based on the UVR_{eff} for solar UVR derived from Equation 3.1 when weighted with the erythemal effectiveness of the CIE.

One UV Index unit is equivalent to 0.025 $W.m^{-2}$ of UVR_{eff}. Alternatively, the UV Index is the biologically effective UVR multiplied by 40. Biologically effective UVR is measured in $W.m^{-2}$ effective and a typical peak value for a summer's day could be 0.30 $W.m^{-2}$. This is equivalent to a UV Index of 12 (0.30 x 40) or alternatively (12 units of UV Index defined as 0.025 $W.m^{-2}$). In terms of SEDs/hr this would be 10.8 SEDs/hr, e.g., 0.30 x 3600 (seconds per hour)/ 100 ($J.m^{-2}$ per SED) = 10.8 SEDs/hr.

Figure 3.4 shows graphically the effects of spectral weighting as applied to solar UVR. The incident solar spectrum at each individual wavelength across the UVR is multiplied by, in this case, the CIE erythemal effectiveness to produce the effect due to that wavelength. The intensity of UVR with wavelength decreases rapidly towards shorter wavelengths in the UVB while the effectiveness of the radiation increases in this region. The combination of these two factors means that the peak of the weighted curve is generally between 300 and 310 nm, in the UVB part of the spectrum.

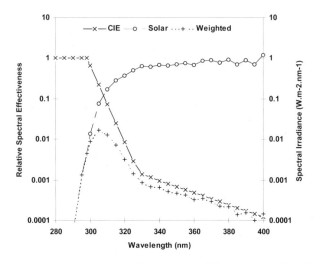

Figure 3.4 The CIE erythemal effectiveness (x: left axis) is multiplied by the spectral irradiance of the solar spectrum at the earth's surface (o: right axis) at each wavelength across the UVR to produce a resultant (+: right axis) weighted curve.

All the wavelength contributions are summed as in Equation 3.1 to give the UVR$_{eff}$, which is equivalent (analogous) to the area under the weighted curve. When the CIE erythemal effectiveness is used as in this case, the UVR$_{eff}$ can be used to calculate T$_{erythema}$, the time to achieve an erythemal dose on a horizontal surface (equivalent to 2 SEDs or 200 J.m^{-2} for fair skin). The times to achieve erythema will be longer for people with skin types less sensitive to UVR, as in Equation 3.3.

$$T_{erythema} \; (seconds) = \frac{200 \quad (J.m^{-2})}{UVR_{eff} \; (W.m^{-2})} \qquad (3)$$

Equation 3.3

It is also possible to spectrally weight the incident solar spectrum with the ICNIRP [5] spectral effectiveness in the same way as in Figure 3.4 and Equation 3.1 and then to calculate the time T$_{max}$ to exceed the ICNIRP exposure limits using Equation 3.2.

On a typical summer's day at mid latitudes around noon, with a UV Index of 12, the time to achieve minimum erythema T$_{erythema}$, at least 2 SED for fair skin, is approximately 11 minutes. The ICNIRP limits would be exceeded in approximately 6 minutes, so complying with these guidelines, which is often difficult, would prevent observable short-term damage due to UVR exposure. Table 3.2 shows the UV Index, the times to exceed the ICNIRP guidelines T$_{max}$ as well as the times to achieve erythema for differing intensities of solar UVR. Also shown for comparison are the equivalent solar UVR intensities in SEDs/hr.

Table 3.2 The variation of time to exceed the ICNIRP [5] guidelines T$_{max}$, time to achieve erythema T$_{erythema}$ and the equivalent SEDs/hr for solar UVR of various UV Indices.

UV Index	T$_{max}$ (mins)	T$_{erythema}$ (mins)	UVR$_{eff}$ (SEDs/hr)
2	39.5	66.6	1.8
4	19.8	33.3	3.6
6	13.2	22.2	5.4
8	9.9	16.7	7.2
10	7.9	13.3	9.0
12	6.6	11.1	10.8
14	5.7	9.5	12.6
16	4.5	8.4	14.4

4. FACTORS AFFECTING SOLAR UVR

4.1 Solar elevation

The single most important factor affecting the amount of solar UVR (for clear skies) is the elevation of the sun in the sky: the higher the sun, the higher the levels of solar UVR. When the sun is low, the path of the radiation through the atmosphere is longer and more of the radiation is absorbed and scattered, as well as being spread over a larger area when it is incident on the surface. Radiation from the sun incident on the top of the atmosphere contains UVC, UVB and UVA. However, due to absorption by oxygen and ozone in the upper atmosphere, no UVC and only a small fraction of the UVB reaches the earth's surface. The height of the sun therefore determines how much UVB penetrates the atmosphere: the lower the sun the less UVB. In winter the sun is low in the sky and contains proportionally less UVB due to absorption and scattering. The same process occurs daily, with the solar UVR around noon being more intense and containing more damaging UVB than early or late in the day. This is why the solar UVR danger period is in the middle of the day and in summer, when the sun is highest in the sky.

Figure 3.5 gives the percentage of the daily total solar UVR within certain time periods. The hours 12 till 2 (1 hour either side of noon: 1 pm daylight savings time) have 31% of the daily total, while almost 60% of this daily total occurs within 2 hours of solar noon (10 am till 2 pm). These percentages will vary for different latitude locations and for different times of year.

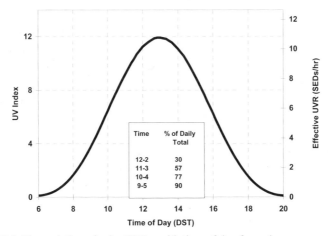

Figure 3.5 The variation of solar UVR$_{eff}$ with time of day for a clear summer day at mid latitude location, showing the relationship between UVR$_{eff}$ in SEDs/hr (right axis) and the UV Index (left axis). The peak UV Index is 12 at solar noon, which is equivalent to UVR$_{eff}$ of 10.8 SEDs/hr.

Geographical location (latitude) is an important factor that determines the position of the sun in the sky. The sun can only be directly overhead between latitudes 23.5°N and 23.5°S. For latitudes further from the equator, the sun will be at its highest at solar noon on December 21st or 22nd for the Southern Hemisphere and on 21st or 22nd June for the Northern Hemisphere. Between September and March, the sun is over the Southern Hemisphere and is higher in the sky there, resulting in higher UVR levels than between March and September, when it is over the Northern Hemisphere. Another factor is that the earth's orbit is elliptical and is at its closest to the sun on January 3rd and at its furthest from the sun on approximately July 4th. This results in about a 3% difference in distance and approximately a 7% higher intensity in January, during the Southern Hemisphere's summer. Coupled with clearer atmospheric conditions and the more significant ozone depletion observed over the Antarctic, this may result in measured ambient UVR which is 12% to 15% higher for geographical locations in the Southern Hemisphere in comparison to similar locations in the Northern Hemisphere [20]. This effect can also be seen in the global UVR climatology discussed in section 4.7.

The yearly variation in solar elevation results in a maximum on December 21/22 and June 21/22 for the Southern and Northern Hemispheres respectively. However, UVR levels are not necessarily a maximum on these days as other factors such as seasonal variations in ozone are also important. For locations inside the tropics, the sun will be directly overhead twice a year. Locations outside the tropics generally show a typical temperate variation in UVR, with solar UVR low in winter and high in summer.

4.1.1 Diffuse and direct UVR

Solar UVR at the earth's surface comes not only directly from the sun but also indirectly from the sky, due to atmospheric scattering. This is called diffuse radiation. Depending on the time of day there can be as much UVR from the sky as there is from the direct sun. Therefore, a person sitting in the shade but being able to view the sky is still exposed to scattered UVR from the sky. People are frequently sunburnt while boating and the assumption is that water is highly reflective and this has increased their UVR exposure. In reality, they are exposed to both direct solar UVR and scattered UVR from the entire sky. It is solar elevation that determines the relative amounts of direct or diffuse UVR. The higher the sun, the shorter the path-length through the atmosphere and the less diffuse and the more direct UVR there is.

Since UVB is scattered more readily than UVA, the diffuse UVB radiation from the sky exceeds the direct UVB from the sun, except for a few hours around solar noon. However, the direct component of UVA is greater than the diffuse for most of the day, with the exception of a few hours in the early morning and evening.

4.2   Effect of ozone on UVR

Total ozone shows a fairly consistent annual cycle but daily variations can be up to 40% of the total. Therefore, while two consecutive days might have the same temperature and cloud cover, the UVR_{eff} hazard could be different by as much as 30% (UV Index 9 vs. 12) due to natural variation in ozone. Generally, ozone levels are lowest in late summer, which usually results in the highest measured UVR_{eff} levels in January (Southern Hemisphere) or July (Northern Hemisphere), even though the sun is higher in the sky in December and June for the respective hemispheres.

4.3   Effects due to clouds

Clouds significantly affect the level of solar radiation measured at the earth's surface, and the effects are wavelength dependent, in that the water vapor attenuates infrared much more than UVR. There is also a small wavelength dependence across the UVR, with UVB being transmitted more readily than UVA [21]. Heavy cloud cover can reduce the levels of UVR to almost zero. However, light cloud cover reduces the levels of UVB by approximately 10% to 50% but it is very dependent on the type of cloud, its thickness and areal coverage. In certain situations, reflected UVR from clouds can actually add to the ambient levels and for short time periods can result in higher UVR than on days with clear sky [22]. There is currently a great deal of research into clouds and their effects on solar UVR [23,24].

Figure 3.6 shows the effect of different cloud conditions on the measured UVR_{eff} for Melbourne, Australia for three days in December 2000. In the absence of cloud the readings for each day would be almost identical, since they are for consecutive days when all other factors affecting UVR are approximately equal. Heavy cloud (Dec 22) reduced UVR to less than 15% of the clear sky value, with a UV Index of only 2.3 and a daily total of 9.6 SED. The scattered cloud (Dec 21) had a variable effect, with the levels rising and falling significantly as clouds passed in front of the sun, while the UV Index was 10.3 with a daily total of 35.9 SED. The clear day (Dec 20) had a UV Index of 10.4 and a daily total of 60.8 SED. While the UV Index was similar for both December 20 and 21 (UV Index 10.3 versus 10.4), indicating that the potential hazard to people was also similar on both days, the total amount of UVR_{eff} incident differed by almost a factor of two. UV

Index ideally represents the potential hazard, while daily total UVR$_{eff}$ describes the overall UVR levels.

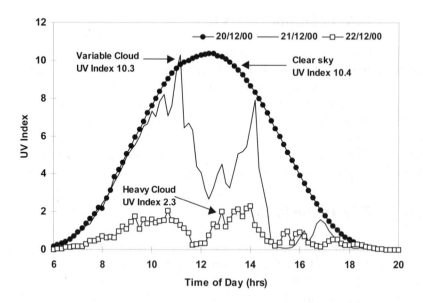

Figure 3.6 The effects of clouds on the levels of solar UVR$_{eff}$ for three consecutive days in December 2000 in Melbourne, Australia.

4.4   Ground surface reflection

Ground reflectance is important because reflected UVR can increase the ambient levels and cause exposure to parts of the body that are normally shaded. If the reflectivity or albedo of the surface is high then these exposures can be significant. The reflectivities of surfaces normally encountered such as lawn grass (reflectance 2–4 %) or asphalt (reflectance 4–8 %) are generally quite low, but beach sand can have a reflectance of 10–15% and fresh snow can be as high as 80–90% [25,26]. On a sunny day the reflected UVR from the fresh snow below can circumvent a person's normal defences against solar UVR from above (for example eyebrows, eye socket, eyelids etc.) and cause sunburn and short-term eye damage. The reflectivities in the UVB part of the spectrum are significantly lower than in the visible.

4.5 Altitude

Solar UVR increases with altitude at a rate of approximately 4% increase in UVR_{eff} for every 300 m [27]. More recently, spectral measurements [28] of solar UVR at two sites in the alps separated by 1 km in altitude showed that the increase in UVR with altitude showed some wavelength dependence. Irradiances at the mountain site at a wavelength of 370 nm were 9% higher than the valley site, increasing to 11% at 320 nm. The UVB increase was 24% at 300 nm, while the UVR_{eff} was 14% higher at the mountain site.

4.6 Air pollution, aerosols, water vapour

Aerosols, small particles suspended in the air, usually occur at altitudes below 2 km above the earth's surface. They can attenuate solar UVR but the effect is generally less than that due to atmospheric scattering.

Absorption by gaseous air pollutants is also a minor factor but the reduction in solar UVR irradiance can be several percent [29]. In exceptional circumstances when the levels of pollutants or dust are very high, solar UVR can be significantly reduced, such as after the 1991 Mount Pinatubo eruption.

4.7 Typical levels of solar UVR

As discussed earlier, when the sun is low in the sky, such as early morning or late afternoon, the UVB/UVA ratio is lower than that at solar noon. For a mid-latitude at solar noon, maximum levels of UVA and UVB are approximately 70 and 2.5 Wm^{-2} respectively in summer and 25 and 0.6 Wm^{-2} in winter. The exact variation between summer and winter UVR levels will depend upon the latitude of the location.

Table 3.3 shows typical maximum summer UV Index values for a number of capital cities around the world. Unless otherwise stated, UV Indices are computed forecasts, but where measured values exist they are also quoted. Many of the forecasts and most of the measurements are freely available on the Internet, and the sites listed beneath the table list or link to this data. The highest UV Indices in this table are generally at locations near the equator and the greatest of these are at locations near the equator and at high altitude (e.g., Mauna Loa, La Paz, and Bogota). While agreement between UV Index forecasting and surface measurements is generally better than 1 to 2 UV index units, considerable work is in progress to further improve this agreement.

Table 3.3 Maximum summer UV Index values for various cities around the world, with a comparison of measured Summer UV Index values where available.

City	Country	UV Index (computed)	UV Index (measured)
Auckland	New Zealand	12-13	12
Lauder	New Zealand	10-11	11
Vienna	Austria	8	7
Barcelona	Spain	9	8
Paris	France	7	7
London	UK	6-7	-
Athens	Greece	10	-
Florence	Italy	9	8
Munich	Germany	7	-
Tokyo	Japan	10-11	-
Hong Kong	China	13	13
Montreal	Canada	8	8
Toronto	Canada	8	8
Los Angeles	USA	11	10
San Francisco	USA	10	-
New York	USA	9-10	-
Miami	USA	13	-
Atlanta	USA	13	9
Houston	USA	12	-
Chicago	USA	9-10	-
Mauna Loa	Hawaii, USA	17-18	16-17
Honolulu	USA	12-13	-
Brisbane	Australia	14	14
Darwin	Australia	16	16
Sydney	Australia	12	12
Melbourne	Australia	12	12
Perth	Australia	13	13
Buenos Aires	Argentina	9	-
Rio de Janeiro	Brazil	11	-
La Paz	Bolivia	19	-
Bogota	Colombia	-	16

NOAA *http://www.srrb.noaa.gov/UV/lindex.html*
COST-713 homepage *http://159.213.57.69/uvweb/wwwcost.html*
World Ozone and UV Data Centre *http://woudc.ec.gc.ca/e/ozone/uv_plots.htm*

A year's solar UVR$_{eff}$ data for Melbourne for July 1998 to June 1999 is shown in Figure 3.7 as a 3D plot. The vertical axis is UV Index while the two horizontal axes are time of day in hours (5 till 19) and day of the year. The effect of clouds on the UVR levels can be seen but the major influence on the shape of the UVR distribution is the position of the sun in the sky, governed by the time of year and time of day. The peak danger period around solar noon in summer is clearly evident and the variation between summer and winter levels is also illustrated.

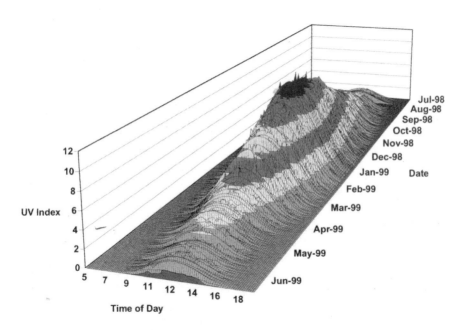

Figure 3.7 A 3D plot of the variation of solar UVR$_{eff}$ for Melbourne, Australia for July 1998 to June 1999.

Surface measurements of yearly total solar UVR$_{eff}$ in SEDs from a number of networks around the world, Australia [30], New Zealand [31], the UK [27,32], Spain [33], the USA [34], Japan [35], Germany [36], Sweden [37] and Holland [38] are shown in Figure 3.8. The latitude gradient of UVR is clearly evident, with locations closer to the equator generally having higher annual levels of UVR than those further from the equator.

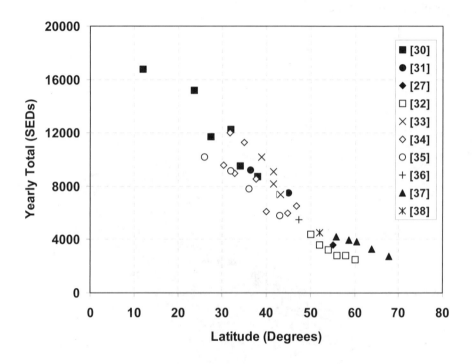

Figure 3.8 Latitude gradient of solar UVR$_{eff}$ in SEDs per year showing measurements from a number of countries around the world ([30] Australia, [31] NZ, [27] the UK (1) and [32] the UK (2), [33] Spain, [34] the USA, [35] Japan, [36] Germany, [37] Sweden, and [38] Holland).

Ground based measurements can provide valuable information on the local ambient solar UVR levels, but the measurements are only valid within a finite distance of the measurement site, approximately 100 kms [39], depending upon local topography and climate. Satellites can observe almost the whole surface of the earth from space and provide UVR climatology data for comparison with surface measurements. Using satellite measurements of ozone and cloud cover, the UVR_{eff} at the earth's surface can be calculated using computer models of UVR transmission through the atmosphere. Comparison with the surface based measurements allows validation of the results. The combination of the two measurement sets is the best way to derive an accurate UVR climatology for an entire country, region, or the world.

Satellite measurements of ozone and derived cloud cover from the Total Ozone Mapping Spectrometer (TOMS) were used in conjunction with surface UVR measurements to examine trends in UVR, ozone and cloud cover and to derive a UVR_{eff} climatology for Australia [40] for 1979 to 1992. As TOMS derived UVR_{eff} data [41] are available for most of the globe, these computations have been extended to generate a UVR_{eff} climatology for the world and are shown in Figure 3.9. The units shown on the plot are SEDs per day averaged over the month of January for the period 1979 to 1992 in (A) and July in (B). The maximum values in January are 70 SEDs per day at a number of locations in the Southern Hemisphere while the maxima for July are 60 SEDs per day in the Northern Hemisphere. The higher levels in the Southern Hemisphere are due to the effects mentioned previously such as the earth being closer to the sun in January and the more significant ozone depletion and clearer atmosphere in the Southern Hemisphere. The computed annual climatology is shown in Figure 3.9 (C) for comparison.

There is widespread concern over the effects of ozone depletion on solar UVR but other factors such as global warming and changes in cloud cover can also change the UVR levels at the earth's surface. A recent study [40] using satellite data found variable trends in the UVR_{eff}, ozone, and cloud cover calculated for the different sub-regions within the Australian region. The main reason for the increases in solar UVR detected in some of the regions (in particular the latitude band 10°S to 20°S) was not ozone depletion but rather changes in cloud cover, which decreased over the north but either remained constant or slightly increased over the south. Therefore, ozone depletion effects vary not only by latitude but also regionally within a latitude band.

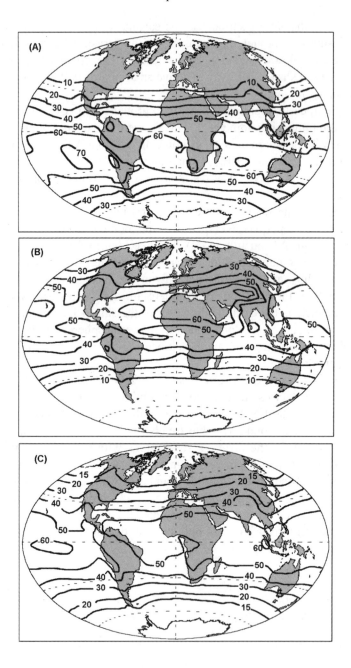

Figure 3.9 Computed UVR climatology for (A) January average, (B) July average and (C) the annual average (units are SEDs/day). Source of satellite data: Laboratory for Atmospheres at the National Aeronautics and Space Administration (NASA) Goddard Space Flight Centre (GSFC).

4.8 Typical personal exposures to solar UVR

Numerous personal exposures studies using a variety of UVR dosimeters but principally polysulphone film have been published. These studies have measured the anatomical distributions of solar UVR or typical exposures for various population groups and many of these are summarized elsewhere [42]. Personal exposure to solar UVR depends on many of the factors that affect solar UVR (e.g., time of day and year, geographical location, local environment), as well as the activity undertaken and protection used. One quantity of interest is the annual UVR exposure of different people and population groups. In the UK about 200 SED per year is estimated as the annual exposure for indoor workers [27,43]. This is of the order of 5% of ambient, mostly obtained from weekend exposures and the remainder from vacations and other outdoor activities. A recent study in the US [44] calculated typical UVR exposures for adults in the US to be 250 SEDs/yr. This study also found, as have a number of previous ones, that males spend more time outdoors and therefore have higher UVR exposures (280 SEDs/yr) than females (220 SEDs/yr). There are very large variations in solar UVR exposures between individuals within any given population, which depend upon personal behavior traits while outdoors [45] and generally result in log normal exposure distributions for the population groups. Certain individuals show consistent behaviour patterns and will consistently have higher or lower UVR exposures compared to the population median [39]. A comparison between similar groups of UK and Queensland school children [45] showed generally higher UVR exposures for Queensland, but with a proportion of the UK subjects having greater exposure than the Queensland group. The median exposure for the Queensland group was twice that of the UK median, while the ambient solar UVR measured during the studies was also higher by a factor of two in Queensland, resulting in the same proportion of exposure relative to ambient for both groups.

Personal exposure to the sun is the important link between the ambient levels of solar UVR and the chronic effects such as skin cancer discussed in more detail in later chapters. Personal UVR exposure is determined by behavior, for example by when an individual chooses to be outside and whether they use protection such as hats, clothing, sunscreens, and sunglasses. The main avenue to reduce personal UVR exposure is through modification of these behavior patterns. Personal exposure studies provide information on the actual UVR exposures as well as guidance in choosing the most appropriate means to reduce the exposures.

5.   ARTIFICIAL SOURCES OF UVR

UVR is used widely in scientific, medical, industrial and domestic fields. Uses include sterilization, photopolymerization, photoactivation processes, psoriasis phototherapy and artificial suntanning. UVR is also inadvertently present in operations such as welding, metal smelting, glass processing and all processes involving incandescent materials. These various sources emit a broad spectrum of UVR. Artificial sources of UVR are described below but are covered in more detail in McKinlay *et al.* [46] and the World Health Organization Environmental Health Criteria 160 [47].

5.1   Incandescent sources

Incandescent sources produce a continuous spectrum of optical radiation by heating a filament, usually tungsten. The surface temperature of the filament determines the shape of the spectrum of radiation emitted: the higher the temperature the more UVR emitted, although the peak of the spectrum is invariably in the infrared. The UVR emissions from a common electric light globe, which operates at about 3000K, are generally negligible [48].

Desk lighting (and also domestic downlighting) involving the use of tungsten halogen (TH) lamps has become increasingly popular over the past 10 years. TH lamps consist of a small quartz bulb containing a tungsten filament and a halogen gas (usually iodine) and emit significant levels of UVR. The presence of the gas minimizes evaporation of tungsten from the filament, thereby prolonging the life of the lamp and allowing it to be operated at a higher temperature than a conventional lamp. The light produced is therefore brighter (for a lower power consumption), but because the operating temperature is higher, the envelope in TH lamps must be quartz. This combination of high filament temperature and quartz envelope (which transmits UVR) results in potentially hazardous levels of UVR emission from the lamp. Surveys of TH lamps [49] found that the ICNIRP UVR exposure limits can be exceeded under certain exposure situations.

The concern with the use of TH lamps in desk lighting is the possibility of skin and short- and long-term eye damage for the user when the lamp is used at relatively short distances for extended periods of time. Since the UVR emission does not contribute to the normal function of these desk lights, it is desirable that it be eliminated and this may be best achieved by the use of a suitable optical filter such as 3 mm window glass, which transmits the visible but substantially absorbs the UVR.

5.2 Low pressure discharge lamps

The mercury lamp in its various forms is used extensively for lighting and as a source of UVR for industrial, medical, and recreational applications. Mercury emission occurs at a number of specific wavelengths, including the UVR wavelengths of 189, 254, 297, 303, 313, 334 and 365 nm. However, for low pressure mercury lamps with quartz envelopes, more than 90% of the energy emitted is at 254 nm, as seen in Figure 3.10, which shows the output from a water purification lamp. This makes them very efficient lamps for use in sterilization and disinfection. If used in rooms where people may be present, such as hospitals or cafeterias, the units need to be shielded to prevent direct viewing or exposure. From Table 3.4 it can be seen that the direct exposure to such a lamp must be limited to less than 3 minutes per day.

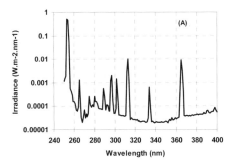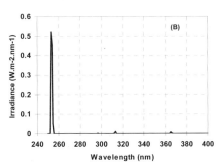

Figure 3.10 The emission spectrum from a germicidal water purification lamp, shown on a logarithmic scale in (A) and linear scale (B). Most of the lamp output is at 254 nm, in the UVC.

Table 3.4 UVR hazards from various types of sources. T_{max} is the time to exceed the ICNIRP [5] UVR exposure guidelines.

Lamp type	T_{max}
Fluorescent lighting	> 8 hrs
Quartz halogen lamps	
No filter	10 mins - 5 hrs
Filter attached	> 8 hrs
Standard lamps 1000W (0.5 m)	20 mins
Mercury discharge lamps	
UVC germicidal lamps	1-3 mins
UVB sunlamps	30 secs
UVA lamps	2-5 hrs
Sunlamps	3 mins
Phototherapy lamps	
Filtered	7 – 400 hrs
Unfiltered	1 min - 300 hrs
Blacklights	5 - 9 hrs
Arc lamps	
Xenon lamps (150 W)	5 hrs
Solar simulator	44 secs
Deuterium lamps	6 mins
Welding	1 - 5 mins
Solar UVR	
Summer mid-latitude	6 mins
Winter, mid-latitude	30 - 40 mins

5.3   Fluorescent lamps

Most low pressure mercury lamps are used for lighting, with a fluorescent phosphor coating on the inside wall which converts the 189 and 254 nm radiation from the arc to visible radiation suitable for illumination. The continuum emission depends upon the phosphor but all lamps generally show the typical mercury emission line structure. These lamps are designed to emit principally in the visible region (see Figure 3.11) although sometimes they emit some UVA. The glass used in the tube generally absorbs wavelengths below 320 nm, so hazardous UVR is virtually eliminated. The diffusers installed on the units also absorb UVR wavelengths and further reduce UVR emissions [50]. Lamp emissions, including UVR, also decrease as the lamps age. A more recent study by NRPB [51] found that while there had been some minor changes in the UVR output of typical fluorescent lamps over the previous 10 years, they still presented neither an acute nor a significant chronic hazard.

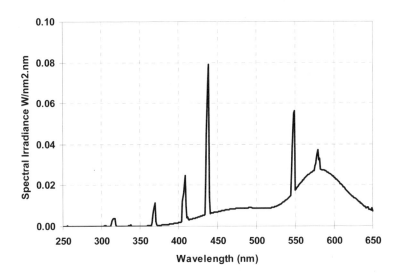

Figure 3.11 The emission spectrum from a typical fluorescent lamp, showing that almost all of the radiation emitted is at wavelengths above 400 nm, in the visible.

Blacklights are used in industry for the detection of flaws and cracks in materials. They emit predominately 366 nm UVR, which causes fluorescence in various dyes that lodge in the cracks of the material under examination. Sometimes the filter used to eliminate the visible may crack and staff can be exposed to some unfiltered UVR, but these lamps are not generally a hazard. Low power blacklights are also used for signature verification and exposures are well below the limits of the ICNIRP exposure guidelines, so they are not a hazard to staff using them or working all day in the vicinity.

Specially designed fluorescent lamps are used in solaria for artificial suntanning [52]. Generally these emit in the UVA with peak emissions at 360 to 370 nm but there is usually some UVB emission as well (generally less than a few percent of the total irradiance), to promote melanin production.

Some tanning lamps have been designed to emit substantial quantities of UVB (see Figure 3.12) but these are extremely hazardous, with maximum exposure times of the order of minutes. Their uncontrolled use can and has resulted in severe erythemal burns on occasion. Standards on the use of solaria for suntanning now exist in a number of countries [53]. These aim to impose controls on solarium exposures and minimize the associated risk. A more detailed discussion on solaria is to be found in Chapter 9. Also shown in Figure 3.12 is a domestic sunlamp. As there are no controls on their use, these domestic sunlamps are potentially dangerous.

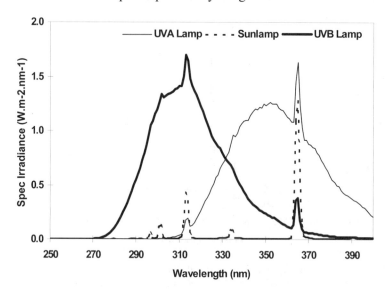

Figure 3.12 The spectral emissions from a UVA solarium lamp, a UVB lamp used in tanning booths and a portable sunlamp for home use. Times to exceed the ICNIRP limits for these lamps are given in Table 4.

5.4   High pressure discharge lamps

Metal halide lamps are generally used in commercial lighting applications but may also be used in photochemical processing and for photographic illumination and studio lighting. High intensity visible radiation is emitted along with substantial amounts of UVR. These lamps have a double envelope, the inner quartz tube containing the mercury-argon vapour discharge, the outer envelope of some form of glass, which generally absorbs the UVR emissions. If this outer envelope is cracked or broken, then the lamps may be a hazard and some metal halide lamps are designed to cease operation if this happens [46].

5.5   Arc lamps

Arc lamps operate at high temperatures and pressures and are intense sources of UVR and often visible radiation. These lamps are filled to very high pressures with mercury vapour or xenon gas or some combination of both. The lamps operate at 6000K, similar to the black-body temperature of the sun, which makes them useful for photographic illumination or as solar simulator sources.

Deuterium arc lamps are used in spectrophotometers to provide UVB and UVC radiation or to calibrate spectroradiometers across the UVB and UVC.

5.6   Welding

Welding falls into two main categories: gas welding or arc welding. The flames in gas welding generally have temperatures of less than 2000K, so UVR emissions are negligible. However, arc welding produces significant levels of UVR, the amounts and spectra depending upon the arc current, the metals being welded and the shielding gas used. Sliney and Wolbarsht [54] provide a comprehensive summary of the emissions from various forms of arc welding and their associated hazards, which can have maximum allowable exposure times for unprotected skin and eyes during an 8-hour working day of the order of seconds. Thus welders and their assistants form one of the largest occupational groups exposed to intense, artificial sources of UVR and optical radiation.

5.7   Occupational exposures

Exposures to industrial sources of UVR should be minimized by procedural and administrative control measures, which limit access of workers to areas and processes utilizing UVR. In addition, simple shielding can further reduce the hazard if one exists or the workers can be issued with protective clothing, eyewear and other items if they must work in the vicinity of a UVR source.

5.8   Medical exposures

Medical exposures to UVR include phototherapy and photochemotherapy. In the treatment of psoriasis using either UVB or UVA plus psoralen, it is expected that the benefits for the patients will outweigh the risks associated with UVR exposures. Sometimes, as with the treatment of hyperbilirubinaemia in newborn babies using blue light (usually 400 to 450 nm), UVR is a by-product of the lamp emission and must be eliminated by using specific plastic shielding which transmits the blue light but blocks the UVR below 400 nm. A more detailed discussion of medical exposures can be found in Moseley [7].

5.9   **Summary of artificial sources**

The hazard associated with the UVR emissions from artificial sources can be determined by applying the spectral weighting shown in Figure 3.5 using the ICNIRP [5] spectral effectiveness for $S\lambda$ in Equation 3.1. The results of this analysis are shown in Table 3.4, where when the maximum allowed exposure time T_{max} is short, it is possible to easily exceed the ICNIRP limits in an 8-hour working day. Such sources are likely to be a UVR hazard and need to be controlled.

UVR exposures due to artificial sources of UVR can be minimized by the application of administrative and procedural control measures. The exception to this is artificial suntanning in solaria, where exposure is by personal choice and can result in significant exposures to a specific section of the population.

CONCLUSIONS

The main focus of this chapter has been to explore the factors affecting solar UVR at the earth's surface. Solar UVR constitutes the source of the largest UVR exposures to the population, is very variable in its intensity and hazard (a hazard that may increase in future due to ozone depletion), and further efforts to reduce this exposure are still required.

Personal exposure to solar UVR depends on many of the factors affecting solar UVR (e.g., time of day and year, geographical location, local environment), as well as the activity undertaken and protection used. Changing people's outdoor behavior is critically important in reducing their solar UVR exposure. Protective measures against solar UVR (such as clothing, sunglasses, hats, and sunscreens) are capable of providing considerable reduction in UVR exposure (an order of magnitude or more), when used appropriately. It is important that outdoor workers have an understanding of their potential for overexposure and that both personal protection measures and structural measures, such as the modification of working hours and the provision of shade, where possible, are invoked.

SUMMARY POINTS

- Solar UVR constitutes the source of the largest UVR exposures to the population.
- Solar elevation, diffuse radiation, ozone levels, effects of clouds, ground surface reflection, geographical location, time of year, and altitude all affect levels of UVR at the earth's surface.
- The organs at risk of UVR damage are the skin and the eyes.
- Changing outdoor behavior is critically important in reducing solar UVR exposure.
- Protective measures against solar UVR such as clothing, sunglasses, hats, and sunscreens are capable of providing considerable reduction in UVR exposure.
- Artificial UVR sources can be extremely hazardous but a range of control measures limits people's exposure.
- Benefits to patients undergoing medical exposures to UVR are expected to outweigh the risks associated with UVR exposure.

IMPLICATIONS FOR PUBLIC HEALTH

People are familiar with and are often unconcerned about exposure to the sun. As a consequence, their solar UVR exposures are significant and constitute a major long-term health problem. The key control to reduce solar UVR exposure is changing behavior. Artificial sources of UVR can be extremely hazardous, much more so than the sun. While people are usually wary about exposure to such artificial sources because they are unfamiliar with them, experience shows these UVR exposures are generally not a major problem because they can be controlled.

ACKNOWLEDGEMENTS

The authors wish to thank the Laboratory for Atmospheres at NASA GSFC for the provision of satellite data on ozone and cloud reflectivities. Thanks also to the staff of the UVR Section at ARPANSA, John Javorniczky, Zina Sofer, Alan McLennan, Stuart Henderson and Sharon Adrain for their invaluable assistance and support.

REFERENCES

1. CIE Research Note (1987) A reference action spectrum for ultraviolet induced erythema in human skin. *CIE J* **6**: 17-22.
2. International Commission on Illumination (1997) *Standard erythema dose, a review*. CIE Technical Report 125. Vienna, Austria: CIE, ISBN 390073481X.
3. IRPA/INIRC (1985) Guidelines on limits of exposure to ultraviolet radiation of wavelengths between 180 nm and 400 nm (incoherent radiation). *Health Phys* **49**(2): 331-340.
4. IRPA/INIRC (1989) Proposed change to the IRPA 1985 guidelines on limits of exposure to ultraviolet radiation. *Health Phys* **56**: 971-972.
5. Matthes R, Bernhardt JH, McKinlay AF, eds. (1999) *Guidelines on Limiting Exposure to Non-Ionizing Radiation*. ICNIRP (International Commission on Non-Ionizing Radiation Protection), ISBN 3-9804789-6-3, pp 207-226.
6. Gibson P, Diffey BL (1989) Techniques for Spectroradiometry and Broadband Radiometry. In: Diffey BL, ed. *Radiation Measurement in Photobiology*. London: Academic Press, pp 71-84.
7. Moseley H (1988) *Non-ionising Radiation: microwaves, ultraviolet and laser radiation*. Bristol: Adam Hilger.
8. Josefsson WAP (1993) Monitoring Ultraviolet Radiation. In: Young AR, Bjorn LO, Moan J, Nultsch W, eds. *Environmental UV Photobiology*. New York: Plenum Press, pp 73-88.
9. Davis A, Deane GHW, Diffey BL (1976) Possible dosimeter for ultraviolet radiation. *Nature* **261**: 169-170.
10. Quintern LE, Horneck G, Eschweiler U, Bucker H (1992) A biofilm used as ultraviolet dosimeter. *Photochem Photobiol* **55**: 389-395.
11. Munakata N, Kazadsis S, Bais A, *et al.* (2000) Comparisons of spore dosimetry and spectral photometry of solar-UV radiation at four sites in Japan and Europe. *Photochem Photobiol* **72**: 739-745.
12. Thakekara MP (1973) Solar energy outside the earth's atmosphere. *Solar Energy* **14**: 109-127.
13. Bird RE, Hulstrom RL, Kliman AW, Eldering HG (1982) Solar spectral measurements in the terrestrial environment. *Appl Optics* **21**: 1430-1436.
14. Farman JC, Gardiner BG, Shanklin JD (1985) Large losses of total ozone in Antarctica reveal seasonal ClOx/Nox interaction. *Nature* **315**: 207-210.
15. United Nations Environment Programme (1998) *Environmental Effects of Ozone Depletion*: 1998 Assessment. ISBN 92-807-1724-3.
16. Lubin D, Jensen EH. (1995) Effects of clouds and stratospheric ozone depletion on ultraviolet radiation trends. *Nature* **377**: 710-713.
17. International Commission on Non-Ionizing Radiation Protection (1995). *Global Solar UV Index*. ICNIRP-1/95.
18. World Health Organization (2002) *Global Solar UV Index: A Practical Guide*. Geneva, Switzerland: WHO.
19. Dixon H, Armstrong B (1999) *The UV Index. Report of a national workshop on its role in sun protection*. Sydney: NSW Cancer Council and Anti-Cancer Council of Victoria.
20. McKenzie RL. (1991) Application of a simple model to calculate latitudinal and hemispheric differences in ultraviolet radiation. *Weather & Climate* **11**: 3-14.
21. Seckmeyer G, Erb R, Abold A (1996) Transmittance of a cloud is wavelength-dependent in the UV-range. *Geophys Res Lett* 23 , 2753-2755.
22. Mims FM, Frederick JE (1994) Cumulus clouds and UV-B. *Nature* **371**: 291.

23. Schafer JS, Saxena VK, Wenny BN, Barnard W, De Luisi JJ (1996) Observed influence of clouds on ultraviolet –B radiation. *Geophys Res Lett* **23**: 2625-2628.
24. Matthijsen J, Slaper H, Reinen HAJM (2000) Reduction of solar UVR by clouds: A comparison between satellite-derived cloud effects and ground-based radiation measurements. *J Geophys Res* **105**: 5069-5080.
25. Sliney D (1994) Epidemiological studies of sunlight and cataract: the critical factor of ultraviolet exposure geometry. *Ophthal Epidem* **1**: 107-119.
26. McKenzie RL, Kotkamp M (1996) Upwelling UV spectral irradiances and surface albedo measurements at Lauder, New Zealand. *Geophys Res Lett* **23**: 1757-1760.
27. Diffey BL (1992) Stratospheric ozone depletion and the risk of non-melanoma skin cancer in a British population. *Phys Med Biol* **37**: 2267-2279.
28. Blumthaler M, Webb AR, Seckmeyer G, Bais AF, Huber M, Mayer B (1994) Simultaneous spectroradiometry; a study of solar UV irradiance at two altitudes. *Geophys Res Lett* **21**: 2805-2808.
29. Frederick JE, Koob AE, Alberts AD, Weatherhead EC (1993) Empirical studies of tropospheric transmission in the ultraviolet: Broadband measurements. *J Appl Meteorol* **32**: 1883-1892.
30. Roy CR, Gies HP, Toomey S (1995) The solar UV radiation environment: measurement techniques and results. *J Photochem Photobiol B: Biology* **99**: 21-27.
31. McKenzie RL, Bodeker JK, Keep DJ, Kotkamp M (1996) UV Radiation in New Zealand: North-to-South differences between two sites, and relationship to other latitudes. *Weather & Climate* **16**: 17-26.
32. Driscoll CMH (1996) Solar UVR measurements. *Rad Prot Dosim* **3**: 179-188.
33. Martinez-Lozana JA, Marin MJ, Tena F, *et al.* (2002). UV Index Experimental values during the years 2000 and 2001 from the Spanish Broadband UV-B Radiometric Network. *Photochem Photobiol* **76**: 181-187.
34. Scotto J, Cotton G, Urbach F, Berger D, Fears T (1988) Biologically effective ultraviolet radiation: Surface measurements in the United States, 1974 to 1985. *Science* **239**: 762-764.
35. Ono, M. (1997) Preliminary Study on Exposure Measurement of Ultraviolet Radiation. In: Sasaki K, Hockwin O, eds. *Cataract Epidemiology*. Dev Ophthalmol. Basel: Karger **27**: 81-88.
36. Seckmeyer G, Mayer B, Bernhard G, Erb R, Jager H, Stockwell WR (1997) New maximum UV irradiance levels observed in central Europe. *Atmos Env* **18**: 2971-2976.
37. Den Outer PN, Slaper H, Matthijsen J, Reinen AJM, Tax R (2000) Variability of ground – level ultraviolet: Model and measurement. *Rad Prot Dosim* **91**: 105-110.
38. Josefson W (1996) *Five years of solar UV-Radiation monitoring in Sweden.* Swedish Meteorological and Hydrological Institute, Norrkoping, Report RMK 71.
39. Gies HP, Roy CR, Toomey S, MacLennan R, Watson M (1995) Solar UVR exposures of three groups of outdoor workers on the Sunshine Coast, Queensland. *Photochem Photobiol* **62**: 1015-1021.
40. Udelhofen PM, Gies P, Roy C, Randel WJ (1999) Surface UV radiation over Australia, 1979-1992: Effects of ozone and cloud cover changes on variations of UV radiation. *J Geophys Res* **104**: 19135-19159.
41. Herman JR, Krotkov N, Celarier E, Larko D, Labow G (1999) Distribution of UV radiation at the Earth's surface from TOMS-measured UV-backscattered radiances. *J Geophys Res* **104**:12059-12076.
42. Gies HP, Roy CR, Toomey S, Tomlinson D (1999) Ambient Solar UVR, Personal Exposure and Protection. *J Epidemiol,* **9**: S115-S121, 1999.

43. European Commission. (1996) Public health and safety at work. *Non-ionizing radiation. Sources, exposure and health effects.* B-1049 Brussels. 1996.
44. Godar DE, Wengraitis SP, Shreffler J, Sliney DH (2001) UV doses of Americans. *Photochem Photobiol* **73**: 621-629.
45. Diffey BL, Gies HP (1998) The confounding influence of sun exposure in melanoma. *The Lancet* **351**:1101-1102.
46. McKinlay AF, Harlen F, Whillock MJ (1988) *Hazards of optical radiation: A guide to sources, uses and safety.* Bristol, Philadelphia: Adam Hilger.
47. World Health Organisation (1994) *Environmental Health Criteria 160: Ultraviolet Radiation.* An authoritative scientific review of environmental and health effects of U.V. with reference to global ozone layer depletion. Joint publication by WHO, UNEP, ICNIRP, Geneva.
48. Pearson AJ, Grainger KJL, Whillock MJ, Drsicoll CMH (1991) Hazard assessment of optical radiation sources used in some consumer products. NRPB Radiolog Prot Bulletin No. 126.
49. Whillock MJ, Pearson AJ, McKinlay AF, Driscoll CMH (1990) Assessment of optical radiation hazards from tungsten halogen lamps. *NRPB Radiolog Prot Bulletin* No. 116.
50. Roy CR, Gies HP, Elliott G (1989) Malignant Melanoma and Fluorescent Lighting: Current Status. *Rad Prot in Australia* **7**(2): 45-49.
51. Pearson A (1998) UVR from fluorescent lamps. *NRPB Radiolog Prot Bulletin* No. 200.
52. Gies HP, Roy CR, Elliott G (1986) Artificial Suntanning: Spectral Irradiance and Hazard Evaluation of Ultraviolet Sources. *Health Phys* **50**: 691-703.
53. Cesarini JP (1999) The French Regulations for Ultraviolet Radiation Sunbeds. *Rad Prot Dosim* **91**: 205-207.
54. Sliney D, Wolbarsht M (1980) *Safety with Lasers and Other Optical Sources.* New York: Plenum Press.

Chapter 4

Stratospheric ozone depletion, UV exposure and skin cancer: a scenario analysis

Harry Slaper[1], Ph.D.; Frank R. de Gruijl[2], Ph.D.
[1]Lab. for Radiation Research, National Institute for Public Health and the Environment (RIVM), Bilthoven, The Netherlands; [2]Dermatology, Leiden University Medical Centre, Leiden, The Netherlands.

Key words: ozone depletion, UV-radiation, skin cancer, risk assessment, Vienna Convention to protect the ozone layer

INTRODUCTION

There is overwhelming evidence, discussed elsewhere in this book, that exposure of the skin to UV-radiation can lead to, or at least contribute to, the development of skin cancer. The sun is the major source of UV-radiation to which the human skin is exposed. Within the earth's atmosphere, ozone serves as a partly protective shield by absorbing most of the effective part of the UV-spectrum and thus preventing a major part of the harmful UV from reaching the earth's surface. Depletion of atmospheric ozone has been observed over large parts of the globe in recent decades, and it was predicted that harmful UV-radiation levels at the earth's surface would have increased. The observed decrease in ozone was thought to be related to the large-scale emissions of halocarbon compounds as a result of human activity [1]. In 1985, in view of the scientific evidence that the emission of halocarbon compounds could lead to ozone depletion, the United Nations Environment Programme (UNEP) initiated the Vienna Convention to protect the ozone

55

D. Hill et al. (eds.), Prevention of Skin Cancer, 55-71.
© 2004 *Kluwer Academic Publishers. Printed in the Netherlands.*

layer. This provided the framework for the discussion and implementation of international restrictions on the production of ozone depleting substances and led to the first international agreement on the reduction of the production of ozone depleting substances in 1987 in the Montreal Protocol. Following scientific evidence that ozone depletion was actually occurring, the Montreal Protocol was strengthened in several later Amendments.

In this chapter we will briefly discuss the process of ozone depletion, and then focus on the changes in ozone and UV-radiation that have been observed. We will then present a scenario analysis of the changes that might be expected to occur in the coming decades as a result of the countermeasures that were agreed upon. This will be followed by an analysis of the consequences of ozone depletion in terms of (future) skin cancer risks and an evaluation of the effectiveness of the countermeasures taken [2]. It should be noted that skin cancer risk is only one of the adverse effects related to increases in UV-radiation levels due to ozone depletion [3].

1.   OZONE LAYER AND OZONE DEPLETION PROCESSES

Oxygen absorbs the most energetic UV radiation (wavelengths below 200 nm) from the sun in the outer reaches of our atmosphere, and ozone, which consists of three oxygen atoms, is formed in the process. Although ozone is rare in our atmosphere, averaging three molecules of ozone for every 10 million air molecules, it absorbs most of the solar radiation with wavelengths below 310 nm, and UV radiation below 290 nm is virtually undetectable at ground level. Solar radiation at these short wavelengths below 300 nm is extremely effective in initiating photochemical reactions, both in the atmosphere and in a wide variety of organic molecules (particularly those with linear repeats of conjugated bonds, or conjugated bonds in ring structures), and is capable of causing damage. Thus, oxygen protects the earth's surface from the most damaging solar UV radiation. However, the small amount of short-wave radiant energy (around 300-310 nm) that seeps through is still capable of causing some damage (e.g., toxic reactions like sunburn in the skin), and life on earth has had to adapt to this continuous challenge.

Most atmospheric ozone is found at an altitude between 15 and 40 km above the earth's surface. This region in the atmosphere is the stratosphere, and the ozone in this layer is referred to as the ozone layer. The absorption of short-wave UV-radiation by the ozone in the stratosphere is a source of heat and this causes the temperatures in the stratosphere to rise with height above the earth's surface. Production and destruction of ozone molecules are normally occurring processes in the stratosphere, but the balance between production and destruction can be changed by an increase of ozone depleting substances containing chlorine and bromine. About 90% of atmospheric ozone is found in the stratospheric ozone layer, and the remainder is found in the lower parts of the atmosphere, the troposphere (lower 10 km). Tropospheric ozone, which is formed as part of photochemical smog in the summer in polluted areas, is a toxic compound and has harmful effects on crop production, forest growth and human health. The direct toxicity of the tropospheric ozone outweighs the fact that tropospheric ozone contributes to the reduction of harmful UV. Environmental policies are therefore aiming at decreasing the tropospheric ozone content and increasing the stratospheric ozone content.

The first concerns over a possible deterioration of the UV-protective ozone layer stemmed from around 1970, and were stirred up by the prospect of a large fleet of supersonic commercial airplanes (Concorde-like) cruising through the stratosphere. It was anticipated that the exhausts of these stratospheric planes would directly inject nitrogen oxides (NO_x) into the ozone layer, which would reduce the concentration of ozone. In the USA, several expert committees were formed for a scientific evaluation [4]. It was concluded that the most likely long-term effect would be an increase in skin cancers. Although scientific data on other potential effects were less firm, it was considered that the effects could be far reaching and that prudence was called for.

At this time the threat of large-scale supersonic transportation had not materialized, but in 1974 Molina and Roland [5] drew attention to the potential effects of man-made chlorofluorocarbons (CFCs), which are very stable and have atmospheric lifetimes of up to more than a century. The molecules can diffuse up into the outer reaches of our atmosphere where high-energy UV radiation breaks them down, releasing reactive chlorine which will diminish the ozone. The long atmospheric lifetime of CFCs and halones implied that the emissions would have an impact on the ozone layer for decades. Model calculations indicated substantial effects, and political pressure mounted to take precautionary action. The use of CFCs in spray cans (for deodorants, shaving cream etc.) was banned. However, it was much harder to eradicate other applications of CFCs, because of the lack of replacements (e.g., for air-conditioning in cars), and/or economic implications (e.g., large disinvestments). Because of the lack of firm scientific data in the form of direct proof, inertia and understandable reservations in industry, the political progress took time, but it received an enormous impetus by the discovery of the "ozone hole" over the Antarctic by Farman et al. in 1985 [6].

2.   THE ANTARCTIC OZONE HOLE

Farman *et al.* [6] found very strong ozone losses in the early spring period over the Antarctic, when comparing the ozone values measured at the ground at Halley Bay before 1980 with those in the early eighties. The ozone observations from ground based and satellite based measurements showed a rapid decline in the early springtime (September-November) ozone column from year to year in the period from 1980-1990. In the period 1990-2000, the total ozone column was reduced by 60% in the period from September to November over large parts of the Antarctic.

The "ozone hole" came as a surprise, since it had not been predicted that ozone depletion would occur to that extent in the polar region during the early Antarctic spring. The observations by Farman *et al.* [6] triggered extensive studies to investigate the precise nature of the processes occurring at the South Pole area. These studies have shown that the area of the Antarctic ozone hole coincides with the region of high chlorine monoxide (ClO), which is the reactive form of chlorine and which is known to break down ozone under the influence of sunlight. The occurrence of the relatively high concentration of chlorine monoxide at the Antarctic is caused by the formation of polar stratospheric clouds in the very cold and stable stratosphere during the Antarctic winter and early spring. These stratospheric clouds catalyze the transformation of chlorine species that do not cause ozone depletion into the reactive chlorine monoxide. The ozone depletion then occurs when the sun reappears in the early Antarctic spring. Later in the spring the Antarctic atmosphere becomes warmer and less stable and the mixing with air from lower latitudes causes a decrease in chlorine monoxide levels and an increase in ozone values over the polar area, and some decreases of ozone over the mid-latitudes.

The question arises as to why a similar depletion is not observed over the Arctic. The Arctic winter is cold enough to form polar stratospheric clouds, but the weather conditions at the Arctic are less stable compared with the Antarctic, and thus the very favorable conditions for the formation of chlorine monoxide, which would be needed to start the rapid destruction of ozone when the sun is reappearing, do not persist into the spring. However, many of the winters in the 1990's have shown persistent extremely low stratospheric temperatures in the Arctic region, leading to enhanced ozone depletion [7]. It is highly uncertain whether this temperature trend will continue as a result of climate change, or whether it will be reversed in coming years. This uncertainty makes it difficult to predict future ozone depletion in the Northern Hemisphere.

The discovery of the Antarctic ozone hole served as a warning and underlined the message "reactive chlorine destroys ozone!" The exceptional atmospheric circumstances at the South Pole in wintertime (a stable, very cold, polar "vortex") taught us that the effect of chlorine was thus far underestimated by neglecting chemical reactions on solid surfaces of stratospheric cloud particles. The relevance of heterogeneous chemistry in stratospheric ozone destruction was also recognized following the volcanic eruption of Mt Pinatubo in 1991. This eruption brought a large load of aerosols into the stratosphere, which had effects on ozone destruction processes similar to the effects of polar stratospheric clouds. In the presence of a high chlorine load (80% of which was of man-made origin), the stratospheric aerosols led to an increase in the transformation of non-reactive chlorine to ozone-depleting reactive chlorine. This enhanced breakdown of ozone would not occur in the absence of man-made chlorine in the stratosphere. As the stratospheric aerosols from volcanic eruptions are removed in 2-5 years, the effects of the Mt Pinatubo eruption on the ozone layer were therefore negligible by the end of the twentieth century.

3.   OZONE TRENDS

Ozone trends have not only been observed in the Polar Regions, but also at mid-latitudes over both hemispheres (see for instance Chapter 4 in [1]). Ground based and satellite based ozone measurements together show that overall year round trends are largest near the poles. No significant trends were observed in tropical regions. In the period 1979 to 1997, the year round downward trends in ozone columns were 3-4% per decade averaged over latitudes from 35-60°N, and less than 1% per decade in the tropical regions. In the Southern Hemisphere, downward ozone trends at mid-latitudes from 35-55°S were 2-3% per decade. From the perspective of UV doses received, it is also important to note that in various regions the ozone depletion shows distinct seasonal dependence: downward trends are usually highest in spring, followed by winter, and lowest in autumn. Furthermore, trends can be substantially higher in certain regions within a particular latitude band.

Trends seem to have weakened over recent years, but in view of the interaction with the diminishing ozone depleting effect of the 1991 Pinatubo eruption, it is too early to conclude that the slowing down is a consequence of countermeasures. Nevertheless, reduced chlorine loads in the troposphere have now been reported and it is expected that chlorine levels in the stratosphere will decrease slowly. Whether this leads to an immediate upward trend in ozone levels remains to be seen, because of possible interactions with effects related to climate change [7]. Temperatures in the stratosphere might further decrease as a consequence of climate change, and this might lead to an increase in the formation of polar stratospheric clouds, which, in the presence of ozone depleting substances, contribute to an enhanced ozone destruction in the polar regions. The expected decrease in the concentrations of ozone depleting substances, caused by the countermeasures that were taken to protect the ozone layer, might thus be counterbalanced by an increased effectiveness of these substances due to polar stratospheric clouds. These consequences for ozone destruction are not restricted to Polar Regions, and, if occurring, will also lead to at least a delay in the recovery of the ozone layer at mid-latitudes. Although highly uncertain, a delay of around twenty years has been estimated [8].

4.   TRENDS IN SURFACE UV-RADIATION

Direct trend measurements of surface UV-radiation levels have been largely lacking over the previous decades [1], simply because long-term monitoring data measured with sufficiently accurate instrumentation is not available. Upward trends for limited periods and under clear sky conditions have now been reported in relation to ozone changes observed. The number of measurement sites has increased in recent years and international comparisons have demonstrated that the accuracy and stability of the instrumentation has improved considerably in recent years [1,9,10]. Nevertheless, it is not possible to derive global UV-trends directly from ground-based UV-measurements. That lower ozone levels lead to higher UV-radiation levels in the shortest wavelengths of the UV-radiation reaching the surface is clear, and can be studied by looking at the changes in UV-radiation in relation to short term changes in ozone. Ozone levels can vary considerably from day to day, and this could be used to analyze UV-radiation levels in relation to ozone changes. It should be noted that ozone mainly absorbs in the UVB (280-315 nm) region of the spectrum, and has hardly any effect on the radiation above 350 nm. Therefore, when considering the effect of ozone changes on UV-radiation it is crucial to analyze the part of the spectrum that is relevant to the effect under consideration, and for many adverse UV-effects this is the UVB part. For many effects, so-called action spectra have been determined, which can be used as a spectral weighting function to identify the effective part of the UV [3]. We are primarily interested in skin cancer risks and therefore use a skin cancer action spectrum (identified as SCUP-h [1]), which has been derived from experiments in hairless mice, and which was transferred to human skin taking into account the difference in optical properties of mouse and human skin [11,12] (see also Chapter 11).

To analyze how ozone changes relate to changes in effective UV doses, we have used five years of UV-monitoring data from the Netherlands to calculate daily sums of weighted UV-doses and of UVA-doses. Taking the ratio of the two diminishes the varying effect of clouds. The effective measured ratio is then divided by a similar ratio obtained by using UV-transfer model calculations with a constant ozone thickness of 350 DU. Figure 4.1 gives the results for this analysis for a large range of measured ozone values covering 230-470 DU. The results clearly demonstrate that lower ozone values lead to higher effective UV-radiation doses, and vice versa. We have also added a line reflecting modeled effective UV-doses using measured ozone values. It can be seen that the UV-transfer model calculations match the measured effective UV-changes in relation to ozone changes very well. This gives some confidence that the UV-transfer model in combination with ozone data can be used to analyse historical trends in effective UV due to ozone depletion.

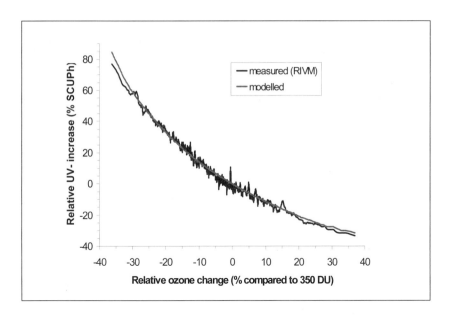

Figure 4.1   Relation between skin cancer weighted UV and the total ozone column, comparing models and measurements from RIVM UV-monitoring system in Bilthoven (52 N), The Netherlands [8]

Using daily ozone measurements from the TOMS-satellite, we calculated the relative trend in effective UV. Figure 4.2 demonstrates that over the period 1980-2000 the trend amounts to an overall increase in effective UV of 6-7% over large parts of Western and Central Europe. The true trend is slightly higher, because due to failure of the instrumentation, the TOMS records are unavailable in some of the years that, according to ground based

data, had the lowest ozone values. The overall change in yearly effective
UV-doses over the previous two decades is 7-10% in the most densely
populated areas of Europe [13,14]. For some years following the Pinatubo
eruption the increases probably have been 10-15% in large parts of Europe
[15].

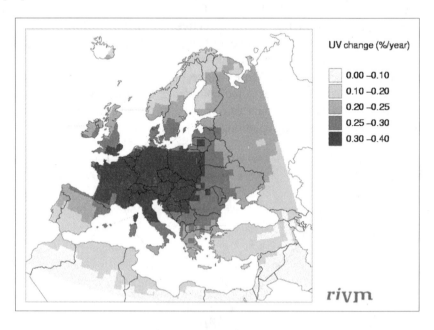

Figure 4.2 UV-trend over the European continent over the period 1980-2000 [14]

5.   SKIN CANCER AND UV-EXPOSURE

5.1   Types of skin cancer

Skin cancer is particularly common in white Caucasians living in tropical
and subtropical areas such as Australia and the USA. In the USA skin cancer
comprises over 30% of cancer cases, with more than 1 million cases per year
[16]. In early epidemiological studies (before 1980) the figures on squamous
cell carcinomas (SCC) and basal cell carcinomas (BCC) were lumped
together and given in the category of "non-melanoma skin cancer" under the
assumption that the etiology of SCC and BCC were very similar. This,
however, proved to be a fallacy, and the impact of solar UV radiation on
these two tumor types needs to be considered separately. BCC, SCC, and

melanoma all show a north-south gradient over the USA, i.e., a positive correlation with ambient UV-radiation, but the relative north-south increases are most substantial for SCC (see Chapter 6).

SCC appears to be most straightforwardly related to the total sun (UV) exposure: these tumors occur on skin areas that are most regularly exposed (face, neck and hands) and the risk goes up with the life-long accumulated UV dose. BCC and melanoma do not show this simple relationship to UV exposure: these tumors appear to be more related to intermittent over-exposure (episodes of sunburn, especially on irregularly exposed skin) and sun exposure in childhood [17,18]. A recent randomized trial [19] showed that 4.5 years use of sunscreen in adulthood lowered the development of SCC, but not of BCC. This would be in line with the finding that UV radiation contributes to the development of SCC at all stages during a lifetime, while UV radiation mostly affects the very early stages of BCC development. Also the level of ambient sun exposure in childhood determines the number of nevi that a person contracts [20], and the number of nevi is a well-established risk factor for melanoma. This further confirms the importance of early life exposure to the risk of melanoma later in life.

5.2   Altered ambient UV radiation and skin cancer incidences

The easiest approach to quantify the effect of an increased UV exposure, such as that caused by a depletion of the ozone layer, is to compare two stationary situations: one with a life-long low UV exposure and the other a life-long high UV exposure. Assuming that the white Caucasian populations in various locations in the USA are sufficiently comparable (in behavior and genetic composition) and in a stationary condition (in relation to UV exposure and skin tumor incidence), one can use the relationship between ambient UV loads and incidence for the assessment. For each percent of ozone depletion, SCC would increase by 3%, BCC by 1.7%, and melanoma by 0.5-1%, if the SCUP-h action spectrum is also applicable to melanoma [12,21,22]. However, such an approach is confounded, in that the incidence rates of BCC and melanoma in particular, are not stationary in the USA and as well, the UV-radiation environment is changing due to changes in the total column ozone.

Transitional changes in incidence rates due to changes in UV exposure are much harder to estimate. This requires much more detailed knowledge, such as whether UV acts early, late, or continuously in the process of skin carcinogenesis. From the above it appears that UV acts throughout the genesis of SCC, but mainly in an early stage of BCC and melanoma development (See Chapter 6). Using a vast body of animal and epidemiological studies in combination with growing knowledge of the biological processes that lead to the development of tumors, we can develop quantitative models that can be used to calculate skin cancer incidence in relation to age and changing UV-exposure over a lifetime (see Chapter 11). Thus, scenario studies of the effects of changes in ozone can be made [2].

6.   SCENARIOS

The Vienna Convention in 1985 was the starting point for international policy agreements on the reduction of halocarbon emissions and provided a framework for the restrictive protocols that followed. The Montreal Protocol (MP) in 1987 provided the first restrictive countermeasures, in which the production of the five major ozone-depleting substances was restricted to 50% of the 1986 production levels by the year 2000. In 1990, the London Amendments to the MP, which aimed for a complete phase out of the primary ozone depleting substances by the year 2000, were agreed upon. Additional restrictions were issued in the Copenhagen Amendments in 1992 where the complete phase out for developed countries was shifted to 1996. Further restrictions were agreed upon in Vienna (1995) and Montreal (1997). Figure 4.3 illustrates the impact of the restrictions on the production of one of the major CFCs (CFC-11) compared to a no-restriction scenario.

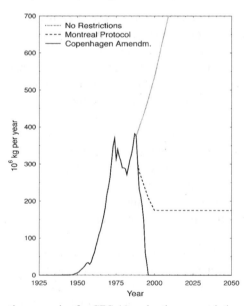

Figure 4.3 Production scenarios for CFC-11 under the no-restrictions scenario, the Montreal Protocol from 1987, and the Copenhagen Amendments.

6.1 Assessment Model for UV Radiation and Risks (AMOUR)

In order to assess the possible future consequences of the various countermeasures, a source-risk model has been developed to evaluate future skin cancer risks in relation to the emission of ozone-depleting substances [2]. Although the model is capable of an evaluation of effects of changes in exposure behavior such as the use of protective clothing and sunscreens, such changes are not included in the scenario analysis presented here. This analysis is focused on ozone changes alone. Although ozone depletion is influenced by climate changes related to greenhouse gas emissions, in this scenario, in line with assumptions made in previous assessments [1,2], we assume that the ozone layer is influenced only by CFC-emissions. We calculate and compare a no-Restriction scenario (NR) with the Montreal Protocol and the Copenhagen Amendments to that Protocol.

In order to evaluate future skin cancer risks in relation to ozone depletion scenarios, the following are required: scenarios for the production and subsequent emissions of ozone depleting substances, the dispersion of the depleting substances into the atmosphere and the subsequent influence on the total ozone column, the consequences of ozone changes on the effective UV-radiation reaching the ground, and finally the dose-time-effect relationships relating skin cancer incidence to UV-exposure. We use the production and emission scenarios in the subsequent Amendments of the Montreal Protocol, assuming global compliance with the countermeasures. CFCs emitted in the lower parts of the atmosphere are not removed from the atmosphere and slowly diffuse to the stratosphere where, under the influence of the intense UV-radiation, a photochemical breakdown releases active chlorine and bromine, which catalyze ozone destruction. The release of active chlorine (and bromine) is analyzed using the methods developed at NOAA [23]. The depletion of ozone in relation to the increase in chlorine loading is based on the historical observations on ozone and chlorine changes. A two dimensional stratospheric chemistry model is used to analyze ozone changes in relation to changes in the chlorine loading and to calculate the saturation levels occurring at high depletion levels.

The relative increase in yearly skin cancer weighted UV-doses for NW-Europe are calculated for three scenarios and presented in Figure 4.4. For comparison, historical changes calculated from ground and satellite based ozone measurement are also shown. The results show that following the strictest countermeasures is likely to return the UV-radiation levels to the 1980 level by approximately 2070. The stratospheric temperature is expected to decrease due to climate change, which could lead to an increase in the number of polar stratospheric clouds, and thus to a more effective depletion of ozone in the Polar Regions. This could also have an impact through transport on ozone at temperate zones. Preliminary analyses indicate that the recovery of the ozone layer might be delayed by ten to more than twenty years [8,24], and it might be that minimum ozone levels and maximum UV-radiation levels are not reached prior to 2020. However, various model studies show large differences, and many uncertainties still exist [7,8].

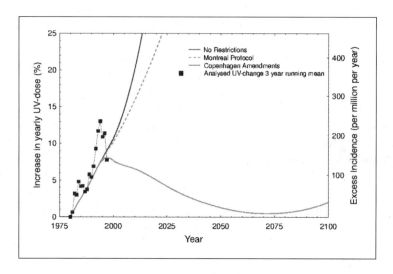

Figure 4.4 UV-radiation changes in NW-Europe in relation to the various scenarios

7.   EXCESS SKIN CANCER RISKS DUE TO OZONE DEPLETION

Without restrictions on ozone depleting substances, skin cancer incidence could quadruple by the end of this century, and even initial restrictions under the Montreal Protocol would still yield a two-fold increase [2]. If the strictest Amendments of the Montreal Protocol are fully and globally adhered to, the future increase in skin cancer risks due to ozone depletion might be restricted to an increase of 5-10% of the present incidence, i.e., 60-100 additional cases per million inhabitants per year. The majority of these would be non-melanoma skin cancers. The additional risk around the year 2000 is no more than a few percent of the incidence around 1980. Thus, it is unlikely that presently reported increases in skin cancer incidence could be attributed to the ozone depletion observed in recent decades. In view of the long latency period between a change in exposure and the change in incidence, one might speculate that present changes relate to changes in behavior towards sun exposure. If behavioral changes towards sun-exposure cause increases in present skin cancer risks it is likely that the estimated future excess skin cancer risks due to ozone depletion are too low. Furthermore, the future risks could be higher due to the above-mentioned effects of climate change. Nevertheless, the results shown in Figure 4.5 clearly demonstrate how important it is to fully comply with the strictest countermeasures agreed upon under the Vienna Convention.

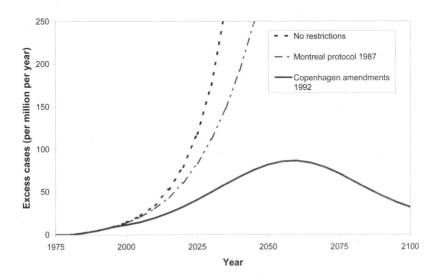

Figure 4.5 Excess skin cancer cases related to ozone depletion, calculated for NW-Europe for three scenarios: no restrictions, implying that no restrictive countermeasures are taken; restrictions according to the Montreal Protocol as agreed upon in 1987 and restrictions according to the Copenhagen Amendments of the Montreal Protocol.

CONCLUSIONS

Ozone depletion has been observed over large parts of the globe, and as a consequence UV-radiation levels have probably increased in Polar Regions and mid-latitudes. The largest ozone depletion occurring in the Antarctic in spring is referred to as the "ozone hole." Ozone depletion has occurred in heavily populated areas in Europe and the USA as well and it is calculated that the UV-doses received increased by 5-15% from 1980 to the mid-1990s.

By combining the epidemiological and animal-experimental data we have derived quantitative tumor-response models for SCC, BCC, and melanoma. These models were used in scenario studies of changes in the thickness of the ozone layer in the stratosphere and corresponding changes in ambient UV radiation at ground level. Thus – based on the assumption that "everything else would remain similar" (*ceteris paribus*) – it was projected that with a minimum ozone level around the turn of the century, the overall skin cancer incidence in the US and NW Europe would show a modest peak with approximately a 10% increase over current levels. If the latest amendments are not met, skin cancer incidence may steadily rise to twice the current levels or more.

The results of the analysis also show that increases in skin cancer incidence presently observed and reported are to a large extent not attributable to the observed changes in the total ozone column. Around the turn of the century, increases that could be attributed to ozone depletion are less than a few percent and would most probably not be distinguishable in present skin cancer statistics. This implies that reported increases are related to other factors, among which changes in behavior towards sun exposure are probably important. If changes in the exposure of the population have led to increases in skin cancer incidence over the past decades this will imply that the excess risks caused by ozone depletion will be higher than the excess risk calculated in the presented scenario studies.

The fact that excess risks due to ozone depletion are presently expected not to exceed around 10% at the most does not mean that protection of the ozone layer is of lower relevance, since it is clearly shown that without countermeasures the skin cancer risks could easily double or quadruple compared to present levels. It remains therefore very important to strictly adhere to the strictest countermeasures agreed upon under the Montreal Protocol. Furthermore, there is considerable uncertainty about future developments, because ozone depletion and recovery can be strongly influenced by climate change. In addition, climate change can lead to changes in cloud patterns and thus to direct changes in UV-radiation received at the ground. In view of these uncertainties it will be important to monitor the UV-radiation and ozone levels globally and regionally in order to establish trends and track changes. Looking at skin cancer risks, the major changes presently observed are related to changes in behavior rather than ozone changes, which stresses the importance of skin cancer prevention programs.

SUMMARY POINTS

- As a consequence of ozone depletion caused by the large-scale emissions of man-made halocarbons, the skin cancer weighted UV-doses increased by 5-15% in heavily populated areas over Europe from 1980 to the end of the twentieth century.

- In 1985 the United Nations Environment Programme (UNEP) provided a framework for international agreements: the Vienna Convention to protect the ozone layer. Countermeasures were agreed to reduce the production and emission of the most important ozone depleting substances in the Montreal Protocol (1987) and subsequent Amendments.

- A scenario analysis illustrates the importance of the countermeasures in limiting the additional cases of skin cancer that are related to decreases in ozone. Without these countermeasures the skin cancer incidence in mid-latitudes (i.e., USA and Europe) would probably have quadrupled by the end of the twenty-first century.

- The scenario shows that adherence to the Montreal Protocol would probably still lead to a doubling of the skin cancer incidence by the end of the twenty-first century but compliance with subsequent stricter amendments will lead to 5-10% increases in skin cancer incidence, peaking in the period 2050-2070.

- Climate change will probably affect future ozone levels, further slowing recovery of the ozone layer despite the countermeasures. In addition climate change might have a direct, location dependent influence on UV-radiation levels through a change in cloud patterns.

- Changes in skin cancer incidence that have been reported over the past decades are probably related to changes in behavior rather than to ozone depletion. Nevertheless, it remains very important to strictly adhere to the countermeasures agreed upon in the Amendments to the Montreal Protocol.

IMPLICATIONS FOR PUBLIC HEALTH

Full global compliance with the countermeasures agreed upon in the strictest Amendments of the Montreal Protocol is vital to avoid large increases in future skin cancer incidences around the globe. Without countermeasures, a fourfold increase in skin cancer incidence could be expected, whereas by following the strictest protocols agreed upon, the future risks might be limited to increases of 10%.

Changes in skin cancer risks follow the changes in UV-exposure, but there is a considerable delay in time, due to the long latency period that occurs between exposure and the occurrence of the skin tumors. Act now to prevent risks much later.

Increases in skin cancer incidence observed in recent decades, are probably related to changes in behavior towards sun exposure rather than the increases in ambient UV-doses observed as a consequence of ozone depletion. This further stresses the importance of public awareness of the risks associated with increases in UV-exposure, and the relevance of skin cancer prevention programs.

The effects of the increases in ambient UV-doses, caused by ozone depletion over the past decades will probably lead to a steady increase in skin cancer risks in the next fifty years.

The interaction between ozone depletion and climate change is highly uncertain and might well cause a delay in the recovery of the ozone layer of around twenty years. In view of the uncertainties it is important to continue and improve monitoring of UV-radiation levels in the coming decades.

ACKNOWLEDGEMENTS

The authors wish to thank the Ministry of Housing, Physical Planning and the Environment ("VROM") and the Dutch Cancer Society ("NKB/KWF") for the financial support of their research.

REFERENCES

1. World Meteorological Organization (1998) *Scientific assessment of ozone depletion.* Global Ozone and Monitoring Project, Report No 44. WMO.
2. Slaper H, Velders GJM, Daniel JS, de Gruijl FR, van der Leun JC (1996) Estimates of ozone depletion and skin cancer incidence to estimate the Vienna Convention achievements. *Nature* **384:** 256-258.
3. United Nations Environment Programme (1998) Environmental Effects of Ozone Depletion: 1998 Assessment. ISBN 92-807-1724-3.
4. CIAP (1975) *CIAP Monograph series,* Vols. 1-6, Grobecker AJ (Ed. in chf), Washington DC: Climate Impact Assessment Program, Department of Transportation
5. Molina MJ, Rowland FS (1974) Stratospheric sink for chlorofluromethanes: chlorine atom catalyzed destruction of ozone. *Nature* **249:** 810-812.
6. Farman JC, Gardiner BG, Shanklin JD (1985) Large losses of total ozone in Antarctica reveal seasonal ClOx/Nox interaction. *Nature* **315:** 207-210.
7. European Commission (2001) European research in the stratosphere 1996-2000, advances in our understanding of the ozone layer during THESEO, EUR 19867, ISBN 92-894-1398-0, Luxembourg.
8. Kelfkens G, Bregman A, de Gruijl FR *et al.* (2002) *Ozone Layer - climate change interactions: Influence on UV levels and UV related effects.* Dutch National Research Program on Global Air Pollution and Climate Change, OCCUR-project (950303), Report 410-200-112, ISBN 90-5851-079-4, RIVM, Bilthoven.

9. Bais AF, Gardiner BG, Slaper H, *et al.* (2001) SUSPEN intercomparison of ultraviolet spectroradiometers. *J Geophys Res* **106** (D12): 12,509-12,526.
10. Kjeldstad B, Johnsen B, Koskela T, eds. (1997) *The NORDIC intercomparison of ultraviolet and total ozone instruments at Izana.* October 1996, Final Report, Meteorological Publications 36, Helsinki: FMI, ISBN 951-697-475-9.
11. De Gruijl FR, Sterenborg HJCM, Forbes PD, *et al.* (1993) Wavelength dependence of skin cancer induction by ultraviolet irradiation of albino hairless mice. *Cancer Res* **53:** 53-60.
12. De Gruijl FR, Van der Leun JC (1994) Estimate of the wavelength dependency of ultraviolet carcinogenesis in humans and its relevance to the risk assessment of a stratospheric ozone depletion. *Health Phys.* **67:** 314-325.
13. Slaper H, Matthijsen J, den Outer PN, Velders GJM (2001) *Climatology of ultraviolet budgets using earth observation (CUBEO): mapping UV from the perspective of risk assessments.* Netherlands Remote Sensing Board (BCRS)_USP-2 report 00-17, ISBN 90-54-11-32-6.
14. Kelfkens G, den Outer PN, Slaper H (2001) Risks and ultraviolet budgets using earth observation (RUBEO): including a non-standard atmosphere and geographic ozone trend differences in risk assessments. Netherlands Remote Sensing Board (BCRS)_USP-2 report 01-33, ISBN 90-54-11-378-2.
15. Slaper H, Velders GJM, Matthijsen J (1998) Ozone depletion and skin cancer incidence: a source risk approach. *J Hazardous Mat* **61:** 77-84.
16. Miller D, Weinstock MA (1994) Nonmelanoma skin cancer in the United States: incidence. *J Am Acad Dermatol* **30:** 774-778.
17. Kricker A, Armstrong BK, English DR, Heenan PJ (1995) Does intermittent sun exposure cause basal cell carcinoma? A case-control study in Western Australia. *Int J Cancer* **60:** 489-494.
18. Holman CD, Armstrong BK (1984) Cutaneous malignant melanoma and indicators of total accumulated exposure to the sun: an analysis separating histogenetic types. *J Natl Cancer Inst* **73:** 75-82.
19. Green A, Williams G, Neale R, *et al.* (1999) Daily sunscreen application and beta-carotene supplementation in prevention of basal cell and squamous cell carcinomas of the skin: A randomized controlled trial. *Lancet* **354:** 723-729.
20. Gallagher RP, McLean DI, Yang GP, Coldman AJ, Silver HK, Spinelli JJ (1990) Suntan, sunburn and pigmentation factors and the frequency of acquired nevi in children. Similarities to melanoma: the Vancouver Mole Study. *Arch Dermatol* **126:** 770-776.
21. Longstreth JD, De Gruijl FR, Kripke ML, Takizawa Y, Van der Leun JC (1995) Effects of increased solar ultraviolet radiation on human health. *Ambio* **24:** 153-165.
22. Scotto J, Fears TR (1987) The association of solar ultraviolet and skin melanoma incidence among Caucasians in the Unites States. *Cancer Invest* **5:** 275-283.
23. Daniel JS, Solomon S, Albritton DL (1995) On the evaluation of halocarbon radiative forcing and global warming potentials. *J Geophys Res* **100:** 1271-1285.
24. Shindell DT, Rind D, Lonergan P (1998) Increased polar stratospheric ozone loss and delayed eventual recovery owing to increasing green-house gas concentrations. *Nature* **392:** 589-592.

Chapter 5

Descriptive epidemiology of skin cancer

Gianluca Severi[1], Ph.D.; Dallas R. English[2], Ph.D.
[1]Division of Epidemiology and Biostatistics – European Institute of Oncology, Milan, Italy;
[2]Cancer Epidemiology Centre, The Cancer Council Victoria, Melbourne, Victoria, Australia

Key words: incidence, skin cancer, time trends, geographic locations, melanoma

INTRODUCTION

The purpose of this chapter is to identify populations and subgroups at high (or low) risk of skin cancer and to discuss time trends in the incidence and mortality of skin cancer that may assist in identifying prevention priorities and in evaluating prevention strategies. We do not discuss genetic factors that may influence susceptibility (other than ethnicity); these are covered in Chapter 7.

Skin cancer is the most common type of cancer in fair-skinned populations. Historically, skin cancers were usually divided into melanoma and non-melanocytic skin cancer (NMSC), which includes a heterogeneous group of skin cancers (see Chapter 2). Basal cell carcinoma (BCC) and squamous cell carcinoma (SCC) account for more than 95% of all NMSC [1,2] and are far more common than melanoma. Melanoma, BCC and SCC differ in terms of incidence, mortality, geographical distribution, age distribution, sex, and association with ultraviolet radiation (UVR).

Most of this chapter is based upon routine reporting of new cases (incidence) and deaths (mortality) from skin cancer. In terms of prevention, incidence is more relevant than mortality because mortality rates are

73

D. Hill et al. (eds.), Prevention of Skin Cancer, 73-87.

influenced not only by incidence rates, but also by survival after diagnosis. For BCC and SCC in particular, survival rates are high, and mortality is a poor proxy for incidence [3-5]. Furthermore, misclassification of cause of death renders the interpretation of mortality very difficult if not impossible for these cancers [4,6]. Thus, we have not discussed mortality from SCC or BCC. However, mortality data are more universally available than incidence data and have generally been collected longer, so for melanoma are useful for studying long-term trends.

Melanoma is included in the incidence data that the International Agency for Research on Cancer (IARC) collects from population-based cancer registries and publishes in the series "Cancer Incidence in Five Continents." The first volume reported data from 1960-1962 while the last included data from 1988-1992 (Volume VII) [7,8]. Although BCC and SCC are more common than melanoma, most cancer registries (including the USA Surveillance Epidemiology and End Results (SEER) registries and the Australian registries) do not routinely report their incidence because of the prohibitive costs of collection. Also, many of those that do report these data do so in different ways – some group BCC and SCC, while others include only SCC and different rules are used for the reporting of multiple primary cancers, which are common features of both types [1,9,10]. Thus, comparisons of rates between different countries could be very misleading. We will report BCC and SCC incidence using data from ad-hoc surveys in Australia [11-13], Finland [2] and the USA [14]. Melanoma mortality data were obtained from the World Health Organization's Mortality Database (*http://www.iarc.fr*).

1.   ETHNICITY

Melanoma is rare in populations of non-European origin. For example, in the first half of the 1960s, the lowest rates among males (below 0.9 per 100,000 per year) were found in USA Blacks, Japanese (resident in Japan and Hawaii), Hawaiians and Filipinos resident in Hawaii, and in India, Singapore, and Puerto Rico [7]. In the 1990s, the differences in rates between populations of European and non-European origin were even greater [8]. Comparisons among different ethnic groups living in the same cities (e.g., Los Angeles) show that the low rates in populations of non-European origin are not due to confounding by place of residence. From the data reported by the Cancer Registries that routinely record other skin cancers [8], and from the USA survey [14], BCC and SCC together are much more common in populations of European origin. Thus, only in

European origin populations are melanoma, BCC, and SCC of public health importance and the remainder of the chapter focuses on such populations.

2. AGE DISTRIBUTION

Figure 5.1 shows data from surveys of BCC and SCC conducted in the USA in the 1970s along with USA SEER registry data on melanoma from the same period. BCC was the most common at all ages and increased steadily with age until around age 60 when the rate of increase slowed. SCC was rare among younger people, showed the greatest increase with age and was concentrated in the elderly. Melanoma was relatively common among the young, but the incidence was reasonably stable after about age 54. Other surveys have also shown that SCC is more concentrated in the elderly than BCC [2,11,14]. More recent data on melanoma and all other cancers (excluding BCC and SCC) from the USA SEER registries are shown in Figure 5.2 (*http://www.seer.cancer.gov*). Melanoma occurred at younger ages than most cancers; its age-specific incidence increased more rapidly than other cancers to about 40 years of age, but then increased more slowly than other cancers. Similar patterns are present for most populations of European origin [8].

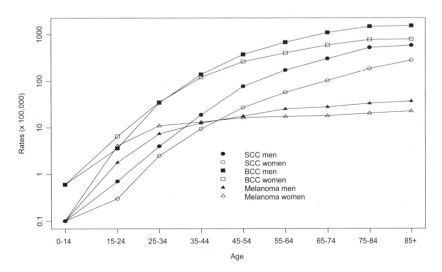

Figure 5.1 Age distribution of BCC, SCC, and melanoma incidence for men and women in the USA (1977-1978). BCC and SCC incidence is from the special NCI survey [14] while melanoma incidence is from the data routinely collected by the SEER program cancer registries (*http://www.seer.cancer.gov*).

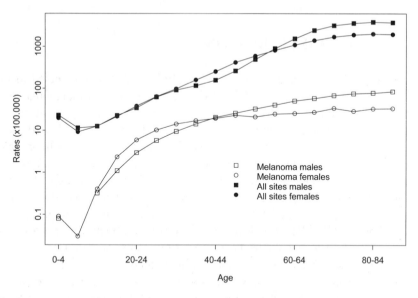

Figure 5.2 Age specific incidence rates separately for melanoma and all cancers (excluding skin cancers other than melanomas). Data are from the SEER program cancer registries (USA) for the period 1991-95 *http://www.seer.cancer.gov*).

3.   GENDER

Differences in melanoma incidence by gender within populations are small and inconsistent. At the beginning of the 1990s, melanoma incidence rates were generally slightly higher in males in Australia, Canada and the USA, while in Europe they were generally slightly higher in females (Table 5.1) [8]. None of these differences is sufficiently large to warrant targeting prevention to one gender.

BCC and SCC incidence rates are substantially higher among men than among women [2,13,14]. The male to female ratio is between 1 and 1.5 for BCC and between 1.6 and 2.7 for SCC.

Table 5.1 Incidence rates of melanoma per 100,000 population in 1960-62 and 1988-92, and the average annual percent increases during the intervening period.

	Males			Females		
	Age standardized incidence rates[c]		Average annual percent increase	Age standardized incidence rates[c]		Average annual percent increase
	1960-62	1988-92		1960-62	1988-92	
Canada, Newfoundland	1.6	3.9	3.2	2.5	5.2	2.6
Canada, Manitoba	1.5	7.1	5.5	2.0	7.0	4.5
Canada, Quebec[a]	1.1	3.7	4.8	1.4	3.3	3.6
Canada, New Brunswick	1.8	8.8	5.7	1.5	8.1	6.1
Canada, Alberta	2.3	7.5	4.2	2.7	7.5	3.6
Canada, Saskatchewan	2.3	8.0	4.3	1.9	7.6	4.9
USA, Hawaii, Caucasian	3.0	19.5	6.6	2.0	12.4	6.4
USA, Alameda County, White[a,b]	3.8	12.3	6.1	3.9	10.8	5.3
USA, Connecticut, White	3.0	13.8	5.4	3.4	11.2	4.2
USA, New York State (less NY City)[b]	2.3	7.8	5.2	2.3	6.0	4.1
Israel, Jews [a]	1.4	9.6	8.1	1.7	9.8	7.3
Slovenia	1.3	4.7	4.6	1.4	5.4	4.7
German Democratic Republic[a]	1.8	5.0	4.1	2.2	5.3	3.7
Hungary, Vas[b]	2.0	4.7	4.5	2.3	4.6	3.5
Poland, Warsaw City[a]	1.4	3.8	4.2	1.3	3.7	4.4
Denmark	1.6	8.8	6.1	2.2	11.7	5.9
Finland	1.9	7.8	5.0	2.1	6.7	4.1
Iceland	0.7	3.7	6.0	1.8	7.2	4.9
Norway	2.7	14.1	5.8	2.6	15.3	6.4
Sweden	2.4	11.0	5.4	2.8	11.1	4.9
UK, Trent (Sheffield)[a,b]	1.0	2.5	4.7	1.5	4.6	5.7
UK, Oxford[a]	1.2	5.8	6.4	2.6	7.6	4.4
UK, South Thames	1.1	4.6	5.1	2.1	6.4	4.0
UK, South Western	1.2	7.3	6.5	2.3	10.3	5.3
UK, Birmingham	0.9	4.5	5.6	1.6	6.1	4.8
UK, Scotland[a]	1.2	6.0	6.8	1.8	8.3	6.3
New Zealand, Non-Maori[a]	6.2	25.0	5.7	9.1	29.8	4.9
Average			5.4			4.8

[a] Initial rates are for 1963-1966
[b] Final rates are for 1983-1987
[c] World Standard population

4.   GEOGRAPHICAL DISTRIBUTION, LATITUDE AND UVR

Within populations of European origin, there are substantial variations in skin cancer incidence (Table 5.1). Generally, melanoma incidence is highest in countries closest to the equator, a phenomenon first recognized by Lancaster [15] in mortality data in the 1950s, although there are exceptions. In Europe, melanoma rates are higher in Norway, Sweden and Finland than in countries of southern Europe such as Spain and Italy [8], which may be due to differences in skin pigmentation. Within Australia and North America, melanoma incidence increases with proximity to the equator [8]. The latitude gradient provided some of the first evidence that melanoma was caused by exposure to sunlight.

BCC and SCC incidence show stronger associations with latitude. During the 1990s, SCC incidence rates in Australia, New Mexico, and Finland were 338, 214 and 7.2 per 100,000 respectively for men and 164, 50 and 4.2 for women [1,2,13]. The corresponding rates for BCC were 849, 1073 and 49 for men and 605, 415 and 45 for women. Within Australia, Finland, and the USA, the incidence of BCC and SCC increase strongly with decreasing latitude [2,13,14]. In the Australian surveys, the incidence in latitudes less than 29°S was approximately 3 times that in latitudes greater than 37°S.

In Figure 5.3, skin cancer incidence in men is plotted against UVB radiation index for the USA [16]. The equivalent graph for women, not presented here, is similar. Incidence rates for SCC increased rapidly with UVB radiation index. The rate of increase was lower for BCC, while melanoma had only a weak association (see also Chapter 6).

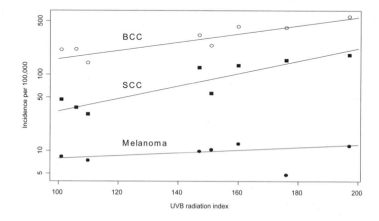

Figure 5.3 Skin cancer incidence by UV index, USA. BCC and SCC data are from a special survey [14] and melanoma data from SEER program cancer registries for 1978-1982. Reprinted with permission from Armstrong and Kricker [16].

5. SOCIOECONOMIC STATUS AND INDOOR/OUTDOOR WORK

Melanoma incidence and mortality rates are generally higher among indoor workers than outdoor workers [17-19] and they are positively associated with socioeconomic status [18,20]. Some studies showed no consistent increase in melanoma risk in indoor workers as compared with outdoor workers of similar socioeconomic status [18,19]. Few studies examining type of work and socioeconomic status have considered body site. In those that did, indoor workers had higher risks for body sites that are usually covered, while on body sites that are usually exposed outdoor workers had higher risks [21,22].

Early reports showed that incidence of NMSC was positively associated with outdoor occupation but none of these studies distinguished between BCC and SCC [23,24]. The evidence from more recent and rigorous descriptive studies is less convincing [12,25].

6. TIME TRENDS

Analysis of trends in incidence is essential for recognizing emerging public health problems and in monitoring the effects of efforts to control skin cancer. From available data, it appears that the incidence and mortality of melanoma increased steadily throughout most of the twentieth century [26,27]. Only in the last twenty years or so has there been evidence of more favorable changes. Given the importance of these trends, we will discuss them in some detail.

Table 5.1 shows incidence rates around 1960 and 1990 for several populations of European origin reported in Cancer Incidence in Five Continents [7,8,28,29]. Within these populations, the average annual increase in incidence was about 5% and ranged from 2% to 8%. No major differences in time trends between males and females were apparent.

An analysis of melanoma incidence in Connecticut from 1950 to 1989 showed that the rate of increase slowed among males, but not females, born most recently [30]. A similar analysis of incidence rates in Canada from 1969 to 1993 showed that age-specific rates started to decrease in younger adults (i.e., age < 55 for women and age < 45 for men) in women born after 1934 and men born after 1944 [31]. Data from Australia, which has the highest incidence rates [8], but which is not included in Table 5.1, are shown in Figure 5.4 for the period 1982-97. The increase in incidence since 1982 has largely been restricted to people at least 60 years of age [32].

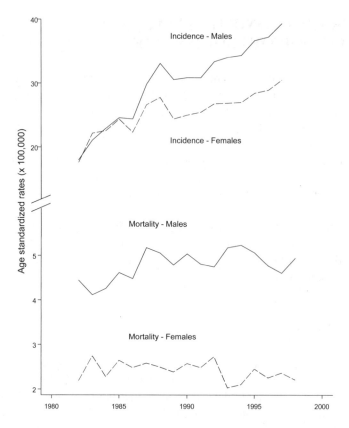

Figure 5.4 Time trends of melanoma mortality and incidence in Australia by gender (1982-1997). Age standardized rates (World Standard population) per 100,000.

Long-term increases in incidence have generally been highest for the trunk and lowest for the head and neck [27]. In some populations, the largest relative increases have been observed on the upper limb [30,31].

A striking feature of melanoma has been the much larger relative and absolute increases in thin melanomas than in thick melanomas [27]. For example, in the USA SEER data, the incidence of thin tumors (< 1 mm) increased substantially between 1986 and 1996, but the incidence of tumors thicker than 4.0 mm was relatively stable [33]. Similarly, in central Europe, the median thickness at diagnosis decreased from 1.2 mm in 1986 to 0.8 mm in 1996 [34]. Interestingly, the median thickness changed little in Queensland during the same period [34].

From 1960 to 1990, the average annual increases in mortality in countries represented by the registries shown in Table 5.1 were substantially less than the corresponding increases in incidence: 3.3% in males and 2.3% in females. Recent decreases in the age-standardized mortality from melanoma have been observed in some countries [35,36] and in more countries, increases in mortality among young persons have slowed, stopped or reversed [27].

In Figure 5.5, mortality rates from 1950-1994 are shown for selected populations separately for younger (30-59 years of age) and older people (60-79). The former experienced average annual increases from 2% or below (USA and Australia) to 9-16% (France, Italy and the former Czechoslovakia). The older group experienced average annual increases from below 5% (women in the USA, Australia, the Nordic countries, and Canada) to 20% or above (France and men in the former Czechoslovakia). In general, in the older group, men had greater increases. These patterns can be divided into three groups [37]. In the first group, increasing rates until generations born around 1930-1935 (or earlier for Australia) were followed by decreasing rates in more recent generations (Australia, the Nordic countries – Sweden, Norway, Finland, and Denmark – and the USA). In the second group, increasing rates until generations born during World War II were followed by flattening or slightly decreasing rates in more recent birth cohorts (the UK and Canada). In the third group a steep, almost linear increase was observed with no major change in this trend (France, Italy, and the former Czechoslovakia).

Before concluding that trends over time in melanoma incidence are real, it is necessary to consider extraneous factors that might affect rates. Two such factors are increasing recognition of thin melanomas and changing management of melanomas. The greater increases in incidence than in mortality and in the incidence of thin as opposed to thick melanomas suggest that some thin melanomas now being identified would once have remained undetected [27,38-41]. Thus, one possible explanation for the increase in incidence of thin melanomas is improved detection of melanomas that have little or no potential for metastasis [39]. However, most authors have concluded that part of the increase is real [27,33,38,42].

While increasing recognition of thin melanomas would inflate the recorded incidence rate, increasing treatment of melanomas in facilities that do not report all cases to cancer registries would have the opposite effect. Cancer registries that rely on hospital notifications alone are most affected. Because the proportion of melanomas treated outside hospitals has increased over time, time trends in melanoma will be underestimated unless notification from laboratories is available. For example, in Washington State USA, where the SEER registry did not use information from pathology laboratories outside hospitals, rates were underestimated by approximately

2% in 1974 and 21% in 1984 [43]. Under-registration in Belgium, which also relies on hospital-based reporting, was even greater [44].

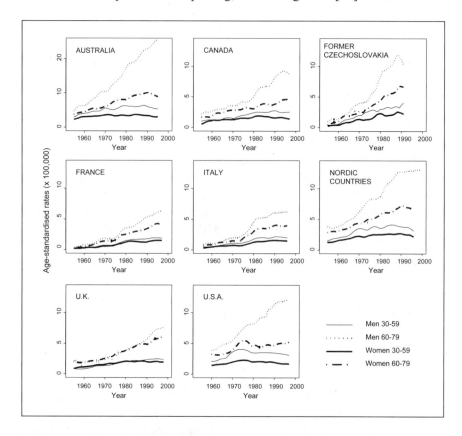

Figure 5.5 Melanoma mortality rates (standardized to the World Standard Population) by age group and gender in selected countries. (Data obtained from the World Health Organization Mortality Database).

Assuming the trends are real, the most recent data suggest that exposure to sunlight, the major cause of melanoma (see chapter 6), has stabilized or declined in some countries. If exposure early in life were important, then one would expect effects of reduced exposure to be seen first among younger people. It may be some time, particularly in populations where exposure has not stabilized, before reductions at all ages can be expected. Although incidence rates may be starting to fall in some populations, they remain much higher than in previous generations, and concerted efforts at prevention are necessary before they will return to the earlier levels.

There is more convincing evidence for mortality than for incidence that in some countries at least, melanoma rates have stabilized or begun to fall. As discussed above, caution is necessary when interpreting mortality trends in terms of incidence, because they are influenced by changes in survival after diagnosis. Indeed, melanoma survival has improved (in the white American population of the SEER program 5 year survival was about 60% at the beginning of the 1960s and almost 90% at the beginning of the 1990s) (*http://www.seer.cancer.gov*). This is presumably because of early detection, since there have been no advances in treatment of melanoma that would explain the increase in survival. The patterns of increasing incidence and mortality in some countries suggest that they have yet to realize the benefits of prevention or early detection.

Much less is known about trends in BCC and SCC. Both BCC and SCC incidence rates appear to have increased, but the rate of increase and particularly the relative increases of BCC and SCC differ from one population to another. In three Australian surveys, performed in 1985, 1990 and 1995, BCC incidence rates increased by 30% for men and 6% for women while SCC incidence rates increased by 100% for men and 87% for women [13]. SCC increased at all ages; BCC rates increased in those over 50 and decreased in those less than 50 years of age [13]. A marked increase in SCC incidence from 1984-1986 to 1990-1992 (52% for men and 113% for women) was found in the Rochester Epidemiology Project database, which contains information on all medical care provided to the residents of Rochester (USA) [45]. In Finland, the increase in rates between the beginning of the 1980s and the early 1990s was around 25% for BCC, SCC for men and women [2].

CONCLUSIONS

Skin cancers are common in populations of European origin, but rare in other populations. BCC and SCC are rarely fatal, but are far commoner than melanoma and may therefore contribute more to health care costs. Men and women have similar risks of melanoma, but men are more likely to develop BCC or SCC. Given the greater mortality from melanoma, equal emphasis on preventing skin cancer in men and women is justified. Melanoma occurs at relatively young ages, and given the importance of early life exposure to sunlight, prevention campaigns that are directed towards the young might be more cost effective. The incidence and mortality rates generally increase with proximity to the equator, but for melanoma at least, this pattern does not hold in Europe, with higher rates in the north (e.g., the Nordic countries) than in the south (e.g., Italy, Spain). These anomalies are likely to be due to a combination of different exposure patterns and different susceptibilities (see Chapters 2 and 7). Melanoma incidence and mortality has been increasing in most populations for many years, and what data there are indicate similar trends have occurred for BCC and SCC. Mortality from melanoma in some countries is now stable or falling in younger adults, but in most populations, there is less evidence that the long-term increases in incidence have abated. However, there is some evidence from Australia and North America that incidence rates have stabilized or started to fall among younger people. One explanation for these falls is that campaigns to prevent skin cancer in these populations are succeeding.

SUMMARY POINTS

- Skin cancers are rare in populations of non-European origin.
- BCC and SCC are far commoner than melanoma but rarely fatal.
- Men and women have similar risks of melanoma but men are more likely to develop BCC or SCC.
- Skin cancer is most common in European populations living closest to the equator.
- Melanoma rates have been increasing steadily for many years, but in some populations there is evidence that the increases have stopped or that rates are starting to fall.

IMPLICATIONS FOR PUBLIC HEALTH

Skin cancer prevention is predominantly an issue for populations of European origin.

The descriptive evidence suggests that exposure to sunlight in such populations is a major cause of skin cancer and that its prevention depends upon successful programs to reduce exposure.

Most countries with populations of European origin have shown long-term increases in melanoma incidence and mortality, presumably because of increases in sun exposure. In some countries, the long-term increases in melanoma have been arrested, suggesting that efforts to prevent it and other skin cancers are succeeding. Nevertheless, their current incidence rates of melanoma are far higher than those of a generation ago and continued efforts to prevent melanoma and other skin cancers are essential.

REFERENCES

1. Hoy WE (1996) Nonmelanoma skin carcinoma in Albuquerque, New Mexico: experience of a major health care provider. *Cancer* **77:** 2489-2495.
2. Hannuksela-Svahn A, Pukkala E, Karvonen J (1999) Basal cell skin carcinoma and other nonmelanoma skin cancers in Finland from 1956 through 1995. *Arch Dermatol* **135:** 781-786.
3. Levi F, La Vecchia C, Te VC, Mezzanotte G (1988) Descriptive epidemiology of skin cancer in the Swiss Canton of Vaud. *Int J Cancer* **42:** 811-816.
4. Østerlind A, Hjalgrim H, Kulinsky B, Frentz G (1991) Skin cancer as a cause of death in Denmark. *Br J Dermatol* **125:** 580-582.
5. Weinstock MA (1997) Nonmelanoma skin cancer mortality. In: Altmeyer P, Hoffmann K, Stucker M, eds. *Skin Cancer and UV radiation.* Berlin: Springer.
6. Weinstock MA, Bogaars HA, Ashley M, Litle V, Bilodeau E, Kimmel S (1992) Inaccuracies in certification of nonmelanoma skin cancer deaths. *Am J Public Health* **82:** 278-281.
7. Doll R, Payne P, Waterhouse JAH (1966) *Cancer Incidence in Five Continents.* Berlin: Springer.
8. Parkin DM, Whelan SL, Ferlay J, Raymond L, Young J (1997) Cancer incidence in five continents, Volume VII. *IARC Scientific Publications* No. 143. Lyon: International Agency for Research on Cancer.
9. Kricker A, English DR, Randell PL, *et al.* (1990) Skin cancer in Geraldton, Western Australia: a survey of incidence and prevalence. *Med J Aust* **152:** 399-407.
10. Karagas MR, Stukel TA, Greenberg ER, Baron JA, Mott LA, Stern RS (1992) Risk of subsequent basal cell carcinoma and squamous cell carcinoma of the skin among patients with prior skin cancer. Skin Cancer Prevention Study Group. *JAMA* **267:** 3305-3310.
11. Giles GG, Marks R, Foley P (1988) Incidence of non-melanocytic skin cancer treated in Australia. *Br Med J* **296:** 13-17.
12. Marks R, Staples M, Giles GG (1993) Trends in non-melanocytic skin cancer treated in Australia: the second national survey. *Int J Cancer* **53:** 585-590.
13. Staples M, Marks R, Giles G (1998) Trends in the incidence of non-melanocytic skin cancer (NMSC) treated in Australia 1985-1995: are primary prevention programs starting to have an effect? *Int J Cancer* **78:** 144-148.
14. Scotto J, Fears TR, Fraumeni JFJ (1983) *Incidence of Nonmelanoma Skin Cancer in the United States.* Bethesda: US Department of Health and Human Services (NIH Pub No 82-2433).
15. Lancaster HO (1956) Some geographical aspects of the mortality from melanoma in Europeans. *Med J Aust* **1:** 1082-1087.
16. Armstrong BK, Kricker A (2001) The epidemiology of UV induced skin cancer. *J Photochem Photobiol B* **63:** 8-18.
17. Holman CD, Mulroney CD, Armstrong BK (1980) Epidemiology of pre-invasive and invasive malignant melanoma in Western Australia. *Int J Cancer* **25:** 317-323.
18. Lee JA, Strickland D (1980) Malignant melanoma: social status and outdoor work. *Br J Cancer* **41:** 757-763.
19. Cooke KR, Skegg DC, Fraser J (1984) Socio-economic status, indoor and outdoor work, and malignant melanoma. *Int J Cancer* **34:** 57-62.
20. Kirkpatrick CS, Lee JA, White E (1990) Melanoma risk by age and socio-economic status. *Int J Cancer* **46:** 1-4.

21. Beral V, Robinson N (1981) The relationship of malignant melanoma, basal and squamous skin cancers to indoor and outdoor work. *Br J Cancer* **44:** 886-891.
22. Vågerö D, Ringbäck G, Kiviranta H (1986) Melanoma and other tumors of the skin among office, other indoor and outdoor workers in Sweden 1961-1979. *Br J Cancer* **53:** 507-512.
23. Blum HF (1948) Sunlight as a causal factor in cancer of the skin of man. *J Natl Cancer Inst* **9:** 247-258.
24. Emmett EA (1973) Ultraviolet radiation as a cause of skin tumors. *CRC Critical Reviews in Toxicology* **2:** 211-255.
25. Teppo L, Pukkala E, Hakama M, Hakulinen T, Herva A, Saxen E (1980) Way of life and cancer incidence in Finland. *Scand J Soc Med Suppl* **19:** 1-84.
26. Swerdlow AJ (1990) International trends in cutaneous melanoma. *Ann N Y Acad Sci* **609:** 235-251.
27. Armstrong BK, Kricker A (1994) Cutaneous melanoma. *Cancer Surv* **19-20:** 219-240.
28. Waterhouse JAH, Doll R (1970) *Cancer Incidence in Five Continents.* Volume II. Berlin: Springer.
29. Parkin DM, Muir CS, Whelan SL, Gao Y-T, Ferlay J, Powell J (1992) Cancer Incidence in Five Continents, Volume VI. *IARC Scientific Publications No. 120.* Lyon: International Agency for Research on Cancer.
30. Chen YT, Zheng T, Holford TR, Berwick M, Dubrow R (1994) Malignant melanoma incidence in Connecticut (United States): time trends and age-period-cohort modeling by anatomic site. *Cancer Causes Control* **5:** 341-350.
31. Bulliard JL, Cox B, Semenciw R (1999) Trends by anatomic site in the incidence of cutaneous malignant melanoma in Canada, 1969-93. *Cancer Causes Control* **10:** 407-416.
32. Australian Institute of Health and Welfare (AIHW) & Australasian Association of Cancer Registries (AACR) (2001) *Cancer in Australia 1998. AIHW cat. no. CAN 12.* Canberra: AIHW.
33. Jemal A, Devesa SS, Hartge P, Tucker MA (2001) Recent trends in cutaneous melanoma incidence among whites in the United States. *J Natl Cancer Inst* **93:** 678-683.
34. Garbe C, McLeod GR, Buettner PG (2000) Time trends of cutaneous melanoma in Queensland, Australia and Central Europe. *Cancer* **89:** 1269-1278.
35. Giles GG, Armstrong BK, Burton RC, Staples MP, Thursfield VJ (1996) Has mortality from melanoma stopped rising in Australia? Analysis of trends between 1931 and 1994. *Br Med J* **312:** 1121-1125.
36. Cohn-Cedermark G, Mansson-Brahme E, Rutqvist LE, Larsson O, Johansson H, Ringborg U (2000) Trends in mortality from malignant melanoma in Sweden, 1970-1996. *Cancer* **89:** 348-355.
37. Severi G, Giles GG, Robertson C, Boyle P, Autier P (2000) Mortality from cutaneous melanoma: evidence for contrasting trends between populations. *Br J Cancer* **82:** 1887-1891.
38. Roush GC, Schymura MJ, Holford TR (1988) Patterns of invasive melanoma in the Connecticut Tumor Registry. Is the long-term increase real? *Cancer* **61:** 2586-2595.
39. Burton RC, Coates MS, Hersey P, *et al.* (1993) An analysis of a melanoma epidemic. *Int J Cancer* **55:** 765-770.
40. Swerlick RA, Chen S (1996) The melanoma epidemic. Is increased surveillance the solution or the problem? *Arch Dermatol* **132:** 881-884.
41. Swerlick RA, Chen S (1997) The melanoma epidemic: more apparent than real? *Mayo Clin Proc* **72:** 559-564.

42. Dennis LK (1999) Analysis of the melanoma epidemic, both apparent and real: data from the 1973 through 1994 Surveillance, Epidemiology, and End Results program registry. *Arch Dermatol* **135:** 275-280.
43. Karagas MR, Thomas DB, Roth GJ, Johnson LK, Weiss NS (1991) The effects of changes in health care delivery on the reported incidence of cutaneous melanoma in western Washington State. *Am J Epidemiol* **133:** 58-62.
44. Brochez L, Verhaeghe E, Bleyen L, Myny K, De Backer G, Naeyaert JM (1999) Under-registration of melanoma in Belgium: an analysis. *Melanoma Res* **9:** 413-418.
45. Gray DT, Suman VJ, Su WP, Clay RP, Harmsen WS, Roenigk RK (1997) Trends in the population-based incidence of squamous cell carcinoma of the skin first diagnosed between 1984 and 1992. *Arch Dermatol* **133:** 735-740.

Chapter 6

How sun exposure causes skin cancer: an epidemiological perspective

Bruce K. Armstrong M.B., B.S., D.Phil.
School of Public Health, The University of Sydney, New South Wales, Australia

Key words: skin cancer, epidemiology, sun exposure, melanoma

INTRODUCTION

It has been widely accepted since early in the 20th Century that sun exposure is a cause of BCC and SCC in humans [1]. That human melanoma is also caused by sun exposure was not suggested until the early 1950s, and is still not accepted by some, or the relationship is described as controversial or complex [2,3]. Nevertheless, an expert working group of the International Agency for Research on Cancer concluded, in 1992, "There is sufficient evidence in humans for the carcinogenicity of solar radiation. Solar radiation causes cutaneous malignant melanoma and non-melanocytic skin cancer" [4].

This chapter will first present the epidemiological evidence that skin cancer is caused by sun exposure in humans. The narrative will then move from "whether" to "how" and try, in the process, to make some sense of the undoubted complexity. A final synthesis will aim to bring out the key facts and principles from the epidemiology of sun exposure and skin cancer that should be borne in mind when designing skin cancer prevention programs.

D. Hill et al. (eds.), Prevention of Skin Cancer, 89-116.

1.   DOES SUN EXPOSURE CAUSE SKIN CANCER?

Much of the epidemiological evidence that sun exposure causes skin cancer is indirect in the sense that it does not make a direct association between exposure of the skin and risk of skin cancer in individual people. This indirect evidence is summarized in Box 6.1. Some of it will be covered in more detail below and some of it is covered in other chapters in this book, particularly Chapters 5 and 7.

Box 6.1 Indirect evidence that sun exposure causes skin cancer.

- Risk of skin cancer is lower in dark-skinned than light-skinned populations (Chapter 5).

- Risk of skin cancer in individuals within a population is higher in people with highly sun-sensitive skin than in those with skin that is less sun sensitive (Chapter 7).

- Incidence of skin cancer in populations generally increases with increasing proximity to the equator and, when measured, increasing ambient solar irradiance (Chapter 5 and Section 1.1).

- The highest or near highest densities of each kind of skin cancer are on body sites that are usually exposed to the sun when outdoors and all skin cancers are rare on sites that are rarely exposed to the sun (Section 1.1).

- People who have benign sun damage in the skin are more likely to develop a skin cancer than those who do not (Section 1.4).

- Incidence of skin cancer in some populations has been observed to fall in a temporal pattern consistent with an effect of increasing efforts to control sun exposure on skin cancer risk (Chapter 5).

Direct evidence that sun exposure causes skin cancer has come mainly from three kinds of epidemiological studies. First, studies have recorded past or usual, self-reported sun exposure of a large group of people, followed them forward in time, recorded newly incident skin cancers, and compared incidence of skin cancer at different levels of sun exposure of individuals in the group. These studies are called "cohort" studies. Second, and equivalently, people with newly diagnosed skin cancer have been asked to recall their sun exposure and this recalled sun exposure has been compared with that of a representative sample of people in the population from which the people with skin cancer came ("case-control" studies). Comparison of sun exposure between these two groups has permitted an estimate of risk of skin cancer in relation to different levels of sun exposure. Third, biological studies in humans have shown direct links between solar UV radiation and some skin cancers. Fourth, subjects have been randomly allocated to receive or not receive special interventions aimed at reducing sun exposure and subsequent risk of skin cancer or precursor lesions has been compared between the two groups. The direct evidence from these sources is summarized in Box 6.2.

Box 6.2 Direct evidence that sun exposure causes skin cancer.

- Risk of SCC increases with increasing lifetime total exposure to the sun, as does risk of melanoma but the evidence for this association is weaker (Section 1.3).

- Risks of BCC and SCC increase with increasing occupational exposure to the sun; paradoxically, that for melanoma falls (Section 1.3).

- Risks of BCC and melanoma increase with increasing non-occupational or "intermittent" exposure to the sun (Section 1.3).

- A history of sunburn to the skin increases risks of BCC, SCC and melanoma, although the evidence that it increases risk of SCC is weak (Section 1.3).

- A UV-specific, tumor suppressor gene mutation is common in BCCs and SCCs and this mutation in *normal skin* has been observed to be associated with BCC in one study (Section 1.5).

- Application of broad-spectrum sunscreen has been observed to reduce the incidence and promote the regression of solar keratoses (precursor lesions to SCC), reduce the incidence of SCC itself, and reduce the incidence of benign melanocytic nevi (precursor lesions to melanoma) in children (Section 1.6).

There are several problems in the cohort and case-control studies, particularly the case-control studies, which have weakened the conclusions that can be drawn from them. Difficulty in gaining accurate recall of sun exposure, particularly in the distant past (when it is probably most relevant), is the biggest problem. Inaccurate recall of exposure could seriously weaken observed relationships between skin cancer and sun exposure. The negative confounding of sun sensitivity with sun exposure is another problem. That is, people whose skin is sensitive to the sun and who may be at greater genetic risk of skin cancer are less likely to expose themselves to the sun. If this confounding effect is not controlled by design or analysis in a study, any observed association between sun exposure and skin cancer will be weaker than it truly is. Inaccurate measures of sun sensitivity in epidemiological studies makes this confounding effect difficult to control.

1.1   Sun exposure inferred from ambient UV

Risk of BCC, SCC, and melanoma in people who migrate from an area of low to an area of high ambient solar irradiance is less than it is in people who were born in the area of high irradiance [5-8]. Risk is greater the earlier a person migrates to the area of high irradiance and little different from that in people born in this area, if migration occurs before about 10 years of age (Figure 6.1). Similarly when individual residence histories are considered and years of life are weighted by estimates of ambient solar irradiance at each place of residence (commonly average annual hours of bright sunlight) and summed over all places of residence, age-adjusted risk of skin cancer increases with increasing irradiance weighted years of life [5,9,10], although less evidently so for BCC than for SCC and melanoma.

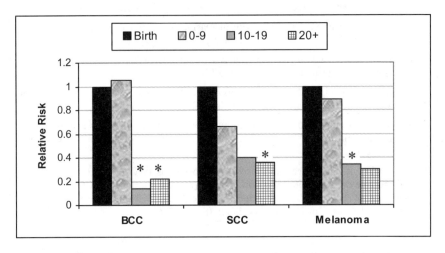

Figure 6.1 Effect of age (years) at arrival in Australia on risk of BCC, SCC and melanoma relative to that in people born in Australia [5-7][†]

[†]An asterisk (*) indicates relative risks for which the 95% confidence interval did not include 1.0. The second two age-at-arrival intervals for melanoma were 10-29 years and 30+ years.

The results by age at migration could suggest, simply, that risk of skin cancer increases with increasing length of residence in an environment with high ambient solar radiation, as do the results based on residence histories, but they can also be taken to suggest that exposure to solar radiation early in life may be particularly important in increasing risk of skin cancer.

1.2 Sun exposure inferred from site of skin cancer

Relative density (incidence per unit area of skin of a specific site relative to incidence per unit area over the whole body) of each of BCC, SCC and melanoma is highest or nearly so on body sites that are usually exposed to the sun when a person is outdoors, less on those that are occasionally exposed and least on those that are rarely exposed (Table 6.1) [1]. SCC, however, differs appreciably from BCC and melanoma in having a much lower density on occasionally exposed sites in both sexes, particularly the shoulders and back, and chest in men. The inference that sun exposure is important in determining body site distribution is made stronger by higher densities of each cancer on the scalp and ears in men than in women, sites that are less covered by hair in men than women [11,12].

Table 6.1 Surface density of BCC, SCC, and melanoma by body site, relative to a density of 1.0 for the whole body, from two whole population series of cases [1,11] (Source: Armstrong *et al.* [1] *Australasian Journal of Dermatology,* used with permission).

	BCC		SCC		Melanoma	
	M	F	M	F	M	F
Usually exposed						
Scalp*, face, neck, ears*	3.9	6.7	6.5	8.9	2.0	2.5
Forearms, backs of hands	1.4	1.3	2.0	3.3	0.5	0.6
Occasionally exposed						
Shoulders, back, chest*	1.8	1.8	0.3	0.2	2.5	1.8
Upper arms, lower limbs	0.4	0.5	0.3	0.4	0.5	1.1
Rarely exposed						
Abdomen, buttocks, scalp†, ears†, chest†	0.0	0.2	0.0	0.4	0.2	0.3

* Men only
† Women only

The relative incidence of different skin cancers by site has varied with time in populations of mainly European origin. In a 1993 review of reports of trends in melanoma incidence by site [13], melanoma of the trunk showed the highest proportional rate of increase in incidence in men in 10 of 13 populations from which data had been reported and melanomas of the face, scalp and neck showed the lowest rate of increase in men in 6 of 13 populations. In women, the highest rate of increase was on the trunk in 5 of 13 populations, on the lower limbs in four and the upper limbs in four; the face, scalp and neck showed the lowest rate of increase in a majority of populations (10 of 13). More recent data on trends in melanoma suggest that the differences in rates of increase in incidence between body sites have diminished and that incidence on the legs in women has begun to fall in some populations [14]. These patterns are generally what would be expected from a number of probable (but not well documented) trends in sun exposure in affluent populations, including increasing recreational exposure of sites previously not much exposed, affecting particularly incidence on the back; falling occupational exposure, affecting trends on the head and neck; and trends in leg-wear in women with greater coverage, affecting trends in incidence on the legs.

There was similar but less distinct variation by site in the rate of increase in incidence of BCC and SCC; while increasing across all sites, relative rates of increase have been generally greater on the trunk and limbs than on the head and neck, particularly for BCC [13,15]. This could be seen as consistent with greater exposure recently of body sites that had previously not been much exposed to the sun.

1.3   Sun exposure recorded or recalled

Because melanoma and possibly BCC are related to pattern as well as amount of sun exposure (see Section 2.1), personal sun exposure is now usually represented in three ways: total exposure, occupational exposure (a more continuous pattern of exposure), and non-occupational or recreational exposure ("intermittent" exposure). History of sunburn is usually recorded also since it is generally thought to indicate a high level of intermittent sun exposure. Each of these may be estimated over the whole or a part of life.

Summary estimates of the relationship between the different types of personal sun exposure and risk of BCC, SCC, and melanoma are given in Table 6.2 [16]. None of the summarized associations is strong. This is probably because of inaccuracy in the recall of past sun exposure and a lack of specificity of measurements for site of the skin cancer in most studies.

Table 6.2. Risk of skin cancer is related to measures of personal sun exposure – summary relative risk estimates from published studies[*] (Source: Armstrong and Kricker [16] *Journal of Photochemistry and Photobiology B,* used with permission).

Type of sun exposure	BCC	SCC	Melanoma
Total	0.98 (0.68-1.41)[†]	1.53 (1.02-2.27)	1.20 (1.00-1.44)
Occupational	1.19 (1.07-1.32)	1.64 (1.26-2.13)	0.86 (0.77-0.96)
Non-occupational or "intermittent"	1.38 (1.24-1.54)	0.91 (0.68-1.22)	1.71 (1.54-1.90)
Sunburn at any age	1.40 (1.29-1.51)	1.23 (0.90-1.69)	1.91 (1.69-2.17)

[*] Values for BCC and SCC are from Armstrong and Kricker [16] and those for melanoma from Elwood and Jopson [66].
[†] Meta-analytic summary of relative risk estimates in the highest exposure categories of the exposure measure (95% confidence intervals in brackets).

BCC is most strongly associated with non-occupational or "intermittent" sun exposure and sunburn, and is weakly associated with occupational exposure. In contrast, SCC is most strongly associated with total and occupational sun exposure, is not associated with non-occupational exposure, and is only weakly related to sunburn. Melanoma shows a pattern more like that of BCC than SCC with quite strong associations with non-occupational exposure and sunburn. It shows some similarity to SCC in being weakly related to total exposure, but is different from both BCC and SCC in its significant *negative* association with occupational sun exposure.

There is moderately strong evidence, then, that each of these cancers is related to one or more measures of sun exposure. The differences in the measures to which they are related suggests that they differ in their relationships to sun exposure, with SCC being most related to the more continuous occupational exposure and BCC and melanoma being more strongly associated with the generally more intermittent non-occupational exposure. These differences are explored further in Section 2.1.

1.4 Sun exposure inferred from other sun-related lesions

Comparable measurements have been made of the associations of BCC, SCC, and melanoma with several measures of benign, sun-related skin lesions: cutaneous microtopography (a measure of loss of skin elasticity due to sun exposure), freckling as a child, solar keratoses (common, benign precursors to SCC), and cutaneous melanocytic nevi (common, benign precursors to melanoma).

Comparing two studies, risks of BCC, SCC, and melanoma increased with increasing grades of cutaneous microtopography; the gradient of increase in risk of BCC and melanoma was threefold from the three lowest grades to the highest [6,17]. The gradient for SCC was not as steep as for BCC and melanoma. In two different studies, each type of skin cancer was significantly and about equally strongly associated with freckling as a child, with about a 60% increase in risk in those with some freckling compared with those with none [18-20]. They were each also significantly associated with presence of solar keratoses, but SCC was much more strongly associated (OR 15.4, 95% CI 8.3-22.8), as might be expected given the precursor relationship, than were BCC (OR 3.9, 95% CI 3.0-5.2) and melanoma (OR 1.9, 95% 1.4-2.5) [6,21]. Only melanoma, however, is at all strongly associated with presence of benign melanocytic nevi [5,6], which have been shown to be associated with sun exposure in children [22], although higher numbers of nevi have been associated with a small increase in risk of BCC in one study [6].

1.5 Sun exposure indicated by biological markers

The "CC to TT" mutation in the TP53 gene of SCC has been described as the "smoking gun" that implicates solar radiation as the cause of SCC. UV radiation produces a number of chemical changes in DNA, the most common of which are cross-links between adjacent pyrimidine bases, cytosine (C) and thymine (T), on a DNA strand. These bases, with two purine bases, adenine and guanine, are the "letters" in the genetic code. If these DNA changes are not repaired before cell division occurs, they may be fixed as mutations, most commonly C to T transitions (i.e., a cytosine base is replaced by a thymine base) where pyrimidine bases are adjacent (a dipyrimidine site) or CC to TT tandem transitions (i.e., two adjacent cytosine bases are replaced by two adjacent thymine bases), which are almost totally specific to UV (see Chapter 11). In 1991, Brash and colleagues [23] reported that 14 of 24 SCCs had mutations in TP53, an important tumor suppressor gene, that three were CC to TT transitions, five were C to T transitions, and all were at dipyrimidine sites. That was the smoking gun.

At last count, TP53 was mutated in over 90% of SCCs, the commonest mutation was a C to T transition at a dipyrimidine site (70%), and 10% of mutations were CC to TT transitions [24]. In an analysis of published TP53 mutations in all skin cancers (mainly SCCs and BCCs) and a wide variety of internal cancers, the prevalence of mutations at dipyrimidine sites was 89% in skin cancers compared with 61% in internal cancers ($P<0.001$) and the prevalence of CC to TT mutations was 19% compared with <1% ($P<0.001$).

A similar pattern of mutations of TP53 is found in BCCs. In a searching analysis of 11 BCCs, 24 different mutations were found in TP53 and all BCCs had at least one. Fifteen mutations were C to T at dipyrimidine sites and two were CC to TT [25]. Risk of BCC has also been shown to be significantly associated with the prevalence of CC to TT mutations in TP53 in normal skin from the mirror image site on the body to that of the BCC, although this prevalence was not correlated with estimates of UV exposure to the site [26]. However, an earlier study had shown that prevalence of CC to TT mutations was higher in skin from exposed than from unexposed body sites in Australian patients.

There is little evidence to suggest that mutation of TP53 is important in causing melanoma. Mutation of another gene, CDKN2A, is strongly associated with risk of melanoma in some high-risk families and is commonly deleted or mutated in melanomas, as well as a wide range of other tumors. In a database of 42 published point mutations of CDKN2A in melanoma tissue or cell lines and 93 internal cancers, 7 mutations in melanoma were CC to TT mutations (16.5%) compared with 1 (1.1%) in the internal cancers [27]. The proportion of mutations at dipyrimidine sites was also said to be higher in melanomas than in internal cancers, but not significantly so.

1.6   Response to changes in personal sun exposure

A number of observational studies have examined the relationship between sun protection measures, including use of hats, clothing and sunscreen, and risk of BCC, SCC, and melanoma. Their results, however, are unreliable because of the great difficulty of controlling negative confounding between sun protection and sun sensitivity and sun exposure (see Chapter 8). One such study, however, suggests a probable effect of sun protection measures in reducing risk of BCC [28]. Patients diagnosed with a BCC were entered into a randomized controlled trial of a synthetic retinoid for prevention of subsequent BCC, and given written recommendations on sun protection. The patients were examined regularly over three years and all suspicious skin lesions removed. Those who reported at the end of follow-up that they had reduced their sun exposure (low exposure group) had an average of 0.2 BCCs in the first 18 months of the study compared with 3.0 in the high exposure group and 1.4 compared with 5.5 in the second 18 months.

Several randomized controlled trials of reduction in sun exposure by daily use of a sunscreen suggest that it can reduce risk of SCC. Two trials showed that daily use of sunscreen over 6 months (one summer) to 2 years (SPF 17 and 29 respectively) can reduce the rate of appearance of new solar keratoses [29,30] and one showed that it increased regression of pre-existing solar keratoses as well [29]. In one trial, SPF 15+ sunscreen applied daily to skin of the head, neck, hands and arms reduced the number of new SCCs diagnosed over 4-5 years from entry into the study by 39% (RR 0.61, 95% CI 0.46-0.81) [31]. This study found no evidence of a reduction in number of new BCCs over the same period, in contradiction of the findings for BCC described above.

One randomized controlled trial of SPF 30+ sunscreen use in school children showed that it might reduce the incidence of new melanocytic nevi [22]; a median of 24 new nevi developed over nearly 3 years in children randomized to sunscreen use compared with 28 in those who were not given sunscreen (p=0.048). While this result might indicate that sunscreen use in childhood reduces risk of melanoma in later life, it says nothing about the effect of sunscreen use by adults on risk of melanoma. The development of new melanocytic nevi appears to be largely confined to the first 15 years of life.

2.   HOW DOES SUN EXPOSURE CAUSE SKIN CANCER?

2.1   Effects of pattern of exposure

The relative density of SCC is low on all body sites except those usually exposed to the sun, while those of BCC and melanoma are moderately high on body sites occasionally exposed to the sun (Table 6.1). If we assume that risk of SCC is a function only of amount of sun exposure, the above differences suggest that an intermittent pattern of sun exposure produces a higher risk of BCC and melanoma than would be expected if their risk were a function only of amount of exposure. In essence, this is the "intermittent exposure hypothesis" about which, when first formulated, it was stated, "High rates of non-melanoma incidence may be associated with cumulative UV exposure, while high melanoma incidence may be associated with brief exposure to high intensity UV radiation. Such an association would explain why skin melanomas are observed on areas of the body which are infrequently exposed such as the trunk in males" [32]. The stronger associations of BCC and melanoma with non-occupational sun exposure than with total and occupational exposure and their associations with sunburn (Table 6.2) also suggest a role for pattern of sun exposure. In contrast, risk of SCC is quite strongly related to occupational and total sun exposure, is weakly related to sunburn and is not at all related to non-occupational exposure.

The effect of pattern of sun exposure on risk of BCC and melanoma is perhaps best conceived by hypothesizing that pattern and amount of sun exposure operate as independent determinants of risk of these cancers, as first suggested by Elwood [33]. This hypothesis is represented graphically in Figure 6.2 and suggests that if pattern is held constant, risk increases monotonically with increasing amount of exposure to solar radiation and if amount is held constant, risk increases monotonically with increasing intermittency of exposure. It also suggests that the slope of increase with amount of exposure is greater for SCC than it is for BCC and melanoma, and that the slope of increase with increasing intermittency is greatest for melanoma, less for BCC and zero for SCC. Straight lines have been used for convenience in representing these trends; while the available evidence favors monotonic trends there is no certain basis for believing that they would be arithmetically linear.

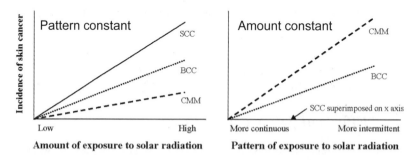

Figure 6.2 The "intermittent exposure hypothesis" for melanoma and BCC represented in terms of the independence of amount and pattern of exposure in determining risk of these skin cancers. In the left hand panel, amount of exposure varies while pattern is held constant; and in the right hand panel, pattern varies while amount is held constant [16]. (Source: Armstrong and Kricker [16] *Journal of Photochemistry and Photobiology B,* used with permission).

If pattern is not held constant as amount of sun exposure increases, increasing amount would probably lead, in most circumstances, to a more constant pattern of exposure that would ameliorate the consequences of increasing amount on risk of BCC and melanoma and could even cause a reduction in risk at high exposure levels [34]. Such an effect might explain the apparently protective effect of high occupational exposure on risk of melanoma shown in Table 6.2 (noting that the reference category here is low *occupational* exposure not low total exposure and could represent highly intermittent exposure). An important practical consequence of this argument for sun protection is the possibility of paradoxical increases in risk of BCC and melanoma, but not SCC, with reduction in sun exposure if intermittency of exposure is allowed to increase as exposure falls (e.g., through introduction of sun protection practices at work but their non-adoption in leisure exposure). This possibility is also suggested by available observations on exposure-response relationships reviewed in Section 2.2.

Why is pattern of sun exposure important in determining risk of melanoma and probably BCC? While it is tempting to answer in terms of acquisition and maintenance of protection by epidermal thickening and pigmentation from a more constant pattern of sun exposure, the fact that there is no evidence that pattern is important in determining risk of SCC makes this explanation insufficient. Gilchrest and colleagues [35] have identified differential susceptibility to apoptosis (cell "suicide") in the face of substantial DNA damage from high-dose sun exposure of relatively unprotected skin as a possible explanation. Their hypothesis, which is supported by some evidence, is outlined in Box 6.3.

Box 6.3 Biological hypothesis to explain the effect of intermittent pattern sun exposure on risk of melanoma and BCC [35].

- The more differentiated keratinocytes, which are probably the cells of origin for SCC, are the most susceptible to apoptosis.

- Thus, only the least damaged of these cells would survive after an episode of high exposure with consequent greater likelihood of successful repair of DNA damage and freedom from mutation.

- Melanocytes, on the other hand, are much less susceptible to apoptosis and therefore more likely to survive high dose exposure, sustain substantial damage and go on to mutation, of which freckles and melanocytic nevi are a visible manifestation.

- The less differentiated basal cells, the presumed cells of origin of basal cell carcinoma, are expected to be less susceptible to apoptosis than the more differentiated keratinocytes because of their lesser differentiation, and are therefore intermediate between them and melanocytes in their susceptibility to effects of high-dose, unprotected sun exposure.

- Against this varying background of susceptibility to mutation in response to high-dose, unprotected exposure, the production of melanin (tanning) and the induction of increased DNA repair capacity provide increased protection of all progenitor cell types against mutation from continuing sun exposure.

2.2   Exposure response relationships

Estimating the functional form and parameters of the relationships between solar UV exposure and the different types of skin cancer is difficult because of inaccurate measurement of sun exposure. Several studies have plotted relative risk of skin cancer as a function of some quantitative measure of sun exposure [9,10,18-20,36,37] and we will use their results descriptively in the hope of developing a conceptual understanding of dose-response patterns that can guide the design of skin cancer control programs.

The published dose-response patterns are summarized in Figures 6.3, 6.4, and 6.5. In preparing them, the exposure-response data were extracted from the published papers (for some this required measurement from printed plots since the numerical data were not published), all scales were converted to arithmetic scales, and the UV exposure measures from the different studies were re-scaled for plotting in a single figure. The rescaling means that the different ranges of exposure in the different studies are represented as equal in the figures. To assist in evaluating the implications of this, the exposure level of the highest category in each study has been footnoted in each figure.

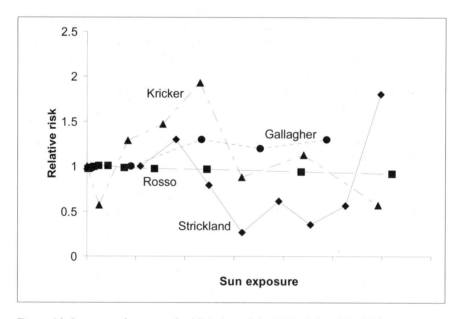

Figure 6.3 Summary of patterns of published trends in BCC relative risk with increasing sun exposure [9,19,36,37].*

*The highest exposure categories in each case were: Strickland ~250 MED per year, Kricker 69,000+ hours of sun exposure of the site of the cancer, Gallagher 280+ whole body equivalent sun exposure hours per year (WBE – the product of actual daytime hours outdoors and proportion of body exposed) and Rosso, 250,000+ hours of sun exposure.

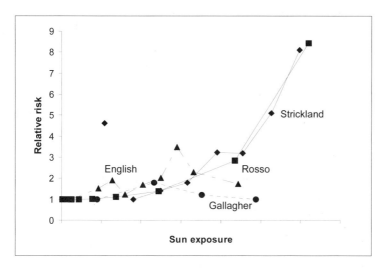

Figure 6.4 Summary of patterns of published trends in SCC relative risk with increasing sun exposure [10,20,36,37].*

*The highest exposure categories in each case were: Strickland ~250 MED per year, Gallagher 280+ WBE per year, Rosso 250,000+ hours of sun exposure, English 90,000+ hours of sun exposure of the site of the cancer.

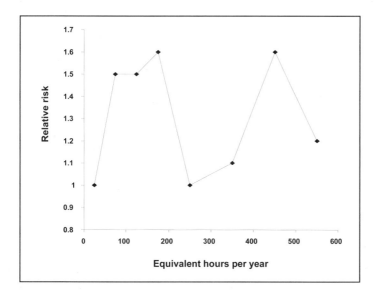

Figure 6.5 Trend in melanoma relative risk with increasing sun exposure in one study [18].*

*The highest exposure category was 500+ WBE per year.

Even without rescaling, the studies would inevitably have been plotted on different scales. They were conducted in areas at different latitudes (ranging from 28° to about 54°) and therefore different ambient UV irradiance, in populations of both southern and northern European origin (with the range of skin types and sensitivity to solar radiation that entails) and several different measures of exposure. The first point in the exposure response relationship recorded by Strickland *et al.* [36] was excluded from their modeled exposure-response for SCC because the four cases that gave rise to it may have arisen in a "hypersusceptible subgroup." We have plotted it but not connected it to the other data points since it is clearly an outlier.

Two contrasting exposure response patterns were observed. The commoner is an initial rise in risk with increasing exposure followed by a plateau or fall in risk. This was the pattern for three of the four studies of BCC, and arguably the fourth if the last data point is ignored as an outlier; two of the four of SCC; and, roughly, the only one of melanoma. The less common pattern is an apparently exponential increase in risk of SCC with increasing exposure in two of the four studies. The pattern for SCC observed by English and colleagues also roughly followed the apparently exponential uptrends of Strickland and Rosso and their colleagues until the last data point.

With these thoughts in mind, and broadly speaking, it appears for BCC and possibly melanoma that there is a point reached after which risk does not increase further with increasing total exposure to the sun and may actually fall. As noted in Section 2.1, this is the exposure-response pattern that might be expected from the combination of dose and pattern effects that is seen in BCC and melanoma and reinforces the need to consider the possibility of a paradoxical increase in risk of skin cancer when exposure is reduced in more heavily exposed populations. Other explanations, in addition to error in measurement of sun exposure, are possible however. For example heavily sun-exposed people might reduce their exposure and possibly their subsequent risk of skin cancer after presenting with sun-related neoplasia or pre-neoplasia [9], as suggested in Figure 6.3 by the data of Kricker and colleagues.

The exposure-response pattern for SCC is less clear. While the apparently exponential relationship seen in two of the populations is what might be expected from dose dependency alone, only two of the four studies showed this pattern. While it could be argued that the highest exposure point from the study of English and colleagues should be ignored, it is probably above the range of true exposure covered by the two studies with exponential curves and so it could indicate a true fall in risk at the highest dose levels. The same, however, probably cannot be said of a similar late downtrend observed by Gallagher and colleagues.

Associations observed between ambient UV irradiance and population risk of skin cancer broadly support these exposure-response patterns based on individual level data. The best population-level data available are still those from the 1977-78 survey of incidence of non-melanocytic skin cancer in the United States [38] and contemporary observations on melanoma incidence by US cancer registries [39]; these data are summarized in Figure 6.6. As might reasonably be expected from the individual-level data (Figures 6.3, 6.4 and 6.5), risk of SCC increased most steeply with increasing ambient UVB radiation.

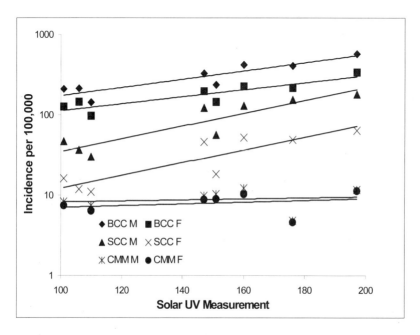

Figure 6.6 Relationship of age-standardized incidence rates of BCC, SCC, and melanoma (CMM) to estimated ambient erythemal UV radiation in ten US populations (Seattle, Minneapolis-St Paul, Detroit, Utah, San Francisco-Oakland, Atlanta, New Orleans, Albuquerque (New Mexico melanoma)) in 1977-78 (BCC and SCC) and 1978-1982 (melanoma) [16] (Source Armstrong and Kricker [16] *Journal of Photochemistry and Photobiology B,* used with permission).

Any expectation regarding the relative rates of change in risk of BCC and melanoma with increasing ambient UVB would be difficult to formulate from the individual-level data (Figures 6.3 and 6.5). In the event, risk of melanoma increased least steeply while that of BCC increased at a rate intermediate between those of melanoma and SCC, suggesting at least that the three main types of skin cancer have different individual-level exposure-response relationships. The detailed interpretation of the population-level exposure-response relationships in terms of individual relationships, however, is complex because of the averaging in the population of many different response patterns, probable uncontrolled confounding of ambient UV with personal sun exposure and cutaneous sun sensitivity, and possible differences between the UV action spectra for the three cancers (see Section 2.4).

2.3   Temporal relationships of exposure to response

The mutagenic capacity of the UV rays in sun exposure makes it probable that sun exposure acts at an early stage in the processes of skin carcinogenesis. The strong association of UV-specific mutations of TP53 with BCC and SCC and a weaker association of these mutations in CDKN2A with melanoma (see Section 1.5) suggest that it does.

The strongest epidemiological evidence for early stage effects of sun exposure in skin carcinogenesis come from studies of migration from areas of low to high sun exposure (Figure 6.1). Risk of all three types of skin cancer in people who migrate to Australia after the first 10 years of life is 40% or less of that in people born there. These results are supported by those of a number of similar studies of melanoma [8]. For melanoma there is also evidence that migration early in life from an area of high risk to an area of low risk is associated with persistence of the high risk [40].

Risk of most cancers is thought to increase as a function of time since first exposure to the initiating agent raised to some power, usually between three and four. This could be sufficient explanation for this apparently very strong effect of early age at arrival on subsequent risk of skin cancer. It could also be, though, that childhood is a period of special susceptibility to the carcinogenic effects of sun exposure. The development of melanocytic nevi in childhood may be an indicator of such susceptibility. Rare at birth, they increase to their maximum density at 9-10 years of age and, thereafter, appear to increase in number only in proportion to growth in skin surface area [41]. There is quite strong evidence that they are caused by sun exposure [22] and they are very strong predictors of subsequent risk of melanoma [5].

Associations between recalled sun exposure in different periods of life and subsequent risks of skin cancer have been described in a number of observational studies. For BCC and SCC, we have reviewed the results of three recent, major studies that present such results.

The studies are consistent in showing a stronger association between BCC and sunburn in childhood than in adulthood or the whole of life [19,37,42,43]. They all also found significant associations between intermittent or recreational sun exposure in childhood or teenage years and BCC. Only one found a similar association with recreational sun exposure in adulthood. This apparently exclusive effect of recreational exposure at less than 20 years of age has also been observed in a recent report of a case-control study in Italy [44].

The results are less consistent for SCC [10,20,37,43]. Two studies were compatible in finding similar effects of child and adult sunburn on risk of SCC, the third found an effect only in childhood. Only two studies compared effects on SCC of estimated total and occupational sun exposure in different periods of life. One found effects of these exposures at all ages with risk higher with total exposure in older age groups; the other found a significant effect only for occupational exposure in the ten years before diagnosis of the SCC. The three studies were consistent in finding little evidence of any effect of non-working day or recreational exposure on risk of SCC at any time in life.

Whiteman and colleagues have recently reviewed the evidence on recalled sun exposure by period of life in studies of melanoma [8]. Summarized over 10 studies, the relative risk of melanoma with a history of sunburn in childhood was 1.8 (95% CI 1.6-2.2) while for sunburn in adulthood it was 1.5 (95% CI 1.3-1.8). For other measures of sun exposure, the pattern was less consistent. In four studies compared for effects of estimated total outdoor exposure, the relative risk was greater in childhood than adulthood in two and the opposite in two (our estimates of summary relative risks – childhood 1.1 95% CI 0.8-1.4, adulthood 1.6 95% CI 1.1-2.4). For beach exposure in six studies, the tallies of relative risks were four greater in childhood and two greater in adulthood (our estimates of summary relative risks – childhood 1.2 95% CI 0.9-1.5, adulthood 1.3 95% CI 0.9-1.9).

Autier and colleagues [45] found that sun protection during sunny vacations in early life was associated with reduced risk of later melanoma, although sun protection in early life could be confounded with sun protection in later life.

In summary, the evidence of these observational studies is that intermittent pattern sun exposure in childhood is more important than the same exposure in adulthood in causing BCC; that sun exposure in adulthood, probably regardless of pattern, is at least as important in causing SCC as is sun exposure in childhood; and that sun exposure in childhood and sun exposure in adulthood may not differ in their effect on risk of melanoma, although the low relative risks suggest that measurement error may be dominant in the melanoma studies.

There is some additional evidence that sun exposure in adult life increases risks of SCC and melanoma. This evidence is summarized in Box

6.4. Undoubtedly the strongest of it is that a program of daily sunscreen use reduced incidence of SCC during a 4-5 year intervention and follow-up period in a randomized controlled trial of daily sunscreen use in Queensland [31]. The previously shown, similar effects of sunscreen on solar keratoses increase the plausibility of this result [29,30]. There was no evidence of a similar effect on BCC in the Queensland trial and there has been no controlled study done to see if there might be such an effect of sunscreen on melanoma

Box 6.4 Evidence that sun exposure near to the time of diagnosis of a skin cancer promotes development of the cancer [1].

- Short-term fluctuations in ambient solar irradiance have been followed within two years by similar short-term fluctuations in incidence of melanoma [46,47].

- The incidence of melanoma varies seasonally with a trough in winter and a peak in spring and summer. This pattern is not confined to sites that are usually clothed in winter [48].

- There is similar seasonal variation in rates of excision of benign melanocytic nevi. Greater inflammation and regression and a higher mean proliferation fraction in those excised in summer than in winter suggests that this variation may be due to sun exposure promoting changes in nevi towards melanoma [49].

- Incidence of melanoma on the more-or-less continually exposed head and neck increases throughout life while that on intermittently exposed sites, such as the legs and back, shows more complex patterns with incidence falling in mid life [50]. Correspondingly, more continually exposed outdoor workers have a higher incidence of melanoma on the head and neck than do indoor workers while the latter have a higher incidence on the more intermittently exposed sites, for which exposure in childhood and early adult life is probably predominant [51,52].

- Sunscreen use reduces the development of new solar keratoses and increases the regression of existing ones [29,30].

- Sunscreen use probably reduces the development of SCC over a period of 4-5 years from beginning to use it [31].

Assuming, as seems reasonable, but not certain on present data, that sun exposure has both early and late effects on risk of SCC, probably melanoma and possibly BCC, a useful conceptualization of their interaction might be in terms that the lifetime potential for skin cancer is determined to a substantial degree by sun exposure in the first 10 years of life and the extent to which this potential is realized is determined by sun exposure in later life. Results obtained by Autier and colleagues [53] support this conceptualization. Indices of mainly recreational sun exposure in childhood and adulthood were each formed into three categories and relative risk of melanoma estimated within all combinations of these categories. Relative risk was 2.0 in each low-high combination (95% CI 0.9-4.5 for the childhood low, adulthood high category and 0.7-5.6 for the adulthood low, childhood high category), with reference to the low-low combination, and the relative risk in the high-high category was 4.5 (95% CI 1.6-12.5) thus suggesting a multiplicative relationship between sun exposure in the two periods of life (Figure 6.7).

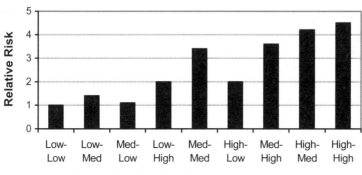

Categories of child and adult sun exposure index

Figure 6.7 Interaction between childhood and adulthood sun exposure (mainly recreational) in determining risk of melanoma [53].

2.4   Spectral response

It is generally believed that the shortest (UV) wavelengths of the spectrum of solar radiation at the surface of the earth are those that cause skin cancer. The UV action spectrum (curve showing the biological effect per unit of exposure) for any biological effect can only be determined rigorously by experiments in which controlled exposures to specific, narrow bands of UV are made and the ensuing responses measured. This has been done for human skin erythema ("sunburn") [54] and, of probably greater relevance to skin cancer, has also been done for the production of pyrimidine dimers in DNA in skin [55], but there is no practical way that the action spectrum for skin cancer can be measured directly in humans.

Inferences can be made about the action spectrum for human skin cancer in several ways. First, there are direct experimental observations of action spectra in experimental animals. The action spectrum of SCC in albino hairless mice [56] shows an initial peak at 293 nm in the UVB range, a trough at 354 nm of between 10^{-4} and 10^{-5} of the effect at the 293 nm peak, and another small peak at 380 nm in the UVA range (still nearly 10^{-4} of the 293 nm peak) after which it again falls. The action spectrum for melanoma has been estimated experimentally in a hybrid of two species of tiny fish, which is prone to melanoma [57], and suggests a peak in the UVA in the vicinity of 365 nm that is about a third of the effect at 302 nm in the UVB. A study of the effect of UVA (320-400 nm with peak at about 370 nm) on induction of melanoma in the South American opossum [58] found it to be effective but less so than would be predicted from the action spectrum in the fish model.

Second, the high proportions of SCCs and BCCs in humans found to have C to T or CC to TT mutations at dipyrimidine sites, the UVB "signature" mutations, in TP53 (see Section 1.5) suggests that the action spectrum for formation of pyrimidine dimers in humans may apply to these cancers. This action spectrum shows a peak at around 300 nm and effectiveness at 366 nm that is about 10^{-4} of the peak, which is similar to the action spectrum for SCC in albino hairless mice (see above) [55]. The evidence that UVB "signature" mutations are also more frequent than expected in CDKN2A in melanoma suggests a role for UVB in melanoma (Section 1.5). These observations in no way exclude an important role for UVA in any of these cancers.

Third, the latitude gradient of incidence of SCC is substantially greater than that of melanoma and, correspondingly, the latitude gradient of UVB is substantially greater than that of UVA [59]. This suggests that melanoma may be less influenced by ambient UVB than is SCC and more influenced by ambient UVA. The latitude gradient for BCC is between the two, but closer to that for SCC than for melanoma.

Fourth, there is accumulating evidence that use of sunbeds and related devices that produce a tan through controlled exposure to UV increases risk of melanoma (see Chapter 9). Relative to ambient levels, UVA emissions from many of the more recent of these devices are much greater than UVB emissions [60]. Given, however, the trend over time towards relatively less UVB and relatively more UVA in the emissions, it is difficult to interpret data on melanoma and use of sunlamps and sunbeds in terms of the action spectrum for melanoma in the absence of data that accurately relate relative risk of melanoma to the period of use of these devices and, therefore, their likely spectral output.

While the epidemiological evidence is weak, taken with the experimental evidence it seems probable that UVB is the main cause of SCC. The epidemiological evidence for melanoma, on the other hand, could indicate a greater role for UVA, and the studies in experimental animals support this possibility. It is not possible on present evidence to draw any conclusion regarding the relative contributions of UVB and UVA to the production of human BCC.

2.5 Modification of effect of sun exposure by sun sensitivity

The apparently strong effect of pattern of exposure on risk of melanoma and the evidence that risk of melanoma may fall with increasing sun exposure (Table 6.2) raise the possibility that acquisition and maintenance of a tan through continuing, steady exposure to the sun (as in occupational exposure) might actually reduce risk of melanoma below what it would have been with lower total sun exposure. Were this to be the case, one might expect to see strong modification of the effect of sun exposure on melanoma risk by skin type with risk falling with increasing exposure in those who tan readily (e.g., skin types III and IV) but increasing in those who tan poorly (e.g., skin types I and II).

Table 6.3 summarizes results of several studies of melanoma that have examined modification by sun sensitivity of risk of melanoma associated with various measures of sun exposure. There is strong evidence from these results that relative risk of melanoma with high non-occupational or recreational sun exposure and high experience of sunburn, relative to low, is greater in people who have high sun sensitivity (generally classified by ability to tan or skin type) than low sun sensitivity. This appears probable also for total and occupational sun exposure, but the evidence is weaker.

Table 6.3 Modification by sun sensitivity of risk of melanoma associated with various measures of sun exposure.

	Summary relative risks* (95% CI) in highest exposure category	
Type of sun exposure	High sun sensitivity	Low sun sensitivity
Total – 3 studies [67,68,53]	2.4 (1.4-4.0)	1.1 (0.7-1.7)
Occupational – 1 study [67]	3.3 (0.8-21)	1.5 (0.6-4.1)
Non-occupational - 3 studies [67,69,70]	4.0 (2.4-6.5)	1.1 (0.7-1.6)
Sunburn – 3 studies [67,70,71]	3.8 (2.5-5.8)	1.2 (0.8-1.9)

* Summary prepared from the relative risks (odds ratios) and their 95% confidence intervals in individual studies by use of standard methods of meta-analysis [66].

For BCC and SCC, there is little evidence to suggest that cutaneous sun sensitivity modifies risk associated with exposure to UV radiation, but little evidence to go on [9,37].

CONCLUSIONS

There is little room for doubt, now, that sun exposure is an important cause of BCC, SCC, and melanoma. We have estimated that sun exposure causes about 65% of cutaneous melanoma worldwide, and this proportion may be as high as 95% in areas of high sun exposure, such as Australia [61]. For BCC and SCC, if we assume, very roughly, that the incidence rate of each in Australia *in the absence of sun exposure* would be the same as it is for all non-melanocytic skin cancer in England and Wales, then 99% are attributable to sun exposure. It is probable, thus, that sun exposure is the main cause of these cancers and it is to the control of sun exposure that the major efforts in skin cancer prevention should be directed.

SUMMARY POINTS

- Sun exposure is an important cause of BCC, SCC, and melanoma.
- Sun exposure in the first 10 years of life determines to a substantial degree the lifetime potential for skin cancer, while sun exposure in later life determines the extent to which this potential is realized.
- Both pattern (more continuous vs. more intermittent) and amount of sun exposure influence the development of skin cancers, with the more continuous pattern occupational exposure associated with SCC, and the more intermittent pattern recreational exposure implicated in the development of BCC and melanoma.
- Messages about sun protection need to be tailored to specific populations at risk. The messages regarding pattern and amount of sun exposure will differ for different groups.
- There is evidence that UVA may play an important role in causing melanoma. It is therefore prudent to promote the use of broad-spectrum sunscreens.

IMPLICATIONS FOR PUBLIC HEALTH

We can draw a number of inferences from the epidemiological observations that would influence decisions about control of sun exposure to prevent skin cancer.

Both pattern and amount of sun exposure should be controlled

The relevance of this issue will depend very much on the nature of the predominant sun exposure. In a population of largely outdoor workers, the main objective will be to reduce sun exposure without increasing intermittency of exposure. That will require implementing sun protection policies and encouraging sun protection practices that reduce sun exposure more or less evenly in both occupational and recreational settings, essentially an all day, every day approach. This approach should apply equally well to BCC, SCC, and melanoma, although the initial gains will probably be more in SCC than the others.

At the other extreme, in a population of largely indoor workers, the main objective will be to reduce intermittency and with it the total amount of sun exposure. Promoting increased protection during recreational sun exposure might be the best way to do this. It would tackle intermittency, have the potential to substantially reduce total sun exposure, and would probably be more credible to this population than the all day, every day approach.

Consideration should be given to targeting sun protection messages more intensively to people who have higher sun sensitivity

This approach has not been favored by health promoters and is contrary to a fundamental principle of disease prevention that favors shifting the population mean exposure to risk factors over targeting people at particularly high exposure or high risk of disease [62]. There are, however, two countervailing issues. First, sun protection messages may be of reduced credibility to people who tan readily and perceive themselves, from their acute response to sun exposure, to be at comparatively low risk. A lower credibility in a sizeable proportion of the population could influence the overall credibility of these messages in the whole population. Second, there is evidence that low and possibly deficient levels of vitamin D are commoner than is generally believed, particularly in those with darker skin and in winter, and even in Australia where ambient UV is generally high [63,64,65]. On these bases, the issue of specific targeting of sun protection messages deserves at least more research if not renewed consideration.

The greatest gains will come from tackling sun exposure early in life

It is clear from the evidence reviewed that sun exposure in early life is very important in determining life-time risk of skin cancer, particularly BCC and melanoma probably. Later life exposure also appears to be important, at least for SCC and probably for melanoma, and we really can't say for BCC. It is only for BCC that there is reasonably clear evidence that the relative effect of sun exposure is greater in childhood than it is in adulthood but no analysis has yet been done that examined the effects of exposure in adulthood conditional on exposure in childhood. Everything we understand, or believe, about multi-stage carcinogenesis would suggest that if sun exposure has both early and late stage effects, the effect of sun exposure in later life will be much greater in someone with much early life exposure than someone with little.

This last point, together with the evidence for effects of early life exposure that are generally as great or greater than those of later life exposure, makes a very strong case on epidemiological grounds for giving priority to the control of early life sun exposure.

Increased protection against sun exposure will prevent skin cancer at whatever age it is applied

This is the message of the Queensland trial showing that daily sunscreen use can reduce risk of SCC over a 4-5 year period. Other sun protection measures would probably also be effective. We don't know, though, with any certainty whether this is true for BCC and melanoma. If sun exposure has late as well as early stage effects in skin cancer production, reduction in sun exposure at the time that skin cancers are common could have a quite dramatic effect on subsequent incidence, especially in people who had substantial early life exposure. The latter point may have motivational value.

Promote the use of broad spectrum sunscreens when sunscreens are used

Sunscreens generally have a narrower spectrum of protection than do neutral density protective measures, such as the wearing of clothes and the use of shade. While it is probable that the action spectrum for all skin cancers has its highest point near 300 nm in the UVB, there is evidence that UVA may be more effective in causing melanoma than SCC. At the levels of effectiveness seen in the hybrid fish model most melanoma could be caused by UVA not UVB because of the much higher ambient solar irradiance in the UVA band. In the absence of full knowledge on these matters, the precautionary principle demands that we should promote and use only sunscreens with sufficiently high effectiveness in the UVA that the natural spectral distribution of solar UV radiation reaching the tissues of the skin is altered minimally if at all.

REFERENCES

1. Armstrong BK, Kricker A, English DR (1997) Sun exposure and skin cancer. *Australas J Dermatol* **38**: s1-s6.
2. Cascinelli N, Marchesini R (1989) Increasing incidence of cutaneous melanoma, ultraviolet radiation and the clinician. *Photochem Photobiol* **50**: 497-505.
3. de Gruijl FR (1993) UV-induced skin cancer: Man and mouse. In: de Gruijl FR, ed. *The Dark Side of Sunlight*. Utrecht: Utrecht University, pp. 111-127.
4. International Agency for Research on Cancer Expert Group (1992) *Solar and Ultraviolet Radiation.* IARC Monographs on the Evaluation of Carcinogenic Risks to Humans, Vol 55. Lyon, France: IARC Press, p. 227.
5. Holman CD, Armstrong BK (1984) Pigmentary traits, ethnic origin, benign nevi, and family history as risk factors for cutaneous malignant melanoma. *J Natl Cancer Inst* **72**: 257-266.
6. Kricker A, Armstrong BK, English DR, Heenan PJ (1991) Pigmentary and cutaneous risk factors for non-melanocytic skin cancer--a case-control study. *Int J Cancer* **48**: 650-662.
7. English DR, Armstrong BK, Kricker A, Winter MG, Heenan PJ, Randell PL (1998) Demographic characteristics, pigmentary and cutaneous risk factors for squamous cell carcinoma of the skin: a case-control study. *Int J Cancer* **76**: 628-634.
8. Whiteman DC, Whiteman CA, Green AC (2001) Childhood sun exposure as a risk factor for melanoma: a systematic review of epidemiologic studies. *Cancer Causes Control* **12**: 69-82.
9. Kricker A, Armstrong BK, English DR, Heenan PJ (1995) A dose-response curve for sun exposure and basal cell carcinoma. *Int J Cancer* **60**: 482-488.
10. English DR, Armstrong BK, Kricker A, Winter MG, Heenan PJ, Randell PL (1998) Case-control study of sun exposure and squamous cell carcinoma of the skin. *Int J Cancer* **77**: 347-353.
11. Green A, MacLennan R, Youl P, Martin N (1993) Site distribution of cutaneous melanoma in Queensland. *Int J Cancer* **53**: 232-236.
12. Buettner PG, Raasch BA (1998) Incidence rates of skin cancer in Townsville, Australia. *Int J Cancer* **78**: 587-593.
13. Kricker A, Armstrong BK, Jones ME, Burton RC (1993) *Health, solar UV radiation and environmental change.* IARC Technical Reports, Vol 13. Lyon, France: IARC Press, pp. 20-44, 52-61.
14. Marrett LD, Nguyen HL, Armstrong BK (2001) Trends in the incidence of cutaneous malignant melanoma in New South Wales, 1983-1996. *Int J Cancer* **92**: 457-462.
15. Karagas MR, Greenberg ER, Spencer SK, Stukel TA, Mott LA (1999) Increase in incidence rates of basal cell and squamous cell skin cancer in New Hampshire, USA. New Hampshire Skin Cancer Study Group. *Int J Cancer* **81**: 555-559.
16. Armstrong BK, Kricker A (2001) The epidemiology of UV induced skin cancer. *J Photochem Photobiol B* **63**: 8-18.
17. Holman CD, Armstrong BK (1984) Cutaneous malignant melanoma and indicators of total accumulated exposure to the sun: an analysis separating histogenetic types. *J Natl Cancer Inst* **73**: 75-82.
18. Elwood JM, Gallagher RP, Hill GB, Pearson JC (1985) Cutaneous melanoma in relation to intermittent and constant sun exposure-the Western Canada Melanoma Study. *Int J Cancer* **35**: 427-433.

19. Gallagher RP, Hill GB, Bajdik CD *et al.* (1995) Sunlight exposure, pigmentary factors, and risk of nonmelanocytic skin cancer. I. Basal cell carcinoma. *Arch Dermatol* **131**: 157-163.
20. Gallagher RP, Hill GB, Bajdik CD *et al.* (1995) Sunlight exposure, pigmentation factors, and risk of nonmelanocytic skin cancer. II. Squamous cell carcinoma. *Arch Dermatol* **131:** 164-169.
21. Bataille V, Sasieni P, Grulich A *et al.* (1998) Solar keratoses: a risk factor for melanoma but negative association with melanocytic naevi. *Int J Cancer* **78:** 8-12.
22. Gallagher RP, Rivers JK, Lee TK, Bajdik CD, McLean DI, Coldman AJ (2000) Broad-spectrum sunscreen use and the development of new nevi in white children: A randomized controlled trial. *JAMA* **283:** 2955-2960.
23. Brash DE, Rudolph JA, Simon JA *et al.* (1991) A Role for Sunlight in Skin Cancer - UV-Induced p53 Mutations in Squamous Cell Carcinoma. *Proc Natl Acad Sci USA* **88:** 10124-10128.
24. Wikonkal NM, Brash DE (1999) Ultraviolet radiation induced signature mutations in photocarcinogenesis. *J Invest Dermatol Symp Proc* **4:** 6-10.
25. Ponten F, Berg C, Ahmadian A *et al.* (1997) Molecular pathology in basal cell cancer with p53 as a genetic marker. *Oncogene* **15:** 1059-1067.
26. Ouhtit A, Nakazawa H, Armstrong BK *et al.* (1998) UV-radiation-specific p53 mutation frequency in normal skin as a predictor of risk of basal cell carcinoma. *J Natl Cancer Inst* **90:** 523-531.
27. Pollock PM, Pearson JV, Hayward NK (1996) Compilation of somatic mutations of the CDKN2 gene in human cancers: non-random distribution of base substitutions. *Genes, Chromosomes & Cancer* **15**: 77-88.
28. Robinson JK, Rademaker AW (1992) Relative importance of prior basal cell carcinomas, continuing sun exposure, and circulating T lymphocytes on the development of basal cell carcinoma. *J Invest Dermatol* **99:** 227-231.
29. Thompson SC, Jolley D, Marks R (1993) Reduction of solar keratoses by regular sunscreen use. *N Engl J Med* **329:** 1147-1151.
30. Naylor MF, Boyd A, Smith DW, Cameron GS, Hubbard D, Neldner KH (1995) High sun protection factor sunscreens in the suppression of actinic neoplasia. *Arch Dermatol* **131:** 170-175.
31. Green A, Williams G, Neale R *et al.* (1999) Daily sunscreen application and betacarotene supplementation in prevention of basal-cell and squamous-cell carcinomas of the skin: a randomised controlled trial. *Lancet* **354:** 723-729.
32. Fears TR, Scotto J, Schneiderman MA (1977) Mathematical models of age and ultraviolet effects on the incidence of skin cancer among whites in the United States. *Am J Epidemiol* **105:** 420-427.
33. Elwood JM (1992) Melanoma and sun exposure: contrasts between intermittent and chronic exposure. *World J Surg.* **16:** 157-165.
34. Armstrong BK (1988) Epidemiology of malignant melanoma: intermittent or total accumulated exposure to the sun? *J Dermatol Surg Oncol* **14:** 835-849.
35. Gilchrest BA, Eller MS, Geller AC, Yaar M (1999) The pathogenesis of melanoma induced by ultraviolet radiation. *N Engl J Med.* **340:** 1341-1348.
36. Strickland PT, Vitasa BC, West SK, Rosenthal FS, Emmet EA, Taylor HR (1989) Quantitative carcinogenesis in man: solar ultraviolet B dose dependence of skin cancer in Maryland watermen. *J Natl Cancer Inst* **81:** 1910-1913.
37. Rosso S, Zanetti R, Martinez C *et al.* (1996) The multicentre south European study 'Helios'. II: Different sun exposure patterns in the aetiology of basal cell and squamous cell carcinomas of the skin. *Br J Cancer* **73:** 1447-1454.

38. Scotto J, Fears TR, Fraumeni JF (1983) *Incidence of Nonmelanoma Skin Cancer in the United States.* Washington: US Department of Health and Human Services.
39. Muir C, Waterhouse J, Mack T, Powell J, Whelan S (1987) *Cancer Incidence in Five Continents* Volume V. Lyon: International Agency for Research on Cancer.
40. Mack TM, Floderus B (1991) Malignant melanoma risk by nativity, place of residence at diagnosis, and age at migration. *Cancer Causes Control* **2:** 401-411.
41. English DR, Armstrong BK (1994) Melanocytic nevi in children. I. Anatomic sites and demographic and host factors. *Am J Epidemiol* **139:** 390-401.
42. Kricker A, Armstrong BK, English DR, Heenan PJ (1995) Does intermittent sun exposure cause basal cell carcinoma? A case-control study in Western Australia. *Int J Cancer* **60:** 489-494.
43. Zanetti R, Rosso S, Martinez C *et al.* (1996) The multicentre south European study 'Helios'. I: Skin characteristics and sunburns in basal cell and squamous cell carcinomas of the skin. *Br J Cancer* **73:** 1440-1446.
44. Corona R, Dogliotti E, D'Errico M *et al.* (2001) Risk factors for basal cell carcinoma in a Mediterranean population: role of recreational sun exposure early in life. *Arch Dermatol* **137:** 1162-1168.
45. Autier P, Dore JF, Lejeune F *et al.* (1996) Sun protection in childhood or early adolescence and reduction of melanoma risk in adults: an EORTC case-control study in Germany, Belgium and France. *J Epidemiol Biostat* **1:** 51-57.
46. Houghton A, Munster EW, Viola MV (1978) Increased incidence of malignant melanoma after peaks of sunspot activity. *Lancet* **1:** 759-760.
47. Swerdlow AJ (1979) Incidence of malignant melanoma of the skin in England and Wales and its relationship to sunshine. *BMJ* **2:** 1324-1327.
48. Schwartz SM, Armstrong BK, Weiss NS (1987) Seasonal variation in the incidence of cutaneous malignant melanoma: an analysis by body site and histologic type. *Am J Epidemiol* **126:** 104-111.
49. Fleming MG, Swan LS, Heenan PJ (1991) Seasonal variation in the proliferation fraction of Australian common nevi. *Am J Dermatopathol* **13:** 463-466.
50. Holman CD, Mulroney CD, Armstrong BK (1980) Epidemiology of pre-invasive and invasive malignant melanoma in Western Australia. *Int J Cancer* **25:** 317-323.
51. Beral V, Robinson N (1981) The relationship of malignant melanoma, basal and squamous skin cancers to indoor and outdoor work. *Br J Cancer* **44:** 886-891.
52. Vagero D, Ringback G, Kiviranta H (1986) Melanoma and other tumors of the skin among office, other indoor and outdoor workers in Sweden 1961-1979. *Br J Cancer* **53:** 507-512.
53. Autier P, Dore JF (1998) Influence of sun exposures during childhood and during adulthood on melanoma risk. *Int J Cancer* **77:** 533-537.
54. McKinlay AF, Diffey BL (1987) A reference action spectrum for ultraviolet induced erythema in human skin. *CIE Journal* **6:** 17-22.
55. Freeman SE, Hacham H, Gange RW, Maytum DJ, Sutherland JC, Sutherland BM (1989) Wavelength dependence of pyrimidine dimer formation in DNA of human skin irradiated in situ with ultraviolet light. *Proc Natl Acad Sci USA* **86:** 5605-5609.
56. de Gruijl FR, Sterenborg HJCM, Forbes PD, Davies RE, Cole C, Kelfkens G (1993) Wavelength dependence of skin cancer induction by ultraviolet irradiation of albino hairless mice. *Cancer Research* **52:** 1-8.
57. Setlow RB, Grist E, Thompson K, Woodhead AD (1993) Wavelengths effective in induction of malignant melanoma. *Proc Natl Acad Sci USA* **90:** 6666-6670.

58. Ley RD (2001) Dose response for ultraviolet radiation A-induced focal melanocytic hyperplasia and nonmelanoma skin tumors in Monodelphis domestica. *Photochem Photobiol* **73:** 20-23.
59. Moan J, Dahlback A, Setlow RB (1999) Epidemiological support for an hypothesis for melanoma induction indicating a role for UVA radiation. *Photochem Photobiol.* **70:** 243-247.
60. Miller SA, Hamilton SL, Wester UG, Cyr WH (1998) An analysis of UVA emissions from sunlamps and the potential importance for melanoma. *Photochem Photobiol* **68:** 63-70.
61. Armstrong BK, Kricker A (1993) How much melanoma is caused by sun exposure? *Melanoma Res* **3:** 395-401.
62. Rose G (1992) *The strategy of preventive medicine.* Oxford: Oxford University Press.
63. Jones G, Blizzard C, Riley MD, Parameswaran V, Greenaway TM, Dwyer T (1999) Vitamin D levels in prepubertal children in Southern Tasmania: prevalence and determinants. *Eur J Clin Nutr* **53:** 824-829.
64. Grover SR, Morley R (2001) Vitamin D deficiency in veiled or dark-skinned pregnant women. *Med J Aust* **175:** 251-252.
65. Pasco JA, Henry MJ, Nicholson GC, Sanders KM, Kolowicz MA (2001) Vitamin D status of women in the Geelong Osteoporosis Study: association with diet and casual exposure to sunlight. *Med J Aust* **175:** 401-405.
66. Elwood JM, Jopson J (1997) Melanoma and sun exposure: an overview of published studies. *Int J Cancer* **73:** 198-203.
67. Dubin N, Moseson M, Pasternack BS (1989) Sun exposure and malignant melanoma among susceptible individuals. *Environ Health Perspect* **81:** 139-151.
68. White E, Kirkpatrick CS, Lee JA (1994) Case-control study of malignant melanoma in Washington State. I. Constitutional factors and sun exposure. *Am J Epidemiol* **139:** 857-868.
69. Weinstock MA, Colditz GA, Willett WC *et al.* (1991) Melanoma and the sun: the effect of swimsuits and a "healthy" tan on the risk of nonfamilial malignant melanoma in women. *Am J Epidemiol* **134:** 462-470.
70. Nelemans PJ, Groenendal H, Kiemeney LA *et al.* (1993) Effect of intermittent exposure to sunlight on melanoma risk among indoor workers and sun-sensitive individuals. *Environ Health Perspect* **101:** 252-255.
71. Cress RD, Holly EA, Ahn DK (1995) Cutaneous melanoma in women. V. Characteristics of those who tan and those who burn when exposed to summer sun. *Epidemiology* **6:** 538-543.

Chapter 7

The role of genetics in the prevention of skin cancer

David Whiteman, B.Med.Sc., M.B., B.S. (Hons), Ph.D.; Rachel Neale, Ph.D.
Population and Clinical Sciences Division, Queensland Institute of Medical Research, Herston, Queensland, Australia

Key words: molecular epidemiology, carcinogenesis, tumor-suppressor genes, risk assessment, genetic counseling

INTRODUCTION

Cancer results from a complex interaction of environmental and genetic factors that impact upon a target cell, eventually leading to uncontrolled growth, invasion of adjacent structures and metastatic dissemination. Recent advances in understanding the mechanisms of carcinogenesis have emphasized the role of molecular pathways leading to cancer, raising expectations among clinicians and the public that many of today's common afflictions will be prevented or definitively treated in the future. This chapter seeks to integrate the findings from the molecular and epidemiological paradigms, and in so doing, highlight salient issues of relevance to the control of skin cancer.

D. Hill et al. (eds.), Prevention of Skin Cancer, 117-139.
© 2004 *Kluwer Academic Publishers. Printed in the Netherlands.*

1.   GENES AND CANCER

1.1   DNA, chromosomes, and genes

The nucleus of every cell in the human body (except for the germ cells - spermatozoa and ova) carries an identical set of detailed instructions on how to function. This "instructional codebook" takes the form of long strands of deoxyribonucleic acid (DNA) that are tightly coiled into the chromosomes that are visible through the light microscope. The DNA code of humans is constructed from more than 3 billion nucleotide base-pairs, the exact sequences of which are crucial for ensuring that a cell functions correctly.

The fundamental unit of heredity is the gene. A gene is a sequence of DNA that encodes a discrete piece of information, usually the code for making a protein, but sometimes carrying other information, in the form of ribonucleic acid (RNA), that regulates the activity or expression of other genes. It is now estimated that the 46 human chromosomes encode around 30,000 genes. Each gene resides at a characteristic location on a particular chromosome, but across the human population there are typically numerous variants of each gene, which differ to some degree in their levels of expression, processing or function of encoded product. These variants are called alleles, and it is this allelic variation which gives rise to the extraordinary diversity of life. For example, the melanocortin 1 receptor gene (MC1R) located on chromosome 16 encodes the receptor for the melanocortin hormone. This receptor plays an important role in regulating the production of melanin in the skin, hair and eyes. Different alleles of MC1R have been associated with blonde, black and red hair respectively.

1.2   Cell division and mutation

Throughout a person's lifetime, cells in the body are constantly replicating through the process of cell division termed mitosis. This highly regulated sequence permits organs to grow, and to replace damaged or aged cells. A second, specialized form of cell division called meiosis occurs only in the gonads to produce germ cells for the transfer of genes to the next generation. Both types of cell division are relevant to the development of skin cancer.

Cell division begins with a "mother" cell copying its entire DNA to ensure that each "daughter" cell has a complete set of genetic information. This process is performed with remarkable fidelity, but, very occasionally, mistakes occur during replication - these mistakes result in changes to the genetic information, and are called mutations. The scope for mutation is enormous - including deletions or insertions of DNA segments, substitution of single base pairs, transposition of fragments of chromosomes and others. Mutations arise by chance, usually at extremely low frequency, when enzymes that repair or copy DNA are inefficient. However, mutations may also arise because of damage to DNA caused by radiation, viruses, chemicals and drugs. Molecular epidemiologists now recognize that exposure of DNA to certain mutagenic agents results in characteristic types of mutations [1]. For example, UVR commonly leads to unique types of mutations at dipyrimidine sites - if one of these mutations is found in a sample of tumor tissue, it may be inferred that the tumor cells were exposed to ultraviolet light at some point in their development.

A mutation that arises during mitosis is called a somatic mutation, and will only be passed on to the daughters of the affected cell. Imagine a keratinocyte in the basement layer of the epidermis being struck by a high-energy photon of UVR. The energy of the collision causes the DNA of the cell to be damaged. When the affected keratinocyte undergoes mitosis, the damaged DNA will be copied into the genome of the two daughter cells. In turn, when these two daughter cells divide, the mutation will be carried in the four "grand-daughter" cells of the original cell. Over the years and many cycles of cell division, potentially thousands of "daughter cells" will be carrying the mutated DNA, however the mutation cannot be passed onto to any other cells except those that are directly descended from the original keratinocyte.

A mutation occurring in a germ cell during meiosis is potentially far more serious, since if the affected germ cell is successfully fertilized, the mutated gene will be present in every single cell in the developing embryo. Such a mutation is called a germline mutation, and is passed down through the generations from parent to offspring. An appreciation of the differences between somatic and germline mutations is fundamental to understanding the likely impact of genetic testing for predicting cancer risks. These concepts will be explored more fully below.

1.3   The genetic origins of skin cancer

In characterizing the role of genes in the development of skin cancer, a distinction may be drawn between genes that act directly within a keratinocyte or melanocyte to initiate carcinogenesis, and the indirect effects of genes that modify a person's risk of developing skin cancer through interactions with other factors in the causal pathway.

1.3.1   Direct effects

The "multistage model of carcinogenesis" has classically described three biologically distinct stages in the development of cancer, termed initiation, promotion and progression [2]. While the latter two terms are gradually falling from use, the concept of the initiation of cancer is still pertinent, whereby a normal cell is irreversibly transformed to a potentially cancerous state following exposure to a carcinogen. In the case of the squamous cell carcinomas (SCC) and basal cell carcinomas (BCC), the initiated cell is an epidermal skin cell; for melanomas, the cell of origin is a melanocyte. Gene mutation is considered to be the fundamental event of cancer initiation. This can be either a somatic mutation arising in a single isolated cell, or a germline mutation present in every cell throughout the body. It is important to recognize that the presence of a mutation in a cell does not inevitably herald the onset of cancer - subsequent mutations must also occur. Indeed, if a single mutation were sufficient to cause cancer, then organisms with germline mutations in key regulatory genes would have literally millions of cancers present at birth.

While no universal genetic target for initiation has been identified for all cancers, three broad classes of "direct effect" cancer causing genes have been described (others will undoubtedly be recognized in the future) - oncogenes, tumor suppressor genes and DNA repair genes. Oncogenes generally function to activate cellular proliferation, either by coding for signal proteins, or through activating DNA transcription. By contrast, tumor suppressor genes act to inhibit cell division; when this inhibition is lost, either through deletion or mutation of the gene, the cell may divide unchecked. The DNA repair genes play a key role in recognizing and repairing damaged sequences of DNA before cells divide [3]. There has been intense activity in the search for these types of direct effect genes as causal agents for skin cancer.

1.3.2   Indirect effects

Genes can influence a person's risk of skin cancer in many ways aside from the direct consequences of a gene mutation in a target cell. A gene (or its protein product) might interact with another causal factor for skin cancer (for example, an environmental carcinogen or another gene) and thus serve to modify a person's susceptibility to the adverse effects of that factor. For example, genes which regulate the production of melanin pigment in a person's skin cells indirectly influence a person's risk of skin cancer, since melanin is the principal means by which epidermal cells are protected from the mutation-inducing photons of solar radiation.

As knowledge of the human genome expands, it is likely that many genes will be identified which are indirectly associated with risk of skin cancer, perhaps encompassing such diverse phenomena as cellular response to injury, metabolism of carcinogenic compounds, immune surveillance for tumor cells and even human behavior. It is becoming increasingly clear that many of these processes will be regulated by numerous genes, each with multiple alleles, and with each allele conferring slightly different levels of susceptibility. In the light of such enormous complexity, our knowledge of the genetic causes of skin cancer is embryonic. Nevertheless, the ways in which genetic knowledge can be applied to the primary prevention of skin cancer may be predicted.

2. GENES AND MELANOMA

2.1 "Direct effect" genes

2.1.1 Familial melanoma

Approximately 10% of people who develop melanoma have one or more family members similarly affected, suggesting a strong genetic contribution among these patients, which may be inherited through the germline. In the early 1990s, genetic epidemiologists around the world began assembling groups of families with a very high incidence of cutaneous melanoma. By comparing the inheritance of chromosome markers with the presence or absence of melanoma, a region was identified on the short arm of chromosome 9 which appeared to be associated with susceptibility to familial melanoma [4-6]. At about the same time, molecular geneticists observed that the same region of chromosome 9 was commonly deleted in cell lines derived from a variety of cancers. The deleted region was identified after screening numerous cancer cell lines [7,8] and found to contain two coding sequences that were very similar to a newly discovered gene involved in regulating cell division [9]. One of these sequences, entitled MTS1 (for Multiple Tumor Suppressor gene 1) encoded a 16 kilodalton protein inhibitor of cyclin dependent kinase 4 [CDK4] known as p16[INK4a.] MTS1 was subsequently renamed CDKN2A.

Studies involving melanoma families from Europe, Australia and North America have since found germline CDKN2A mutations in many affected individuals [10-12]. Mutant p16[INK4a] proteins derived from tumors have also been demonstrated to have reduced or absent biological activity in functional assays [12,13], further underscoring the causal role of this gene-product in a subset of melanomas.

Since fewer than half of the melanoma families studied have mutations in the CDKN2A gene [12,14], additional candidates for familial melanoma genes have been sought among other regulators of cell division. To date, three melanoma families have been identified with mutations in the CDK4 gene [15]. Two other interesting candidate genes have been intensely investigated for possible causal associations with familial melanoma. One of these genes, P14ARF, actually overlaps the CDKN2A gene and shares some of the same sequence, leading to speculation that this gene may also play a role in melanoma development. Despite this promising finding, there is as yet no convincing evidence that P14ARF is causally associated with familial melanoma [16]. The other candidate gene, CDKN2B, lies very close to the CDKN2A locus, and shares a similar mechanism of action. Nevertheless, there have been no melanoma families yet identified carrying a germline mutation in CDKN2B [16-18].

The p53 gene product is a multifunctional protein involved in transcription, cell cycle regulation, apoptosis and DNA repair. Mutations in the TP53 gene are one of the most common gene defects, found in over 50% of all human cancers. In UV radiation-induced epidermal skin cancer, TP53 mutations have been found in 90% of all squamous cell carcinomas and ~50% of all basal cell carcinomas. The majority of these mutations were C→T or CC→TT transitions, the signature mutations of UV radiation exposure. Alterations in the TP53 gene or in TP53 expression are also involved in melanoma formation, but to a lesser extent than in epidermal skin cancer (see also Chapter 6).

2.1.2   Other high risk groups

Two other groups of melanoma patients have been studied on the premise that they may have an inherent susceptibility to develop melanoma, but again, the proportion of cases identified with mutations in "direct effect" genes has been low. Between 5-15% of patients with multiple primary melanomas but without a family history of the disease have germline mutations in the CDKN2A gene [19,20]. In the only study of children who developed cutaneous melanoma before the age of 15 years, one case out of 30 had a germline CDKN2A mutation [21]. A similarly low prevalence of germline CDKN2A mutations was observed in a sample of North American melanoma patients diagnosed before age 40 years [22].

Several other inherited cancer syndromes are associated with an increased risk of melanoma. Patients with xeroderma pigmentosum (XP) have a markedly reduced ability to repair DNA that has been damaged by UVR, and as a consequence, they develop cutaneous melanoma at more than one thousand times the rate of the normal population [23]. Interestingly, the tumors occur in the same anatomical distribution as the general population, suggesting a common etiology. Cowden disease is another autosomal dominant syndrome, caused by mutation of the PTEN gene. Affected individuals predominantly develop breast and thyroid cancer, but also melanoma. There is no evidence that germline PTEN mutations account for cases of melanoma outside of this syndrome however [24].

2.1.3   "Sporadic" melanoma

Far and away the majority of melanomas occur in people with no family history of this tumor, and these are usually referred to as "sporadic" melanomas. Published estimates of the prevalence of germline mutations of the CDKN2A gene among people with sporadic melanoma are few, presumably because of the a priori assumption that sporadic cases are not due to inherited factors, and there is, therefore, little to be gained in searching for germline mutations in direct effect genes. This assumption appears well founded, since a large, population-based study in Queensland, Australia found no germline CDKN2A mutations among 201 cases of sporadic melanoma [25]. In contrast, a Canadian study of 254 patients reported an overall prevalence of germline CDKN2A mutations of 3.2% [26]. This figure is almost certainly an over-estimate due to selection bias, since the patients in that study were recruited from specialized pigmented lesion clinics, and included people with a strong family history of melanoma, as well as those with early onset disease, multiple primaries or atypical nevus syndrome.

Evidence for somatic mutations in direct effect genes as a cause for melanoma has been sought from uncultured tissue from sporadic tumors, but overall, findings have been inconsistent across studies and difficult to interpret. For example, mutations in CDKN2A, TP53, N-RAS and PTEN have all been observed at varying frequencies in melanomas, but none of these genes appear to be necessary or sufficient in causing melanoma.

Recently, the emphasis of scientific inquiry has shifted from merely observing the frequency of mutations in these direct effect genes to identifying those factors that are associated with their abnormal expression. For example, a case-control study which combined assessments of molecular expression with epidemiological techniques [27] found that melanomas which stained positively for p53-protein were more common on exposed anatomical sites, and in people with sun sensitive phenotype and a past history of epidermal skin cancer. In contrast, people with p53-negative melanomas had higher nevus counts and a greater propensity to freckling. Similar observations have been made with other genes. UV-specific mutations of N-RAS are more common in melanomas from sun-exposed sites than from unexposed sites [28,29], and are more common among melanomas from Australia than Europe [29]. Together, these findings suggest that cutaneous melanomas arise through different causal pathways, characterized by somatic mutations of direct effect genes. Clearly, more work is required in this area, which may have important implications for primary prevention programs.

2.2   "Indirect effect" genes

The search for constitutional genes that confer an increased risk of melanoma through indirect effects on the target cell has largely been driven by the candidate gene approach. That is, genes known to be involved in a cellular pathway of potential relevance to skin cancer, or which are associated with a phenotypic attribute known to be risk factor for melanoma, are selected as candidates for further research. Alternative strategies for gene discovery (using segregation or linkage studies) have limited power for identifying "indirect effect" genes, since the genotypes are typically common and the vast majority of people with the genotype do not have disease.

Several candidate genes have been postulated as "risk factors" for melanoma; typically these candidates have involved either the genes controlling levels of pigmentation in the skin or genes coding for DNA repair or detoxifying enzymes. Few have been conclusively demonstrated to have any measurable effect.

Most interest has focused on the MC1R gene, which encodes a receptor for the melanocyte-stimulating hormone (MSH). It has been known for many years that among mammals, differences in coat color between individual members of the same species are determined by variations in the relative proportions of eumelanins (black pigments) and pheomelanins (red-yellow pigments). These proportions, in turn, are governed by variants of the MSH receptor, and it seemed likely that the same was true for humans in respect to skin color. Following identification of the human MC1R gene in 1992 [30], researchers set about characterizing allele frequencies in human populations. Valverde *et al.* [31] provided the first evidence that human MC1R genotype was related to pigmentation phenotype, identifying several variants associated with both hair color and skin type among British subjects. Variant alleles of the MC1R gene were identified among 82% of those with red hair, 33% of those with fair or blonde hair but less than 20% of those with brown or black hair. The association of MC1R genotype with skin type was even more pronounced - 52% of those with skin type I had variant alleles, compared with 26% of those with skin type II and 3% and 0% for those with skin types III and IV, respectively. Similar associations with hair color have since been reported among Irish [32] and Australian [33] populations, although associations with skin type have been less conclusive.

Because MC1R genotype is associated with red hair color and fair skin type, and because these pigmentation phenotypes are both associated with risk of melanoma, a logical extension is to assess whether MC1R genotype is associated with risk of melanoma. Several studies have sought evidence for such an association, although only one study to date has ascertained a population-based sample of incident cases and community controls for comparison [34]. This study was conducted in the high incidence population of Queensland. It was found that people carrying one of three particular variants of MC1R had a 2-fold increased risk of melanoma, even after adjusting for hair and eye color. Those with two or more variants of MC1R had a 4-fold increased risk of melanoma. These associations appeared to be modified by pigmentation type, since a stratified analysis restricted to those with darker complexions found that MC1R variants conferred a 10-fold increased risk of melanoma, whereas a similar analysis restricted to fair-skinned people found no association with MC1R. The authors suggest that one explanation for these findings is that whilst these MC1R variants increase risk of melanoma primarily by determining fair skin type, these variants also confer risk through alternative (direct) mechanisms, such as through other signals within the melanocyte.

An earlier study conducted among patients in northern England [35] found only weak evidence of an association between MC1R genotype and risk of melanoma. These data are difficult to interpret since the control participants in the English study all had a diagnosis of basal cell papilloma, possibly diminishing the power of the study to find an association.

Ultraviolet A radiation is thought to contribute indirectly to ultraviolet-induced carcinogenesis by causing oxidative stress. Thus there are justifiable grounds for proposing that genes of the glutathione S-transferase (GST) gene family, which produce enzymes that detoxify products arising as a result of oxidative stress, may be indirectly involved with the development of melanoma. While there is some experimental evidence in human subjects that the level of glutathione S-transferase activity confers protective effects against the inflammatory effects of sun exposure [36], no conclusive associations with risk of melanoma have been found [37].

3.   GENES AND EPIDERMAL SKIN CANCERS

3.1   Direct effect genes

3.1.1   Inherited skin cancer syndromes

There are two well-characterized inherited disorders which predispose to epidermal skin cancers, nevoid basal cell carcinoma syndrome (NBCCS), also known as Gorlin's syndrome [38] and xeroderma pigmentosum (XP).

Approximately 90% of people with NBCSS develop at least one basal cell carcinoma (BCC) by 40 years of age, and most of these lesions occur on sun-exposed skin [39]. Sufferers of NBCCS also have a high incidence of internal cancers such as ovarian fibroma, cardiac fibroma and meningioma, as well as characteristic phenotypic abnormalities including pitting of the palms and soles, coarse facial features and malformations of brain, spine, ribs and teeth [40].

NBCCS is now known to arise from germline mutations in the PTCH gene, located on chromosome 9q22.3 [41,42]. This gene is the human homologue of the *patched* gene, first identified in the fruit fly. The human PTCH gene is a critical component of an important signaling pathway and is thought to act as a tumor suppressor by inactivating various genes that have complex roles in cell growth and differentiation [43]. Despite the high morbidity experienced by sufferers, NBCSS is a rare cause of BCC, accounting for fewer than 0.5% of all cases.

As for melanoma, patients with XP have a markedly increased risk of developing SCC or BCC very early in life. Among XP patients less than 20 years old, the incidence of skin cancer is approximately 1000 times higher than in the normal population [23].

3.1.2   Sporadic epidermal skin cancers

The overwhelming majority of skin cancers arise in people with no known germline mutations in "direct effect" genes, but are rather thought to be due to somatic mutations in other direct effect genes resulting from environmental insults. Of these, TP53 is the most frequently mutated gene in SCC and BCC. This tumor suppressor gene is located on the short arm of chromosome 17 and encodes a protein known as p53. This protein plays a critical role in control of the cell cycle and cellular growth. If the TP53 gene in a cell is deleted or mutated (for example, by UVR), the cell will have a reduced capacity to repair further DNA damage. Additional mutations can then accumulate to enable the cell to continue its progression down the carcinogenic pathway.

Somatic mutations in the TP53 gene have been detected in approximately 50% of BCCs and over 90% of SCCs [44-46]. They also occur commonly in solar keratoses, suggesting that TP53 mutations are an early carcinogenic event. UVR causes characteristic mutations, the most common being the formation of dimers between adjacent pyrimidines on the same DNA strand, and almost all the TP53 mutations seen in skin cancers are of this signature type. Recent studies have focused on the role of polymorphisms of TP53 (particularly codon 72) as conferring increased risks of SCC, but there is no consistent evidence of a disease-associated effect [47].

There has been speculation that the XP genotype may serve as another model for how sporadic skin cancer develops. Whereas patients with XP carry a germline mutation that reduces the ability of all of their cells to repair UV-induced DNA damage, it is possible that sporadic skin cancers may develop from individual keratinocytes that have lost the capacity to repair DNA. Alternatively, people carrying alleles of DNA repair genes that have a reduced (but not absent) DNA repair capacity may be at increased risk for SCCs or BCCs. So far, the epidemiological data are conflicting with respect to any association between DNA repair capacity and sporadic skin cancers. One study demonstrated a lower DNA repair capacity in the cells of patients with BCC than in controls [48]; another showed that this association was restricted to patients with psoriasis [49], while in an Australian study there was no difference in the mean DNA repair capacity [50]. Future work may identify specific polymorphisms in repair genes that increase susceptibility to carcinogens: to date these have not been isolated [51].

Bi-allelic inactivation of the PTCH gene, resulting from two somatic mutations, has also been implicated in the carcinogenesis of sporadic BCCs. The proportion of sporadic BCCs in which both copies of the gene are inactivated ranges from approximately 20% [52] to 38% [53]. This is almost certainly an underestimation as the method used to detect mutations is thought to be only 50% sensitive [54]. UVR "signature mutations" account for approximately 50% of PTCH gene mutations in sporadic tumors, although additional non-signature mutations could also be caused by UVR [53,54]. Because allelic loss of PTCH is also common in BCCs, and since UVR does not typically cause deletion of genetic material, other, as yet unknown, environmental agents may also be responsible for inactivation of PTCH.

3.2   Indirect effect genes

It is well recognized that people with red hair, blue eyes and fair skin which burns rather than tans have a higher risk of keratinocyte cancers than people with more pigmented skin. This is thought to be due largely to the increased passage of UVR through the skin to the susceptible keratinocytes in deeper skin layers. As described above, polymorphisms in pigmentation genes such as MC1R regulate the quantity and type of melanin in the skin, thus having an indirect effect on the development of skin cancer. Nevertheless, identifying particular allelic variants which confer an increased susceptibility to BCC has been relatively unsuccessful so far. Indeed there is some evidence that the MC1R variants examined thus far may actually be associated with the number of tumors that a person develops (that is, multiplicity), rather than the risk of an initial BCC [55].

Polymorphisms at a number of GST loci, for example GSTM1 and GSTT1, have been shown to influence outcome among patients with an initial BCC; for example the GSTT1 null genotype was associated with a decreased time to the next BCC presentation (reviewed in [56]. Null genotypes at the GSTM1 and GSTT1 loci are found in 50% and 20% of Caucasian populations respectively.

4.   GENES AND PREVENTION OF SKIN CANCER

The preceding sections have given an overview of the current state of knowledge regarding the genetic causes of melanoma, SCC and BCC. While several key genes have been identified as playing a directly causal role in the development of cancers of the skin, it is apparent that even among individuals with a very strong family history of melanoma, an identified gene mutation is found only in the minority. Other, as yet unidentified, genes must be involved in these heritable cancers, and it is likely that their number will be many and their prevalence low. For the vast majority of "spontaneous" or "sporadic" cancers of the skin, the causal pathway involves a complex interplay of environmental factors and somatic mutations in genes which directly affect cellular behavior, as well as the effects of modifying genes, sometimes far removed from the target cell, but which nevertheless contribute to the initiation or promotion of the cancer. Given this complex web of causality, the question arises as to how genetic knowledge can be applied to prevent new cases of skin cancer and, more generally, reduce the public health burden of these diseases.

At present, the principal strategies through which genetic knowledge might be applied to prevent skin cancer are limited to various forms of genetic screening. In the future, when the function of genes and their protein products will have been characterized with greater precision, there are prospects for early detection, treatment for preneoplastic conditions, gene therapy and even vaccination to prevent the development of skin cancers.

4.1   Current recommendations for genetic screening

The term "genetic screening" broadly describes the process of identifying people whose genetic constitution confers an increased risk of cancer. The international Melanoma Genetics Consortium, comprising oncologists, dermatologists, molecular geneticists and epidemiologists, recently issued a consensus statement regarding genetic screening for melanoma susceptibility genes [57]. The Consortium concluded that genetic screening was rarely indicated outside the research setting, and should not be in routine clinical use. This policy was reiterated at the 5th World Conference on Melanoma in Venice (March, 2001). Reasons for rejecting genetic screening as a clinical tool, even among high-risk families, include the uncertainty of prevalence and penetrance estimates in this setting, but also relate to the practical considerations of managing risk. These issues are explored in greater detail in the following section.

The clinical care of members of melanoma-prone families extends to educating them about the dangers of exposure to sunlight, the need for routine skin examinations from the age of 10 years and the removal of suspicious skin lesions. The Consortium holds the view that the preventive strategies of education and surveillance should apply to all members of an affected family, not just those with the affected genotype. This is because there is a high incidence of melanoma even among non-carriers of the genotype in many families. In other words, a negative genetic screening test result provides no basis for complacency in a high-risk setting. Clearly, screening for melanoma susceptibility genes among the general population is not viable given current levels of knowledge.

The utility of genetic screening as a tool for the prevention of SCC and BCC is even less clear than for melanoma. Aside from the very rare families with mutations in PTCH or one of the XP genes (fewer than 1 in 100,000 people), the causal pathway for SCC and BCC involves interactions between the principal environmental carcinogen (sunlight) and many genes indirectly involved in skin pigmentation, DNA repair and detoxification of reactive oxygen species. Identifying combinations which confer a higher risk, and are therefore suitable for screening, is unlikely in the foreseeable future. Identification of particular allelic polymorphisms among patients with BCC may assist in identifying those likely to experience further skin cancers, or the time until the next lesion. However, the costs and benefits of genetic screening in comparison with regularly examining the skin of affected people need to be determined.

4.2   Exploring the issue of genetic screening

The foregoing sections have drawn an arbitrary but conceptually helpful distinction between genes which directly or indirectly cause skin cancer, and then drawn a further distinction between germline and somatic mutations. For the foreseeable future, genetic screening will be restricted to testing for germline mutations of high-risk "direct effect" genes, or for disease-associated alleles of "indirect effect" genes, since these are carried by all cells in the body and hence will be detectable in a sample of cells from the blood or buccal mucosa. Screening tests for somatic mutations, while technically feasible, are likely to be of limited clinical utility in the short term.

There are a range of clinical scenarios whereby a doctor or a patient might consider testing for the presence of genes which predispose to melanoma or the more common types of skin cancer, and there have even been suggestions that population-based genetic screening may be a future measure for cancer control [58,59]. Genotype screening of individuals and populations are two separate issues, although they share common features in determining their utility. Thus, notwithstanding the ease of obtaining a DNA sample, there are several parameters which must be established before any kind of genetic screening test can be implemented. Since the genetics of familial melanoma have been studied with greater intensity than other types of skin cancer, the following discussion will largely feature examples from the melanoma literature.

In determining the feasibility of a screening test to detect a specific genotype in a target population, three fundamental questions arise, namely:

- What proportion of people carry the genotype of interest?
- What proportion of gene carriers go on to develop melanoma?
- Are there any interventions which reduce the risk of melanoma among gene carriers? [60]

The parameters which address the first two queries are the prevalence and the penetrance of the gene, respectively. The prevalence is simply the likelihood of identifying a mutation of the specified gene in whichever group is being targeted for screening (for example, members of high-risk families, patients with multiple primary melanoma, or even the general population). Once a mutation has been identified in a person, clinical management will focus on the chances of that person developing melanoma. The penetrance, defined as the absolute risk of developing the disease within a given time period among those with the genotype of interest, answers this latter question. A penetrance of 100% indicates that all mutation carriers will eventually develop melanoma, whereas a penetrance of 50% means that only half the mutation carriers will develop melanoma. Both the prevalence and penetrance of each genotype must be estimated with reasonable precision before undertaking genetic screening, to ensure that appropriate risk assessments and constructive counseling can be offered to identified gene carriers.

Thirdly, and arguably most importantly, the rationale underlying a genetic screening program is that by identifying those with a genotype that places them at higher than average risk for a disease, some intervention can take place which either reduces the risk of developing the disease (primary prevention), or in some other way reduces the burden of morbidity or mortality associated with the disease (secondary prevention).

All of these components of a genetic screening test (prevalence, penetrance and risk reduction) can be combined into a single parameter called the number needed to screen (NNS). This parameter can be estimated for various scenarios under which a screening program might be contemplated, and is the number of people who have to be screened in a target population in order to prevent one case of the disease (or prevent one death, depending upon the context). Clearly, the NNS is influenced by the prevalence of the genotype, the risk associated with that genotype, and also by the risk reduction which can be effected by intervention. These issues are explored below.

4.2.1 Prevalence of susceptibility genes for skin cancers

Current estimates of the prevalence of CDKN2A mutations in "high-risk" families range between 20-40%, based upon research studies of melanoma kindreds from around the world [61]. These figures are likely to be overestimates however, as the ascertainment of affected families has seldom been population-based, but rather determined by ad hoc referral patterns to various research centers. Indeed, a rather lower prevalence of CDKN2A mutation has been observed in the largest population-based study of familial melanoma yet undertaken. Among Queensland families categorized as "high-risk" (defined as those as being above the 95th percentile of risk compared with all other families in Queensland), the prevalence of CDKN2A mutations was 10% [25]. The implication for a screening program targeted towards high-risk families is that between 60-90% will have no detectable mutations, yet by definition, members of these families are at very high risk of melanoma. For families with less dense clustering of melanoma, the likelihood of identifying CDKN2A mutations is very low. Overall, it was estimated that 0.2% of melanomas in that population were attributable to mutations in the CDKN2A gene.

Little is known about the prevalence of genotypes which indirectly cause melanoma or skin cancer by increasing susceptibility. The best-studied gene to date is MC1R. Various alleles of the MC1R have been associated with modestly elevated risks of melanoma in some studies, and the combined prevalence of these low-risk alleles is around 30% in Caucasian populations [34,35].

4.2.2   Penetrance of susceptibility genes for skin cancers

Current estimates of the penetrance of melanoma among CDKN2A mutation carriers are based on relatively small numbers of families, for whom some degree of ascertainment and surveillance biases are probably inescapable. While figures of 60% [62] or higher [63] have been suggested in the literature, the validity of these estimates is unknown. There is some evidence that melanoma is becoming more common, and with younger onset, among more recent generations of mutation carriers [63], in line with general population trends in melanoma incidence. Estimates of penetrance are also confounded by the occurrence of melanoma in members of CDKN2A-mutation families who are not themselves CDKN2A mutation-carriers (phenocopies), highlighting the difficulties of estimating penetrance in some populations [16]. Finally, because of the small samples for statistical analysis, researchers have grouped all CDKN2A mutation-carriers together when estimating penetrance, even though protein-binding assays indicate that different types of CDKN2A mutations result in differing levels of functional activity of the expressed p16 protein. Further research with larger datasets should resolve this important issue of heterogeneity in penetrance.

The penetrance of indirect effect genes such as MC1R has not been established. Based on relative risk estimates between 2 and 4 for carriers of one or more MC1R variants [34], a very crude estimate of penetrance may be calculated as the product of the relative risk by the baseline risk in the population at large. In Queensland, the lifetime risk for cutaneous melanoma has been estimated at 1 in 14 [64]; a doubling of risk among carriers of MC1R variants suggests a lifetime penetrance for melanoma as high as 1 in 7. Clearly, the penetrance would be expected to be lower among populations with a lower incidence of melanoma.

4.2.3   Numbers needed to screen

Table 7.1 presents the NNS for a given genotype to prevent one melanoma event (either a new case of the disease, or death) under a range of assumptions. The left-side column lists the prevalence of the genotype to be screened; this will vary according to the population being targeted for screening. The next column provides a range of penetrance estimates within each band of prevalence, to accommodate the uncertainty of the data at present. Penetrance estimates in the range 0.5 to 0.9 have been used, as these appear reasonably robust for CDKN2A and melanoma. The greatest uncertainty is in the area of risk reduction, that is, the degree to which a person's risk of melanoma can be reduced based upon a knowledge of a person's genotype. At present, there are no data to address these issues. Nevertheless, one might predict that risk reductions in the interval 20% to 80% could be achieved, with a halving of risk a reasonable "middle-ground" estimate. Thus, NNS have been estimated for these conditions. The table suggests that screening of the general population for high-risk genes such as CDKN2A is unlikely to be adopted, simply because the prevalence of mutations is too low. In targeted populations where the prevalence of the genotype is much higher, the NNS becomes more manageable. Perhaps the most difficult issues will revolve around genetic screening for the low-penetrance, indirect effect genes, where estimates of penetrance are likely to show considerable allelic variation, and will be very difficult to obtain. Moreover, the figures presented in this table are estimates of lifetime risk, and the risk reductions are also calculated over a lifetime. Such long-term interventions may be unsustainable and risk reductions may be lower than those anticipated here. Nevertheless, the figures present a general guide to the magnitude of any proposed genetic screening program.

Table 7.1 Number needed to screen (NNS) to prevent one case of melanoma under various scenarios, assuming a causal association between genotype and disease.

Prevalence of genotype	Penetrance	Number needed to screen		
		Magnitude of risk reduction		
		20%	50%	80%
5 per 10,000				
Population-at-large -	0.5	20,000	8,000	5,000
estimate of CDKN2A	0.7	14,286	5,714	3,571
prevalence	0.9	11,111	4,444	2,778
10 per 100				
Familial melanoma -	0.5	100	40	25
lower estimate of	0.7	71	29	18
CDKN2A prevalence	0.9	56	22	14
50 per 100				
Familial melanoma -	0.5	20	8	5
upper estimate of	0.7	14	6	4
CDKN2A prevalence	0.9	11	4	3
30 per 100				
Population-at-large -	0.14 (Qld)	119	48	30
estimate of MC1R	0.08 (Vic)	208	83	52
prevalence	0.04 (US)	417	167	104

NNS = 1/(prevalence x penetrance x relative risk reduction)

4.3   Genetic treatment of pre-cancerous mutations

While genetic screening is unlikely to play a major role in skin cancer control in the near future, there is considerable optimism that soon, treatments will be delivered directly onto the skin to specifically repair damaged genes. This is an example of primary prevention which occurs after exposure to the causal agent. For example, T4 endonuclease V is an enzyme which recognizes and repairs gene mutations caused by UVR. Experimental systems have been developed which carry this enzyme into the skin, and have been shown to double the rate of removal of cyclobutane pyrimidine dimers from DNA [65]. A randomized clinical trial comparing daily application of an active liposomal formulation with placebo in patients with XP demonstrated significant reductions in the rate at which new solar keratoses developed in the active group [66]. Despite these promising results, the widespread application of treatments of this type should be viewed in the context of population interventions. Firstly, DNA repair enzymes would almost certainly need to be applied from a young age to prevent the accumulation of mutations that contribute to skin cancer later in life, particularly in heavily sun-exposed populations. The long-term safety of these preparations therefore needs to be determined. Secondly, if regular, long-term use of topical preparations is necessary to prevent skin cancer (a pattern of use similar to topical sunscreens), then it is likely that their application might face many of the same behavioral barriers as currently limit the use of sunscreen.

CONCLUSIONS

The vast majority of skin cancers are caused by the interaction of sun exposure and genetic susceptibility. It is becoming increasingly evident that genetic susceptibility is conferred by many different types of genes, including genes controlling the cell-cycle, DNA repair and pigmentation.

As only very few people carry germline mutations in high risk genes for skin cancer, it is unlikely that population screening for genes will ever be implemented as a skin cancer control strategy. However, novel genetic therapies may be one option for treatment of skin cancer in the future.

SUMMARY POINTS

- Skin cancers arise predominantly through the combined effects of sun exposure and genetic susceptibility
- "Hereditary" or "familial" cases of skin cancer typically herald the presence a germline mutation in a key regulatory gene in every cell of the body.
- "Sporadic" cases of skin cancer result from one or more somatic mutations of regulatory genes in individual skin cells. These mutations usually result from ultraviolet radiation exposure of the target cell.
- Screening for high-risk skin cancer genes is currently not recommended outside of the research setting. It is highly unlikely that widespread screening for high-risk skin cancer genes will ever be adopted as a population strategy for skin cancer control, although it may be applicable in certain clinical settings.
- Gene therapy for pre-cancerous lesions of the skin offers potential for non-invasive treatment.

IMPLICATIONS FOR PUBLIC HEALTH

Counter to the optimism of some commentators for the disease preventive potential of the human genome project, those with a background in public health may view these claims with some caution. Undoubtedly, the genetic and genomic revolutions herald enormous scope for changes in the way cancers are diagnosed and treated, but their impact upon cancer prevention appears more limited. Notwithstanding the appeal of controlling skin cancer through gene technology, this is clearly an over-simplification of the process of carcinogenesis, and ignores the enormous contribution of the environmental, behavioral and socio-cultural factors to the burden of skin cancer in populations. Epidemiological studies clearly indicate that the major cause of the common skin cancers is exposure to sunlight, and while methods for reducing exposure are proving difficult to implement across the population, there is little reason to suspect that primary prevention strategies based upon gene technology will be more effective.

We have seen that genetic screening for high-risk "direct effect" genes is likely to be of limited assistance as a preventive tool, and is of no benefit to the general community. Variants of low-risk "indirect effect" genes are very common in the population, and the cumulative magnitude of their effect at the population level is likely to be very great. These effects remain to be quantified in the general population. Combining all of the risk information, both from genes and other risk factors, into a single algorithm which can be used in the clinical setting is a challenge facing researchers. While epidemiological research into conditions such as cardiovascular disease has led to the development of individual risk prediction charts [67] which are highly acceptable in the primary care setting [68], it is not yet clear whether similar approaches will work for the prevention of melanoma. The key difference between cardiovascular diseases and skin cancers is the number and type of interventions which can be used to prevent disease. Whereas for cardiovascular diseases there are pharmacological agents for reducing blood pressure and lipids, for improving systolic function, for preventing thrombosis and controlling diabetes, as well as behavioral programs for stopping smoking, modifying diet and increasing levels of physical activity, the range of interventions for the primary prevention of skin cancer is essentially limited to avoidance of sunlight. Thus, from the perspective of public health, the question is not "how do you counsel genotype-positive people?", but rather, "how do you counsel the genotype-negative people?" Until more is known about the various causal pathways leading to these diseases, the general advice to all fair-skinned people should be to minimize exposure to sunlight, regardless of genotype.

REFERENCES

1. Harris CC (1996) p53 tumor suppressor gene: at the crossroads of molecular carcinogenesis, molecular epidemiology, and cancer risk assessment. *Environ Health Perspect* **104:** Suppl 3:435-439.
2. Pitot HC (1993) The molecular biology of carcinogenesis. *Cancer* **72:** 962-970.
3. Kolodner RD (2000) DNA repair: guarding against mutation. *Nature* **407:** 607-609.
4. Petty EM, Gibson LH, Fountain JW, *et al.* (1993) Molecular definition of a chromosome 9p21 germ-line deletion in a woman with multiple melanomas and a plexiform neurofibroma: implications for 9p tumor-suppressor gene(s). *Am J Hum Genet* **53:** 96-104.
5. Cannon-Albright LA, Goldgar DE, Meyer LJ, *et al.* (1992) Assignment of a locus for familial melanoma,MLM, to chromosome 9p13-p22. *Science* **258:** 1148-1152.
6. Nancarrow DJ, Mann GJ, Holland EA, *et al.* (1993) Confirmation of chromosome 9p linkage in familial melanoma. *Am J Hum Genet* **53:** 936-942.
7. Kamb A, Gruis NA, Weaver-Feldhaus J, *et al.* (1994) A cell cycle regulator potentially involved in genesis of many tumor types. *Science* **264:** 436-450.
8. Nobori T, Miura K, Wu DJ, Lois A, Takabayashi K, Carson DA (1994) Deletions of the cyclin-dependent kinase-4 inhibitor gene in multiple human cancers. *Nature* **368:** 753-756.
9. Serrano M, Hannon GJ, Beach D (1993) A new regulatory motif in cell-cycle control causing specific inhibition of cyclin D/CDK4 [see comments]. *Nature* **366:** 704-707.
10. Gruis NA, van der Velden PA, Sandkuijl LA, *et al.* (1995) Homozygotes for CDKN2 (p16) germline mutation in Dutch familial melanoma kindreds. *Nature Genetics* **10:** 351-353.

11. Hussussian C, Struewing JP, Goldstein AM, *et al.* (1994) Germline p16 mutations in 153familial melanoma. *Nature Genetics* **8**: 15-21.

12. Harland M, Meloni R, Gruis N, *et al.* (1997) Germline mutations of the CDKN2 gene in UK melanoma families. *Hum Mol Genet* **6**: 2061-2067.

13. Koh J, Enders GH, Dynlacht BD, Harlow E (1995) Tumour-derived p16 alleles encoding proteins defective in cell-cycle inhibition. *Nature* **375**: 506-510.

14. Soufir N, Avril MF, Chompret A, *et al.* (1998) Prevalence of p16 and CDK4 germline mutations in 48 melanoma-prone families in France. The French Familial Melanoma Study Group [published erratum appears in Hum Mol Genet 1998 May;7(5):941]. *Hum Mol Genet* **7**: 209-216.

15. Zuo L, Weger J, Yang Q, *et al.* (1996) Germline mutations in the p16INK4a binding domain of CDK4 in familial melanoma. *Nat Genet* **12**: 97-99.

16. Flores JF, Pollock PM, Walker GJ, *et al.* (1997) Analysis of the CDKN2A, CDKN2B and CDK4 genes in 48 Australian melanoma kindreds. *Oncogene* **15**: 2999-3005.

17. Platz A, Hansson J, Mansson-Brahme E, *et al.* (1997) Screening of germline mutations in the CDKN2A and CDKN2B genes in Swedish families with hereditary cutaneous melanoma. *J Natl Cancer Inst* **89**: 697-702.

18. Liu L, Goldstein AM, Tucker MA, *et al.* (1997) Affected members of melanoma-prone families with linkage to 9p21 but lacking mutations in CDKN2A do not harbor mutations in the coding regions of either CDKN2B or p19ARF. *Genes Chromosomes Cancer* **19**: 52-54.

19. Mackie RM, Andrew N, Lanyon WG, Connor JM (1998) CDKN2A germline mutations in U.K. patients with familial melanoma and multiple primary melanomas. *J Invest Dermatol* **111**: 269-272.

20. Monzon J, Liu L, Brill H, *et al.* (1998) CDKN2A mutations in multiple primary melanomas [see comments]. *N Engl J Med* **338**: 879-887.

21. Whiteman DC, Milligan A, Welch J, Green AC, Hayward NK (1997) Germline CDKN2A mutations in childhood melanoma. *J Natl Cancer Inst* **89**: 1460.

22. Tsao H, Zhang X, Kwitkiwski K, Finkelstein DM, Sober AJ, Haluska FG (2000) Low prevalence of germline CDKN2A and CDK4 mutations in patients with early-onset melanoma. *Arch Dermatol* **136**: 1118-1122.

23. Kraemer KH, Lee MM, Andrews AD, Lambert WC (1994) The role of sunlight and DNA repair in melanoma and nonmelanoma skin cancer. The xeroderma pigmentosum paradigm. *Arch Dermatol* **130**: 1018-1021.

24. Boni R, Vortmeyer AO, Burg G, Hofbauer G, Zhuang Z (1998) The PTEN tumour suppressor gene and malignant melanoma. *Melanoma Res* **8**: 300-302.

25. Aitken J, Welch J, Duffy D, *et al.* (1999) CDKN2A variants in a population-based sample of Queensland families with melanoma. *J Natl Cancer Inst* **91**: 446-452.

26. Ung-Juurlink C (1999) American Academy of Dermatology 1999 Awards for Young Investigators in Dermatology. The prevalence of CDKN2A in patients with atypical nevi and malignant melanoma. *J Am Acad Dermatol* **41**: 461-462.

27. Whiteman DC, Green A, Parson PG (1998) p53 Expression and risk factors for cutaneous melanoma:a case-control study. *Int J Cancer* **77**: 843-848.

28. van-'t-Veer LJ, Burgering BM, Versteeg R, *et al.* (1989) N-ras mutations in human cutaneous melanoma from sun-exposed body sites. *Mol Cell Biol* **9**: 3114-3116.

29. van-Elsas A, Zerp SF, van-der-Flier S, *et al.* (1996) Relevance of ultraviolet-induced N-ras oncogene point mutations in development of primary human cutaneous melanoma [see comments]. *Am J Pathol* **149**: 883-893.

30. Chhajlani V, Wikberg JE (1992) Molecular cloning and expression of the human melanocyte stimulating hormone receptor cDNA. *FEBS Lett* **309**: 417-420.

138

Chapter 7

31. Valverde P, Healy E, Jackson I, Rees JL, Thody AJ (1995) Variants of the melanocyte-stimulating hormone receptor gene are associated with red hair and fair skin in humans. *Nature Genetics* **11:** 328-330.
32. Smith R, Healy E, Siddiqui S, *et al.* (1998) Melanocortin 1 receptor variants in an Irish population. *J Invest Dermatol* **111:** 119-122.
33. Box NF, Wyeth JR, O'Gorman LE, Martin NG, Sturm RA (1997) Characterization of melanocyte stimulating hormone receptor variant alleles in twins with red hair. *Hum Mol Genet* **6:** 1891-1897.
34. Palmer JS, Duffy DL, Box NF, *et al.* (2000) Melanocortin-1 receptor polymorphisms and risk of melanoma: is the association explained solely by pigmentation phenotype? *Am J Hum Genet* **66:** 176-186.
35. Ichii-Jones F, Lear JT, Heagerty AH, *et al.* (1998) Susceptibility to melanoma: influence of skin type and polymorphism in the melanocyte stimulating hormone receptor gene. *J Invest Dermatol* **111:** 218-221.
36. Kerb R, Brockmoller J, Reum T, Roots I (1997) Deficiency of glutathione S-transferases T1 and M1 as heritable factors of increased cutaneous UV sensitivity. *J Invest Dermatol* **108:** 229-232.
37. Heagerty AHM, Fitzgerald D, Smith A, *et al.* (1994) Glutathione S-transferase GSTM1 phenotypes and protection against cutaneous tumours. *Lancet* **343:** 266-268.
38. Gorlin R (1987) Nevoid basal-cell carcinoma syndrome. *Medicine* **66:** 98-113.
39. Evans D, Ladusans E, Rimmer S, Burnell L, Thakker N, Farndon P (1993) Complications of the naevoid basal cell carcinoma syndrome: results of a population based study. *J Med Genet* **30:** 460-464.
40. Gorlin R (1995) Nevoid basal cell carcinoma syndrome. *Dermatological Clinics* **13:** 113-125.
41. Johnson R, Rothman A, Xie J, *et al.* (1996) Human homolog of patched, a candidate gene for the basal cell nevus syndrome. *Science* **272:** 1668-1671.
42. Hahn H, Wicking C, Zaphiropoulos P, *et al.* (1996) Mutations of the human homologue of Drosophila patched in the nevoid basal cell carcinoma syndrome. *Cell* **85:** 841-851.
43. Brash DE, Ponten J (1998) Skin precancer. *Cancer Surv* **32:** 69-113.
44. Brash D, Rudolph JA, Simon JA, *et al.* (1991) A role for sunlight in skin cancer: UV-induced p53 mutations in squamous cell carcinoma. *Proc Natl Acad Sci USA* **88:** 10124-10128.
45. Rady P, Scinicariello F, Wagner RF Jr, Tyring SK (1992) p53 mutations in basal cell carcinomas. *Cancer Res* **52:** 3804-3806.
46. Campbell C, Quinn A, Ro Y, Angus B, Rees J (1993) p53 mutations are common and early evens that precede tumor invasion in squamous cell neoplasia of the skin. *J Invest Dermatol* **100:** 746-748.
47. Bastiaens MT, Struyk L, Tjong-A-Hung SP, *et al.* (2001) Cutaneous squamous cell carcinoma and p53 codon 72 polymorphism: a need for screening. *Mol Carcinogen* **30:** 56-61.
48. Wei Q, Matanoski G, Farmer E, Hedayati M, Grossman L (1993) DNA repair and aging in basal cell carcinoma: a molecular epidemiologic study. *Proc Natl Acad Sci USA* **90:** 1614-1618.
49. Dybdahl M, Frentz G, Vogel U, Wallin H, Nexo B (1999) Low DNA repair is a risk factor in skin carcinogenesis: a study of basal cell carcinoma in psoriasis patients. *Mutation Res* **433:** 15-22.
50. Hall J, English D, Artuso M, Armstrong B, Winter M (1994) DNA repair capacity as a risk factor for non-melanocytic skin cancer - a molecular epidemiologic study. *Int J Cancer* **58:** 179-184.

51. Benhamou S, Sarasin A (2000) Variability in nucleotide excision repair and cancer risk: a review. *Mutation Res* **462:** 149-158.

52. Unden A, Holmberg E, Lundh-Rozell B, *et al.* (1996) Mutations in the human homologue of Drosophila patched (PTCH) in basal cell carcinomas and the Gorlin Syndrome:Different in vivo mechanisms of PTCH inactivation. *Cancer Res* **56:** 4562-4565.

53. Gailani M, Stahle-Backdahl M, Leffell D, *et al.* (1996) The role of the human homologue of Drosophila patched in sporadic basal cell carcinomas. *Nat Genet* **14:** 78-81.

54. Evans T, Boonchai W, Shanley S, *et al.* (2000) The spectrum of patched mutations in a collection of Australian basal cell carcinomas. *Human Mutat* **16:** 43-48.

55. Jones F, Ramachandran S, Lear J, *et al.* (1999) The melanocyte stimulating hormone receptor polymorphism: association of the V92M and A294H alleles with basal cell carcinoma. *Clinica Chimica Acta* **282:** 125-134.

56. Lear T, Smith A, Strange R, Fryer A (2000) Detoxifying enzyme genotypes and susceptibility to cutaneous malignancy. *Br J Dermatol* **142:** 8-15.

57. Kefford RF, Newton-Bishop JA, Bergman W, Tucker MA (1999) Counseling and DNA testing for individuals perceived to be genetically predisposed to melanoma: A consensus statement of the Melanoma Genetics Consortium. *J Clin Oncol* **17:** 3245-3251.

58. van-Ommen GJ, Bakker E, den-Dunnen JT (1999) The human genome project and the future of diagnostics, treatment, and prevention. *Lancet* **354 Suppl 1**: SI5-S10.

59. Collins FS (1999) Shattuck Lecture - Medical and societal consequences of the Human Genome Project. *N Engl J Med* **341:** 28-37.

60. Vinei P, Schultc P, McMichael AJ (2001) Misconceptions about the use of genetic tests in populations. *Lancet* **357:** 709-712.

61. Piepkorn M (2000) Melanoma genetics: an update with focus on the CDKN2A(p16)/ARF tumor suppressors. *J Am Acad Dermatol* **42:** 705-722.

62. Harland M, Holland EA, Ghiorzo P, *et al.* (2000) Mutation screening of the CDKN2A promoter in melanoma families. *Genes Chromosomes Cancer* **28:** 45-57.

63. Battistutta D, Palmer J, Walters M, Walker G, Nancarrow D, Hayward N (1994) Incidence of familial melanoma and MLM2 gene. *Lancet* **344:** 1607-1608.

64. MacLennan R, Green AC, McLeod GRC, Martin NG (1992) Increasing incidence of cutaneous melanoma in Queensland, Australia. *J Natl Cancer Inst* **84:** 1427-1432.

65. Yarosh DB, O'Connor A, Alas L, Potten C, Wolf P (1999) Photoprotection by topical DNA repair enzymes: molecular correlates of clinical studies. *Photochem Photobiol* **69:** 136-140.

66. Yarosh D, Klein J, O'Connor A, *et al.* (2001) Effect of topically applied T4 endonuclease V in liposomes on skin cancer in xeroderma pigmentosum: a randomised study. *Lancet* **357:** 926-929.

67. Jackson R (2000) Updated New Zealand cardiovascular disease risk-benefit prediction guidc. *Br Med J* **320:** 709-710.

68. Isles CG, Ritchie LD, Murchie P, Norrie J (2000) Risk assessment in primary prevention of coronary heart disease: randomised comparison of three scoring methods. *Br Med J* 320:690-691.

Chapter 8

Sunscreens: can they prevent skin cancer?

Richard P. Gallagher[1,2], F.A.C.E., M.A.; Tim K. Lee[1,3], Ph.D.;
Chris D. Bajdik[1,2], Ph.D.
[1]Cancer Control Research Program, B.C. Cancer Agency, Vancouver, BC, Canada;
[2]Department of Health Care and Epidemiology, University of British Columbia, Vancouver, BC,
Canada; [3]School of Computing Services, Simon Fraser University, Burnaby, BC, Canada

Key words: melanoma, non-melanoma skin cancer, prevention, sunscreens

INTRODUCTION

Skin cancer is the most common malignancy in humans [1]. Furthermore, Armstrong and Kricker [2] have calculated that in white populations over 90% of cutaneous malignant melanomas are caused by sun exposure. Similar proportions of both basal cell carcinoma and squamous cell carcinoma of the skin are likely attributable to sunlight exposure [3]. Because of the high proportion of skin cancer caused by sunlight, prevention programs have become increasingly common not only in high incidence areas such as Australia [4,5], but also in lower incidence countries such as Canada [6], the US [7,8] and the UK [9].

Most of these programs have focused on decreasing solar exposure either by sun avoidance, by time-shifting activities to avoid periods of high insolation, or by increasing the use of protective clothing in the sun. Sunscreens have also been employed in many of these prevention initiatives; but only as a "last resort" where shade or protective clothing is not an

D. Hill et al. (eds.), Prevention of Skin Cancer, 141-156.
© 2004 Kluwer Academic Publishers. Printed in the Netherlands.

alternative [10]. The reason for this is that although they have been demonstrated to be effective at preventing sunburn, little high quality human evidence has been available until recently that sunscreens may prevent skin cancer. This chapter will review the available evidence for the three major types of skin cancer; cutaneous malignant melanoma (CMM), squamous cell carcinoma (SCC) and basal cell carcinoma (BCC). The recent information about behavioral aspects of sunscreen use which suggests that use of these agents has encouraged rather than attenuated the rising incidence of cutaneous melanoma will also be discussed.

1.   DEVELOPMENT OF SUNSCREENS

Use of sunscreens to prevent sunburn was first reported in 1928 [11]. During World War II, the need to maintain Allied troops' health in high sunlight areas such as the South Pacific led to the use of red petrolatum to prevent severe sunburn which would otherwise have adversely affected light-skinned soldiers. During the 1960's para amino benzoic acid (PABA) became a very popular sunscreen, and during the late 1960s and the 1970s achieved widespread use in North America, and to a lesser extent in Europe. However reports of contact sensitization [12] led to concerns about its long-term use. Furthermore this compound is water-soluble and its ability to provide adequate sun protection quickly declined with heavy sweating or bathing. Most of the sunscreens developed during the period up to the 1980's were designed to prevent sunburn and thus primarily filtered UVB (280-315 nm). Concerns about the erosion of the earth's stratospheric ozone layer, which surfaced in the 1980s, however, sensitized the public to the carcinogenic potential of solar radiation, and led to demands for both a higher UVB sun protection factor (SPF) and UVA protection. More recently, experiments with the Xiphophorus fish model have led to the hypothesis that longer wavelength UVA radiation might be involved in the genesis of melanoma [13]. This in turn has resulted in sunscreen manufacturers providing formulations which attenuate a much broader band of UV wavelengths than previously. Current broad-spectrum sunscreen formulations contain a number of active agents, each of which attenuates different parts of the UV spectrum affording good filtering of both short wavelength UVB (280-315 nm), and longer UVA (315-400 nm) wavelengths.

2. SUNSCREENS AND CUTANEOUS MALIGNANT MELANOMA (CMM)

Evidence of the potential effects of sunscreen use on risk of CMM comes from the case-control studies summarized in Table 8.1. No randomized trials of sunscreen and melanoma have been conducted although a single trial of sunscreens in attenuating nevi in children has been conducted [14] and this will be described later.

The Norwegian study of Klepp and Magnus [15] evaluated the use of "sun lotions and oils" and subsequent risk of melanoma. They found an elevated risk of melanoma among males (but not females) who used these agents "sometimes", "often" or "almost always" as compared with subjects who did not use them. This hospital-based study was followed by that of Graham *et al.* [16] which also demonstrated an increased risk only in males using sunscreens. The population-based study carried out in New York [17] demonstrated a significantly increased risk on univariate analysis, but this decreased to a non-significant level with control for "tendency to sunburn" and "participation in water sports."

The large case-control studies conducted in Western Canada [18], Western Australia [19] and Denmark [20] showed no elevated risk with long-term or consistent use of sunscreens. Interestingly the Canadian study showed a significantly elevated risk, however, in those using sunscreens "only for the first few hours" in the sun.

The first study to show a significantly decreased risk of CMM with consistent sunscreen use was that of Holly *et al.* [21], conducted among women age 25-59 in the San Francisco Bay area. Two studies of melanoma among sun-resistant Mediterranean populations [22,23] both demonstrated reduced risk of CMM in those using sunscreens although both studies were relatively small; and the quality of information on sunscreen use in the latter investigation was relatively poor.

Two well-conducted studies in Sweden [24,25] and a large European study [26,27] showed elevated risks of CMM with use of sunscreens. Substantially higher elevated risks were seen in those using sunscreens in order to tan or in order to spend more time sunbathing [25,26,27].

Table 8.1 Case control studies of sunscreens and risk of cutaneous malignant melanoma [1]

Country/date	Type of cases/controls	No. cases/controls	Exposure	RRa (95% CI)	Comments	Reference
Norway 1974-75	Hospital cases Other cancer controls	78 cases 131 controls	Sometimes, often or almost always use sun lotion/oil	M 2.8^b (1.2-6.7) F 1.0^b (0.42-2.5) T 2.3^b (1.3-4.1)	Elevated risks among males only. Sunscreens not differentiated from "sun lotions".	Klepp & Magnus [15]
USA 1974-80	Hospital cases Other cancer controls	404 cases 521 controls	Used sunscreen, Used suntan lotion	M 2.2^b (1.2-4.1) M1.7 (1.1-2.7) F "No added risk"	Elevated risks among males only	Graham et al. [16]
USA 1977-79	Population cases and controls	324 male trunk melanoma cases 415 controls	Always used "suntan lotion"	2.6^b (1.4-4.7) Not significant after control for tendency to sunburn, and water sports	"Suntan lotions" and "sunscreens" not differentiated in questionnaire	Herzfeld et al. [17]
Sweden 1978-83	Hospital cases Population controls	523 cases 505 controls	Often used sun protection agents	1.8^b (1.2-2.7)		Beitner et al. [46]
Canada 1979-81	Population cases and controls	369 trunk and lower limb melanomas 369 controls	Used sunscreen "almost always"	1.1 (0.75-1.6)	Highest risk in those using sunscreen "only for first few hours" RR=1.62 (1.04-2.52)	Elwood & Gallagher [18]
Australia 1980-81	Population cases and controls	507 cases 507 controls	Used sunscreens ≤ 10 years	1.1 (0.71-1.6)		Holman et al. [19]
USA 1981-86	Population cases and controls	452 cases 930 controls	Always used sunscreens	All cutaneous melanoma 0.62s^b (0.49-0.83) Superficial Spreading Melanoma (SSM) 0.43 (CI not available)	Study involved only women aged 25-59 at diagnosis. CI estimated RR for SSM adjusted for host factors and sun exposure	Holly et al. [21]
Denmark 1982-85^a	Population cases and controls	474 cases 926 controls	Always used sunscreens	1.1^b (0.8-1.5)		Osterlind et al.[20]

Country/date	Type of cases/controls	No. cases/controls	Exposure	RRa (95% CI)	Comments	Reference
Australia 1987-94	Population cases Controls from same school	50 cases 156 controls all children < 15	Always used sunscreens	2.2 (0.4-12) on holidays 0.7 (0.1-6.0) at school		Whiteman et al. [47]
Sweden 1988-90	Population cases and controls	400 cases 640 controls (1.1-3.7)	Almost always used sunscreens	Trunk 1.4 (0.6-3.2) Other sites 2.0	No information on duration of use	Westerdahl et al. [24]
Spain 1989-93	Hospital cases Hospital visitors	105 cases 138 controls	Always used sunscreens	0.2 (0.04-0.79)		Rodenas et al. [22]
Spain 1990-94	Hospital cases and controls	116 cases 235 controls	Used sunscreen	0.48 (0.34-0.71)	Inadequate description of sunscreen use	Espinoza-Arranz et al. [23]
Europe 1991-94	Hospital cases Neighborhood controls	418 cases 438 controls	Ever use psoralen sunscreens Ever use sunscreens	2.3 (1.3-4.0) 1.5 (1.1-2.1) M 1.8 (1.1-2.7) F 1.3 (0.87-2.0)	Highest risk in those sun-sensitive subjects using sunscreens to tan: RR, 3.7 (1.0-7.6)	Autier et al. [26]
Austria 1992-94	Hospital cases and controls	193 cases 319 controls	Often used sunscreen	3.5 (1.8-6.6)		Wolf et al. [48]
Sweden 1995-97	Population cases and controls	571 cases 913 controls	Always used sunscreen Used sunscreens to spend more time sunbathing	8.7 (1.0-75) 8.7 (1.0-76)		Westerdahl et al. [25]
Italy 1992-1995	Hospital cases and controls	542 cases 538 controls	Always used sunscreen Used low SPF Used medium SPF Used high SPF	0.8 (0.54-1.17) 0.96 (0.52-1.77) 0.90 (0.63-1.28) 1.41 (0/85-2.35)		Naldi et al. [28]

[1] Adapted from: IARC Handbooks of Cancer Prevention, Vol. 5: *Sunscreens*; IARC Lyon, 2001

a Relative risk estimates adjusted for phenotype and sun-related factors where possible

b Crude relative risk ratio only available

The most recently published investigation was conducted in Italy [28]. The study recruited a total of 542 cases and compared their sunscreen use with that of 538 patients admitted to the same hospitals as the cases. After adjustment for host susceptibility factors no significant differences in risk between users and non-users was found. Further analysis showed that cases using the highest SPF sunscreens had a higher risk of melanoma (relative risk, RR = 1.41; 95% confidence interval, CI = 0.85-2.35) than cases using minimal or medium SPF preparations, although this difference was not statistically significant. Of interest is the lower risk for melanoma seen in sunscreen users with freckles (RR = 0.50; 95% CI = 0.29-1.17) and those in the highest tertile of nevus counts (RR = 0.78; 95% CI = 0.44-1.78); groups traditionally at high risk of melanoma.

Most of the studies noted above, particularly those prior to the 1990's, were conducted primarily to investigate the association between sunlight exposure, pigmentary characteristics and melanoma risk. The data collected on sunscreen use therefore were often sketchy with relatively poor information on the frequency with which they were applied. For the most part no data was collected on actual quantities used. Thus several factors needed to truly evaluate whether sunscreens might prevent melanoma are absent either because questions were not asked or because subject recall is inadequate. Additional information needed includes whether a high SPF (15+) formulation was used, whether adequate sunscreen was applied to reach the sunscreen's advertised SPF value, and whether it was re-applied periodically. Without this information it is likely that data on inadequate use will dilute data on efficacious use and any protective effect will be missed.

In addition to the quality of the information available, serious potential problems with uncontrolled confounding due to host susceptibility factors are likely to be present. Sunscreens are most commonly used by those whose skin is highly susceptible to sunburn. These people are also at the highest risk of CMM due to their sensitivity. Unfortunately, accurate measures of skin sensitivity (used to control for this variable when evaluating sunscreen use) are difficult to obtain. For this reason, evaluation of the association between CMM and sunscreen use is very likely confounded by sun sensitivity [1]. Finally, review of epidemiologic data indicates that childhood and adolescence may be a period of particular solar susceptibility [29] to initiation of melanoma. If this is true, and effective sunscreens were not available or were not utilized during this period, then correctly reported sunscreen use subsequent to this period and prior to diagnosis, will suggest a positive relationship between use and melanoma risk.

Clearly these problems present major difficulties in drawing conclusions about whether sunscreens protect against CMM, and the problems are unlikely to be addressed with case-control or retrospective cohort studies, no matter how competently they are carried out. A randomized trial is of course the optimum method for evaluating sunscreen efficacy, but such trials have not been conducted for reasons of cost and study duration.

One randomized trial has been conducted to evaluate whether sunscreen use can inhibit nevus formation [14]. This is a potentially important question, as up to 50% of CMMs are thought to originate in pre-existing nevi. The study was carried out in Vancouver, Canada among school children age 6-7 and 9-10 years and their parents/guardians. All children had their nevi counted and were then randomized into two groups. The intervention group received 2 containers of SPF-30 sunscreen each year, along with instructions for parents to apply the agent any time when the children were expected to be outside in the sun for 30 minutes or more. The other group of children and their parents received no sunscreen and continued to apply sunscreen in a self-directed manner. The children were closely followed for 3 years and at the end of this time, had their nevi counted again. Children in the sunscreen group had fewer new nevi than those in the non-sunscreen group. An interaction effect was also detected between sunscreen group and freckling, suggesting that use of sunscreen was more important in preventing new nevi among subjects who freckled easily. Examination of reported sun behavior during the course of the trial showed no difference between the 2 study groups in cumulative exposure, although the children in the non-sunscreen group reported more episodes of "unprotected" (no sunscreen on sun-exposed sites) exposure. A lower mean frequency of sunburns and a lower sunburn severity score (6.8 vs. 7.4) among children in the sunscreen group were seen although the differences were not statistically significant. These data suggest that short-term protection was afforded by the sunscreen.

3.   SUNSCREENS AND SQUAMOUS CELL CARCINOMA (SCC) OF THE SKIN

Several studies have been conducted to evaluate use of sunscreens in the prevention of SCC, including one randomized trial [30]. In addition there are several randomized trials evaluating use of sunscreens in prevention of actinic keratosis (AK) a known precursor of SCC [31,32]. These are summarized in Table 8.2.

Table 8.2 Randomized trials of sunscreen and risk of skin cancer, actinic keratoses (AK), or melanocyte nevi

Country/ Date	Type of lesion	Cohort / Subjects	Duration of follow-up	Exposure	Rate Ratio or RR (95% CI)	Reference
Victoria, Australia 1991-92	Actinic keratoses	Cohort of 588 subjects age 40+ **Sunscreen Arm:** 333 new AK in 210 subjects **Non-Sunscreen Arm:** 508 new AK in 221 subjects **Sunscreen Arm:** Old lesion regression 28% **Non-Sunscreen Arm:** Old lesion regression 20%	6 months	Daily sunscreen to head, neck and hands vs daily placebo use	0.62 (0.54-0.71) in sunscreen arm vs non-sunscreen arm Rate of regression in sunscreen arm 1.53 (1.29-1.80)	Thompson *et al.* [31]
Texas USA 1987-1990	Actinic keratoses	Cohort of 50 subjects age 39-78 **Sunscreen Arm:** 13.6 AK per year in 25 subjects **Non-sunscreen Arm:** 27.9 AK per year in 25 subjects	2 years	Daily sunscreen application vs daily placebo use	0.48 (calculated crude) ratio 36% adjusted* reduction in sunscreen arm	Naylor *et al.* [32]
Nambour Australia 1992-1996	Squamous cell carcinoma Basal cell carcinoma	Cohort of 1383 subjects age 20-69 **Sunscreen Arm:** 28 SCC in 22 subjects **Non-sunscreen Arm:** 46 SCC in 25 subjects **Sunscreen Arm:** 153 BCC in 65 subjects **Non-sunscreen Arm:** 146 BCC in 63 subjects	4 years	Daily sunscreen to head neck arms and hands vs self-directed sunscreen use	SCC lesions: 0.61 (0.46-0.81) SCC subjects 0.88 (0.50-1.60) **BCC Lesions:** 1.0 (0.82-1.30) **BCC Subjects:** 1.03 (0.73-1.50)	Green *et al.* [30]
Vancouver, Canada	Benign melanocytic nevi	Cohort of 458 children age 6-7, 9-10	3 years	Sunscreen on all sun-exposed sites when in the sun for 30+ minutes vs self-directed sunscreen use	Median counts Sunscreen arm: 24 Non-sunscreen arm: 28 Relative rate 0.85§	Gallagher *et al.* [14]

* Naylor *et al.* - Adjusted reduction takes into consideration an imbalance of risk factors at study entry between the 2 groups
§ Gallagher *et al.* - Data showed a strong interaction between sunscreen arm and degree of freckling. Being assigned to sunscreen arm was more important in children who freckled.

The study of Green *et al.* [30] was conducted in Nambour, Queensland, Australia. A total of 1621 study subjects age 20-69 were randomized into 4 study groups; sunscreen plus oral β-carotene, sunscreen plus oral placebo, oral β-carotene without sunscreen, and no sunscreen plus oral placebo. Participants were instructed to apply sunscreen to their head and neck, arms and hands every morning and after heavy sweating, bathing, or long solar exposure. Those randomized to no sunscreen were asked to continue their normal use pattern. Subjects were followed for 4.5 years during which time new skin lesions were tracked and pathology reports were obtained. At the end of the observation period 1383 subjects remained in the study. Subjects randomized to daily sunscreen (regardless of β-carotene status) showed significantly fewer new SCCs (RR = 0.61; 95% CI = 0.46-0.81) than those randomized to no sunscreen. Furthermore, the data suggested that fewer subjects in the sunscreen arms reported new SCCs than subjects in the no sunscreen trial arms (RR = 0.88; 95% CI = 0.50-1.60), although this was not statistically significant. A potential concern in a trial is that being in the intervention arm might modify behavior enough to result in fewer hours in the sun, and hence a lower risk of SCC. However data showed that changes in pattern of exposure were no more frequent in the sunscreen group than in the no-sunscreen group [33]. As might be expected in this trial of older subjects, relatively few sunburns were reported, however, the sunscreen group had fewer than the no-sunscreen group, indicating the expected short-term benefits of use.

The trials of Thompson *et al.* [31] in Australia and Naylor *et al.* [32] in the US likewise demonstrated reduced risk for the appearance of new actinic keratoses with daily use of high SPF sunscreen. These studies are perhaps less convincing than the Nambour trial for several reasons. First of all the numbers of subjects enrolled in the trials were small, and the duration of the trials was shorter. Secondly, the effect of sunscreen was only seen on a precursor of SCC; rather than SCC itself. Nevertheless, the results are supportive of the findings from the Nambour trial.

In an observational study, the effect of sunscreens on risk of SCC was investigated among 191 cases occurring in a cohort of 107,900 female nurses [34] in the U.S. No protective effect was seen for sunscreen use among women who had spent 8 hours or more per week outdoors over the 2 years prior to diagnosis compared to women with the same outdoor exposure who did not use sunscreen (RR = 1.1; 95% CI = 0.83-1.7).

A case-control study of 132 SCC cases and 1031 controls [35], was conducted within a cohort of 4103 subjects age 40-64 originally recruited in 1987 in Geraldton, Western Australia [36]. No significant difference was seen between those using sunscreen of SPF>10 "half the time or more" and those not using it, for 3 different age periods of life; (Age 8-14 RR = 0.61,

95% CI = 0.08-4.7; Age 15-19 RR = 1.9, 95% CI = 0.82-4.4; Age 20-24 RR = 0.99, 95% CI = 0.44-2.2).

Foote *et al.* [37] evaluated sunscreen use and risk of development of SCC among 918 actinically damaged (≥ 10 actinic keratoses) residents of Arizona USA, recruited as a control group for a trial designed to evaluate whether oral vitamin A would prevent non-melanocytic skin cancer. Of these 918 subjects, followed for a mean of 57 months, 129 developed an SCC. Analysis indicated that those who "always" used sunscreens had a non-significantly elevated risk for SCC (RR = 1.42; 95% CI = 0.79-2.55) compared to those who did not use sunscreens. After adjustment for all relevant factors, older age, male gender, red hair color and adult residence in Arizona for 10+ years were the factors which independently predicted the appearance of SCC. Extrapolation from findings in this unusual group are difficult, as at recruitment they all had lesions which are known to be precursors of SCC.

A further investigation in a less sun-sensitive population of Spain [38] analyzed all non-melanocytic cancers together, and no separate data is available on SCC.

4.   SUNSCREENS AND BASAL CELL CARCINOMA (BCC) OF THE SKIN

Limited information is available on sunscreens and risk of BCC. The Nambour randomized trial [30] noted earlier also examined the incidence of new BCCs among the 1383 Australian subjects after 4.5 years of follow-up. No protective effect was seen for either the number of new BCCs (RR = 1.05, 95% CI = 0.82-1.34) among the sunscreen users, or for the number of sunscreen subjects who developed new BCCs (RR = 1.03, 95% CI = 0.73-1.46) by comparison to those in the non-sunscreen arms.

Hunter and his colleagues [39] analyzed data on women diagnosed with BCC during their participation in a large U.S. cohort study of 73,366 female nurses. A total of 771 cases were available for analysis, and those who reported that they usually used sunscreen when outdoors during the summer had a significantly elevated risk of BCC (RR = 1.4; 95% CI = 1.2-1.7), compared to nurses who did not use sunscreen. The authors noted that the relative risk for sunscreen use declined after adjustment for childhood sun-sensitivity, hair color, and history of sunburn, and attributed the remaining elevated risk in those using sunscreen to unmeasured confounding.

Foote *et al.* [37] studied sunscreen use and incidence of first BCC in a group of 918 subjects with sun-damaged skin originally recruited as a control group for a vitamin A study as noted above. A total of 164 BCCs were seen in the study subjects in the mean 57 months of follow-up. Those who used sunscreens "always" had an increased risk of BCC (RR = 1.55; 95% CI = 0.94-2.54) by comparison with those who never used them. When adjustment was made for all factors, only increased age independently predicted BCC.

Case control studies conducted in Spain and Australia compared sunscreen use among skin cancer patients and controls [38,36] but the Spanish study did not report separately on BCC. The investigation of Kricker *et al.* [36] compared SPF>10 sunscreen use among 226 BCC cases and 1021 controls age 40-64 who had been recruited into the Geraldton cohort study in Western Australia. Those who reported sunscreen use more than one-half the time in the 9 years prior to diagnosis had an increased risk of BCC (RR = 1.8; 95% CI = 1.1-2.9). No increased risk was seen in those using sunscreen for 10 years or more prior to diagnosis.

5.   ISSUES CONCERNING SUNSCREEN USE

Several behavioral issues require comment before summarizing knowledge to date on the relationship between sunscreen use and skin cancer risk. A number of retrospective case-control studies have shown a positive association between use and melanoma risk. Those studies which have analyzed reasons for use, and have acquired more detail on use [24,25,26] have however, shown some unusual trends in their findings. Autier *et al.* [26] showed that use of sunscreens among those who sunbathed resulted in higher risk than in those who did not report sunbathing. Similarly, Westerdahl and colleagues [25] demonstrated very high risks of melanoma in those who used sunscreen to enable them to spend more time sunbathing (RR = 8.7; 95% CI = 1.0-75.8). This may suggest that inappropriate use of sunscreens to purposely maximize time in the sun without burning may overpower the sunscreen's ability to afford protection to melanocytes, even though no sunburn appears to result from the exposure. A randomized trial of SPF-10 versus SPF-30 sunscreen was conducted by Autier *et al.* among 87 French and Swiss students age 18-24 who were intending to go on holidays for at least 15 days in the 2 months after recruitment [40]. Study subjects were unaware of which sunscreen they had been allocated, and were asked to keep daily records of their outdoor exposure. Results of the study showed that those randomized to the SPF-30 group had mean holiday duration similar to those allocated to the SPF-10 group. Similarly, the volume of sunscreen used in the two study groups was the same, as was the number of sunburns experienced by the participants. However, subjects randomized to the SPF-30 sunscreen spent significantly more hours per day in the sun than those randomized to the SPF-10 group. A trial of similar design by Autier and his colleagues using UVB and UVA personal dosimeters instead of self-reported data to determine solar exposure showed similar results [41]. Those using SPF-30 sunscreens spent more time sunbathing than those using the SPF-10 preparation. Further, the differences between the participant groups using the two different sunscreens were maximal in those subjects reporting no sunburn. These results suggest that attempts to increase the sun protection factor in sunscreens may have the effect of inducing subjects to increase their time spent in the sun in the absence of sunburn. If a sunscreen can be "overpowered", with significant damage to melanocytes in the absence of visible sunburn, the excess time in the sun may result in a higher risk of melanoma.

It is useful to note that in the Nambour sunscreen trial [33], which demonstrated a protective effect of sunscreens against SCC, the solar exposure of those in the sunscreen arm did not differ from that in the control arm. A similar finding was observed in the trial of Gallagher and colleagues [14], which demonstrated a protective effect against new nevi in children. The participants' behavior in these protective trials therefore is not typical of the subjects who use sunscreens to maximize their sun exposure in order to develop a suntan. Further research is needed on this phenomenon.

CONCLUSIONS: SUNSCREENS AND SKIN CANCER PREVENTION

At the present time, the place of sunscreens in primary cancer prevention programs is problematic. There is mounting evidence that sunscreens can prevent SCCs [30], as well as actinic keratoses [31,32], which are known to be precursors of SCC. However, in each of these studies, it appears that the sunlight behavior of those randomized to the sunscreen arm did not differ from that of the controls in the non-sunscreen arm. Perhaps the protective effect seen against SCC and its precursor lesion may not have been seen had the subjects been using sunscreens to deliberately increase exposure.

In the case of CMM, a number of studies have suggested a positive association between sunscreen use and melanoma risk. It is difficult to speculate how such a result could occur except through uncontrolled confounding or through inappropriate use of sunscreens by subjects in order to maximize solar exposure. If the latter explanation were responsible for these results, however, it might be expected that the advent of high SPF (SPF 15+) sunscreens in the 1980s would have spurred a continued increase in melanoma incidence among young and middle age subjects (those who sunbathe most). However, in most countries with high risk white populations, incidence of melanoma, particularly in the younger age groups appeared to have peaked around the mid 1980s, and may be dropping [42,43,44] at least in women. The United States may be an exception, as incidence appears to have peaked only for shallow melanomas in males born since 1950 [45].

It seems unlikely that the question of whether sunscreen use reduces or increases risk of melanoma will be answered by further case-control studies, as subject recall and confounding will continue to be major concerns with currently available retrospective methods. Primary prevention programs will then, of necessity, continue to focus on ways of reducing exposure to the sun in susceptible populations by sun avoidance methods, including shifting outdoor activities away from times of maximum insolation, and encouraging use of protective clothing.

SUMMARY POINTS

- There is mounting evidence that sunscreen use can prevent SCCs, as well as actinic keratoses, but no evidence that use can prevent basal cell carcinoma.
- Retrospective case-control studies of melanoma and sunscreen use may be hindered by accuracy of subject recall and confounding effects. Results from these studies need to be interpreted with great care.
- Public health messages should focus on reducing excessive exposure by use of clothing or sun avoidance until more is learned about the effectiveness of sunscreens in reducing cancer risk

IMPLICATIONS FOR PUBLIC HEALTH

Specific recommendations concerning the use of sunscreens have been given in the recent IARC monograph on sunscreens [1] and are appropriate for re-statement here. They are:
1. Sunscreens should not be the first choice for skin cancer prevention, and should not be used as the sole agents for sun protection.
2. Sunscreens should not be used as a means of extending the duration of solar exposure, such as prolonged sunbathing, and should not be used as a substitute for clothing on usually unexposed sites such as the trunk and buttocks.
3. Daily use of sunscreens with a high sun protection factor (SPF-15+) on usually exposed skin is recommended for residents of high solar insolation areas who work outdoors or enjoy regular outdoor recreation.

4. As adequate solar protection is more important during childhood than at any other time in life, the first two recommendations should be assiduously applied by parents and school managers.

REFERENCES

1. International Agency for Research on Cancer Expert Group (2001) *Sunscreens.* IARC Handbooks of Cancer Prevention, Vol. 5. Lyon, France: IARC Press.
2. Armstrong BK, Kricker A (1993) How much melanoma is caused by sun exposure? *Melanoma Res* **3:** 395-401.
3. International Agency for Research on Cancer Expert Group (1992) *Solar and Ultraviolet Radiation.* IARC Monographs on the Evaluation of Carcinogenic Risks to Humans Vol 55. Lyon, France: IARC Press, pp.1-316.
4. Hill D, White V, Marks R, Borland R (1993) Changes in sun-related attitudes and behaviors, and reduced sunburn prevalence in a population at high risk of recurrence of melanoma. *Eur J Cancer Prev* **2:** 447-456.
5. Dobbinson S, Borland R, Anderson M (1999) Sponsorship and sun protection practices in lifesavers. *Health Promot Int* **14:** 167-175.
6. Rivers JK, Gallagher RP (1995) Public education projects in skin cancer. Experience of the Canadian Dermatology Association. *Cancer* **75** (Suppl): 661-666.
7. Weinstock MA, Rossi JS, Redding CA, Maddock JE (1998) Randomized trial of intervention for sun protection among beachgoers (Abstract) *J Invest Dermatol* **110:** 589.
8. Geller AC, Hufford D, Miller DR, *et al.* (1997) Evaluation of the ultraviolet index: Media reactions and public response. *J Am Acad Dermatol* **37:** 935-941.
9. Hughes BR, Altman DG, Newton JA (1993) Melanoma and skin cancer: Evaluation of a health education programme for secondary schools. *Br J Dermatol* **128:** 412-417.
10. Marks R (1996) The use of sunscreens in the prevention of skin cancer. *Cancer Forum* **20:** 211-215.
11. Shaath NA (1997) Evolution of modern sunscreen chemicals. In: Lowe NJ, Shaath NA, Pathak MA, eds. *Sunscreens, Development, Evaluation and Regulatory Aspects*, 2nd Ed. (Cosmetic Science and Technology Series, Vol 15), New York: Marcel Dekker, pp.3-33.
12. Kligman AM (1966) The identification of contact allergens by human assay. 3. The maximization test: A procedure for screening and rating contact sensitizers. *J Invest Dermatol* **47:** 393-409.
13. Setlow RB, Grist E, Thompson K, Woodhead AD (1993) Wavelengths effective in induction of malignant melanoma. *Proc. Natl Acad Sci. USA* **90:** 6666-6670
14. Gallagher RP, Rivers JK, Lee TK, Bajdik CD, McLean DI, Coldman AJ (2000) Broad spectrum sunscreen use and the development of new nevi in white children: A randomized controlled trial. *JAMA* **283:** 2955-2960
15. Klepp O, Magnus K (1979) Some environmental and bodily characteristics of melanoma patients. A case-control study. *Int J Cancer* **23:** 482-486.
16. Graham S, March J, Haughy B, *et al.* (1985) An inquiry into the epidemiology of melanoma. *Am J Epidemiol* **122:** 606-619.
17. Herzfeld PM, Fitzgerald EF, Hwang SA, Stark A (1993) A case control study of malignant melanoma of the trunk among white males in upstate New York. *Cancer Detect Prev* **17:** 601-608.

18. Elwood M, Gallagher RP (1999) More about: Sunscreen use, wearing clothes, and number of nevi in 6 to 7 year old European children. *J Natl Cancer Inst* **91:** 1164-1166.

19. Holman CDJ, Armstrong BK, Heenan PJ (1986) Relationship of cutaneous malignant melanoma to individual sunlight exposure habits. *J Natl Cancer Inst* **76:** 403-414.

20. Osterlind A, Tucker MA, Stone BJ, Jensen OM (1988) The Danish case-control study of cutaneous malignant melanoma. II, Importance of UV light exposure. *Int J Cancer* **42:** 319-324.

21. Holly EA, Aston DA, Cress RD, Ahn DK, Kristiansen JJ (1995) Cutaneous melanoma in women. I. Exposure to sunlight, ability to tan, and other risk factors related to ultraviolet light. *Am J Epidemiol* **141:** 923-933.

22. Rodenas JM, Delgado-Rodriguez M, Herranz M, Tercedor J, Serrano S (1996) Sun exposure, pigmentary traits, and risk of cutaneous malignant melanoma: A case-control study in a Mediterranean population. *Cancer Causes Control* **7:** 275-283.

23. Espinosa-Arranz J, Sanchez-Hernandez JJ, Bravo Fernandez P, *et al.* (1999) Cutaneous malignant melanoma and sun exposure in Spain. *Melanoma Res* **9:** 199-205.

24. Westerdahl J, Olsson H, Masback A, Ingvar C, Jonsson N (1995) Is the use of sunscreens a risk factor for malignant melanoma? *Melanoma Res* **5:** 59-65.

25. Westerdahl J, Ingvar C, Masback A, Olsson H (2000) Sunscreen use and malignant melanoma. *Int J Cancer* **87:** 145-150.

26. Autier P, Dore J-F, Schifflers E, *et al.* (1995) Melanoma and use of sunscreens: An EORTC case-control study in Germany, Belgium & France. *Int J Cancer* **61:** 749-755.

27. Autier P, Doré JF, Cesarini JP, Boyle JP (1997) Should subjects who used psoralen suntan activators be screened for melanoma? Epidemiology and Prevention Subgroup, EORTC Melanoma Cooperative Group EORTC Prevention Research Division. *Ann Oncol* **8:** 435-437.

28. Naldi L, Gallus S, Imberti GL, Cainelli T, Negri E, LaVecchia C (2000) Sunscreens and cutaneous malignant melanoma: An Italian case-control study. *Int J Cancer* **86:** 879-882.

29. Whiteman DC, Whiteman CA, Green AC (2001) Childhood sun exposure as a risk factor for melanoma: a systematic review of epidemiologic studies. *Cancer Causes Control* **12:** 69-82.

30. Green A, Williams G, Neale R, *et al.* (1999) Daily sunscreen application and beta-carotene supplementation in prevention of basal cell and squamous cell carcinomas of the skin: A randomized controlled trial. *Lancet* **354:** 723-729.

31. Thompson SC, Jolley D, Marks R (1993) Reduction of solar keratoses by regular sunscreen use. *New Engl J Med* **329:** 1147-1151.

32. Naylor MF, Boyd A, Smith DW, Cameron GS, Hubbard D, Neldner KH (1995) High sun protection factor sunscreens in the suppression of actinic neoplasia. *Arch Dermatol* **131:** 170-175.

33. Green A, Williams G, Neal R, Battistutta D (1999) Betacarotene and sunscreen use (Author's reply). *Lancet* **354:** 2163-2164.

34. Grodstein F, Speizer FE, Hunter DJ (1995) A prospective study of incident squamous cell carcinoma of the skin in the nurses' health study. *J Natl Cancer Inst* **87:** 1061-1066.

35. English DR, Armstrong BK, Kricker A, Winter MG, Heenan PJ, Randell PL (1998) Case-control study of sun exposure and squamous cell carcinoma of the skin. *Int J Cancer* **77:** 347-353.

36. Kricker A, Armstrong BK, English DR, Heenan PJ (1991) Pigmentary and cutaneous risk factors for non-melanocytic skin cancer - a case-control study. *Int J Cancer* **48(5):** 650-662.

37. Foote JA, Harris RB, Giulliano AR, *et al.* (2001) Predictors for cutaneous basal and squamous cell carcinoma among actinically damaged adults. *Int J Cancer* **95:** 7-11.

38. Suarez-Varela MM, Gonzales AL, Caraco EF (1996) Non-melanoma skin cancer: A case-control study on risk factors and protective measures. *J Environ Pathol Toxicol Oncol* **15:** 255-261.
39. Hunter BR, Colditz GA, Strampfer MJ, Rosner B, Willett WC, Speizer FE (1990) Risk factors for basal cell carcinoma in a prospective cohort of women. *Ann Epidemiol* **1:** 13-23.
40. Autier P, Dore J-F, Negrier S, *et al.* (1999) Sunscreen use and duration of sun exposure: A double blind randomized trial. *J Natl Cancer Inst* **91:** 1304-1309.
41. Autier P, Dore J-F, Reis AC, *et al.* (2000) Sunscreen use and intentional exposure to ultraviolet A and B radiation: a double blind randomized trial using personal dosimeters. *Br J Cancer* **83:** 1243-1248.
42. Marrett L, Nguyen HL, Armstrong BK (2001) Trends in the incidence of cutaneous malignant melanoma in New South Wales, 1983-1996. *Int J Cancer* **92:** 457-462.
43. Bulliard JL, Cox B (2000). Cutaneous malignant melanoma in New Zealand: trends by anatomic site 1969-1993. *Int J Epidemiol* **29:** 416-423.
44. Bulliard JL, Cox B, Semenciw R (1999) Trends by anatomic site in the incidence of cutaneous malignant melanoma in Canada. *Cancer Causes Control* **10:** 407-416.
45. Jemal A, Devesa SS, Hartge P, Tucker MA (2001) Recent trends in cutaneous melanoma incidence among whites in the United States. *J Natl Cancer Inst* **93(9):** 678-683.
46. Beitner H, Norell SE, Ringborg U, Wennersten G, Mattson B (1990) Malignant melanoma: Aetiological importance of individual pigmentation and sun exposure. *Br J Dermatol* **122**: 43-51.
47. Whiteman DC, Valery P, McWhirter W, Green AC (1997) Risk factors for childhood melanoma in Queensland, Australia. *Int J Cancer* **70:** 26-31.
48. Wolf P, Quehenberger F, Mülleger R, Stranz B, Kerl H (1998) Phenotypic markers, sunlight-related factors and sunscreen use in patients with cutaneous melanoma: An Austrian case-control study. *Melanoma Res* **8:** 370-378.

Chapter 9

Issues about solaria

Philippe Autier, M.D., M.P.H.
Centre for Research in Epidemiology and Health Information Systems, Luxembourg

Key words: sunbed, sunlamp, artificial tanning, skin cancer

INTRODUCTION

The fashion of using artificial sources of ultraviolet radiation (i.e., sunlamps, sunbeds, solaria, tanning beds, indoor tanning, tanning parlors) for cosmetic or recreational purposes is widespread among fair skinned communities, particularly in countries where sunny, hot weather is infrequent (e.g., Northern Europe, Canada). Exposure to solar radiation is recognized as the major environmental risk factor for cutaneous melanoma [1], particularly when sun exposure is intentional, i.e., motivated by the willingness to get a tan or to stay in the sun for recreational purposes [2]. Ultraviolet radiation (UV) is deemed to represent the part of the solar spectrum involved in the genesis of melanoma. Therefore, it has been suggested that exposure to sunlamps/sunbeds could contribute to the melanoma incidence in Caucasian populations. Fears have focused on melanoma, as sunbed exposure resembles the type of sun exposure most associated with that malignancy.

This chapter reviews the evidence gathered so far on a possible implication of sunlamp/sunbed exposure in melanoma occurrence.

D. Hill et al. (eds.), Prevention of Skin Cancer, 157-176.
© 2004 *Kluwer Academic Publishers. Printed in the Netherlands.*

1.   HISTORICAL BACKGROUND

In the 1920s, the first "artificial sky" made with fluorescent lamps was commercialized to treat various skin conditions such as psoriasis and dermatitis. In the forties and fifties, mercury lamps were popular in Northern Europe and North America. Typically, they were portable devices equipped with a single UV lamp, sometimes accompanied by infrared lamps (to heat the skin). Exposure to these lamps was of short duration but could lead to the development of erythema, burns and blistering. These tools were primarily used in children, for helping the synthesis of vitamin D3. Some adults used them for getting a tan. Since these UV lamps were primarily intended for domestic use, many were still in use after most nations had put a ban on their commercialization.

In the sixties, with the growing fashion of tanning, alternative sources of ultraviolet radiation were invented for fair skin populations living in areas where bright sunlight is available only during a few periods of the year. These units generally comprised three to six short fluorescent lamps, and tanning of the whole body required the subject to expose one body part after another.

In the seventies, ultraviolet B radiation (UVB, 280-320 nm) was recognized as the most carcinogenic part of the solar spectrum, and a shift in usage occurred towards low-pressure fluorescent tubes emitting essentially in the ultraviolet A range (UVA, 320-400 nm). With the advent of low-pressure long fluorescent tubes, body size tanning units usually called sunbeds or solaria became commercially available.

2.   EXPOSURE TO SUNLAMPS/SUNBEDS

The indoor tanning fashion spread in the eighties. Before 1980, less than 5% of the adult population in Belgium, France and Germany seemed to have ever used a sunlamp for tanning purposes [3]. Another 5% had been exposed to artificial UV sources for medical or occupational reasons. In 1995, about one third of the adult population of these countries had ever used sunbeds. Surveys in Europe and North America indicate that between 15 and 35 % of women, and between 5 and 10% of men 15 to 30 years old have used sunbeds [3-5]. In Sweden, after 1995, 70% of females and 50% of males 18 to 50 years old reported sunbed use [6-8]. In the late nineties, the indoor tanning fashion rapidly extended in Mediterranean areas like the north of Italy [9,10], and in countries with an emerging economy such as Argentina [11]. In the State of Victoria, Australia – a sunny area with high records of skin cancers – 9% of subjects 14 to 29 years old reported sunbed use in the past year [12]. A substantial proportion of sunbeds are used in private facilities, and in Germany or Nordic countries, home-made solaria are not uncommon.

In Scotland, a population known for its particular susceptibility to sunlight, 17% of sunbed users had more than 100 sessions per year [13], and duration of a tanning session is typically of 15 to 20 minutes. A market survey done in Denmark in 1996 (AC Nielsen-AIM, Copenhagen, 1997 – unpublished data) showed that 11% of subjects, 13 years old or more, reported use of sunbeds less than once per month, 8% used sunbeds 1 to 3 times per month, and 5% used sunbeds at least once every week. Taken together with data from other surveys, the latter figures give evidence that a proportion of sunbed users may accumulate annual exposure durations exceeding 20 hours.

3.   PHOTOBIOLOGICAL ASPECTS

During a sunny day on the Mediterranean coast, the solar ultraviolet (UV) spectrum at noon contains 4-5% of UVB, and 94-95% of UVA. UVB is far more efficient than UVA for inducing the synthesis of melanin, and for producing a deep, persistent tan. UVB is also more erythemogenic than UVA. For sunburns caused by sun exposure, solar UVB contributes about 80% towards sunburn, and solar UVA contributes to the remaining 20% [2].

The "solar sky" available before World War II emitted in the UVA range. In the forties until the sixties, the ultraviolet spectrum off mercury lamps consisted of about 20% ultraviolet C radiation (UVC, 100-280 nm – a radiation that does not reach the Earth's surface) and 30 to 50% of UVB [14]. In the eighties, before regulations were enforced, UVB could represent up to 5% of the UV output of sunbeds. In the eighties and nineties, with the growing concern about the carcinogenic potential of UVB, the UV output of low-pressure fluorescent lamps was shifted to the UVA, yielding the so-called "UVA-tanning." More recently, high-pressure lamps producing large quantities of long wave UVA (>335-400 nm) per unit of time were marketed; these can emit 10 times more UVA than is present in the sunlight. Some sunbeds combine high-pressure long wave UVA lamps with classic low-pressure fluorescent lamps.

Hence, in large powerful tanning units, the UVA irradiation intensity may be several times higher than that of the midday sun. However, the term "UVA tanning" often used is misleading, as the output of a sunbed equipped with low pressure fluorescent lamps always contains some UVB (around 1 to 2% of the UV spectrum), which is critical for the induction of a deep, persistent tan.

In the nineties, regulations in some countries (e.g., Sweden, France) limited to 1.5% the maximum proportion of UVB in the UV output. However, in the real world, the UV output and spectral characteristics of sunbeds vary considerably. Surveys in the UK on sunbeds operated in public or commercial facilities revealed substantial differences in UV output, mainly for UVB, for which 60-fold differences in output were observed [13,15] and the proportion of UVB in UV output could vary from 0.5 to 4%. These differences are due to sunbed design (e.g., the type of fluorescent tubes used as sources, the materials composing filters, the distance from canopy to the skin), to sunbed power, and to tube aging. Sunbeds in commercial facilities seem to have a greater output in the UVB range [16], as consumers are more satisfied by the fast and deep tan they have paid for. With tube aging, the output of fluorescent lamps decreases, and the proportion of UVB decreases more rapidly. Hence, non-replacement of lamps may lead to a need for longer or more frequent tanning sessions, or to non satisfaction of consumers.

In the nineties, UVA became suspected of being involved in the induction of melanoma. UVA was also recognized as the wavelength responsible for skin aging. Because of uncertainties about the UV wavelength(s) implicated in melanoma occurrence, and concerns that high UVA doses were a cause of premature skin wrinkling, in the late nineties a new trend was to equip sunbeds with fluorescent lamps having a UV output, in both wavelength and energy, comparable to midday sun in a sunny, hot area (e.g., the "Cleo Natural Lamps" of Philips Cy, Eindhoven, The Netherlands). These lamps emit a larger proportion of UVB (around 4%). The rationale for solar-like sunbeds is that with a correct UV energy dosage, sunbed sessions resemble habitual sun exposure without imbalances between total UV, UVB or UVA [17].

4.   WHY SUNBED USE, AND WHAT DO CONSUMERS KNOW ABOUT SUNLAMPS/SUNBEDS?

The popularity of indoor tanning is rooted in the perceived cosmetic and psychological benefits of acquisition or maintenance of a healthy, attractive look [18]. There is also a widespread belief that acquisition of a pre-vacation tan may protect against the harmful effects of the sun. Many subjects report improved well-being as a strong motive for sunbed use. UV exposure (especially high UVA doses) can induce a sensation of well-being, mediated by the synthesis of enkephalin in the skin, that enters the blood stream and then influences the central nervous system [19]. In North European countries, and Canada, commercial advertising may advocate sunbed use from November to March to combat the so-called "winter depression" or "seasonal depression", associated with the absence of days with bright sunshine and long nights. However, light therapy using white fluorescent lights is as effective for the treatment of seasonal depression [20].

5. DATA ON THE RELATIONSHIP BETWEEN SUNLAMP/SUNBED USE AND SKIN CANCER

5.1 Clinical data

Numerous clinical reports have been published about the deleterious effects of exposure to sunlamps/sunbeds on the skin (for a review, see Spencer & Amonette, 1995 [21]), and on the eye [22]. Severe skin burns may be seen in subjects who used photosensitizing drugs or skin lotions to foster their tanning ability (e.g., the psoralens) [23].

5.2 Skin erythema

Skin erythema or burns are reported by 18 to 44 % of sunbed users, mainly by subjects with a poor ability to tan [3,4,6,8,21,24]. UVB is one thousand times more erythemogenic than UVA, but in many studies, skin erythema occurred after exposure to modern sunbeds. It is known that high fluxes of UVA (which are commonly encountered in modern high power tanning machines) are capable of inducing skin erythemal reactions [25].

5.3 Interpretation of results from epidemiological studies

In the absence of a valid animal model for human melanoma, epidemiological studies are mandatory for producing the most convincing documentation of an association between sunbed use and melanoma. Epidemiological investigation of this issue faces the challenging issue of how to recognize *now* a current exposure that could become recognized as a carcinogenic hazard in the future.

In that respect, five aspects must be carefully borne in mind. First, if sunlamp/sunbed exposure has an initiation effect on melanoma occurrence, the latency period between exposure to a potentially carcinogenic agent and melanoma occurrence may be 30 years or more. Sunbed use has become a frequent exposure only during the last twenty years. Therefore, in the case of initiation effect, the impact on melanoma incidence will probably not be detectable before the year 2010. If sunlamp/sunbed exposure had rather a promoter effect on melanoma occurrence, then the eventual influence on melanoma could be measurable now.

Secondly, the existence of a latency period may lead to an underestimate of the actual association between indoor tanning and melanoma. Because the carcinogenic effect of more recent exposures is not yet detectable, a lack of distinction between previous and recent exposures may mask the actual increase in risk.

Thirdly, sunbed users have a greater propensity than average to engage in intentional sun exposure [26]. In that respect, examining the possible melanoma risk associated with sunbed use is somewhat comparable to the tough exercise of examining the additional risk of lung cancer attributable to a new type of cigarette. Hence, epidemiological investigations on the sunbed-skin cancer association should carefully collect data on sun exposure history, and statistical analysis of epidemiological data should always adjust risk estimates for intentional sun exposure.

Fourthly, the UV output of sunlamps/sunbeds has changed over time. If the UVB were the wavelength mainly implicated in melanoma occurrence, then an association between sunlamp/sunbed exposure and melanoma could be observed for exposure to older types of sunlamps, in the forties until the sixties. Exposure to more recent tanning machines could only have a marginal impact, given that their output in the UVB range is lower than for the midday sun. In the latter case, it is probable that the influence of sun exposures will always supersede the eventual influence of sunbed use. If UVA played a significant role in melanoma occurrence, then exposure to sunlamps/sunbeds that took place after 1980 could emerge as a risk factor for melanoma.

Fifth, it has been calculated that significant exposure to sunlamps/sunbeds (i.e., >10 to 20 hours per year) entails annual total doses of UV comparable to annual doses received during holiday sunbathing in Mediterranean areas [27,28]. However, UV output of modern sunbeds is not similar to the midday sun, and therefore the biological impact of sunbed radiations may differ from the biological impact of the midday sun. Sweden is a country with a high proportion of sun-sensitive subjects with the highest exposure level to sunlamps/sunbeds ever recorded in the world. A recent large survey in the Stockholm area suggests that, overall, one sunburn or skin reddening episode out of ten is due to exposure to sunlamps/sunbeds, and the remaining nine to sun exposure (e.g., during sunbathing) [8]. An association between sunburn and melanoma has been found in most epidemiological studies. If sunburns are markers of the occurrence of biological events possibly leading to melanoma, then the low proportion of sunburn or skin reddening induced by sunlamps/sunbeds may indicate that at population level, in spite of the high amounts of UV radiation that can be received through sunlamp/sunbed use, sun exposure remains the most important factor implicated in melanoma occurrence.

5.4   Results from epidemiological studies on cutaneous melanoma

At least twenty-two epidemiological investigations have looked at the association between cutaneous melanoma and exposure to sunlamps/sunbeds. Most of these studies just examined whether at least one exposure to sunlamps/sunbeds was associated with cutaneous melanoma. Analysis of these "ever/never" type of questions is not informative, among other reasons because of the masking effect of recent sunbed exposures.

Six epidemiological case-control studies explored in more detail the relationship between exposure to sunlamps/sunbeds and cutaneous melanoma (Tables 9.1 and 9.2) [3,7,29-32]. Four of these studies addressed sunlamp/sunbed use before 1990, when the indoor tanning fashion was in its early phase.

The following results suggest a positive association between sunlamp/sunbed exposure and melanoma:

1. In three out of four studies that distinguished between earlier and more recent first sunbed exposure, the melanoma risk was higher in subjects who had their first exposure many years before the diagnosis of melanoma, as compared with subjects who reported only recent exposures (Table 9.2). However, because relatively few subjects had earlier exposures, most risk estimates did not reach statistical significance. The two Swedish studies [7,31] did not perform an analysis by time period.

2. In the European Organization for Research and Treatment of Cancer (EORTC) study [3], subjects who reported skin erythemal reactions caused by tanning sessions and more than 10 hours of sunlamp/sunbed exposure, displayed a seven-fold increase in melanoma after adjustment for natural sun susceptibility and recreational sun exposure. The wide 95% confidence interval of 1.7 to 32.3 indicates the estimate was imprecise. No other study collected appropriate data on sunbed-induced skin erythema.

3. In the most recent Swedish study [7], "regular" sunbed users had a melanoma risk significantly increased by 20 to 170%. Regular sunbed users represented 25% of control subjects less than 36 years, 14% of control subjects 36-60 years, and 5% of control subjects older than 60 years. In the three age groups, after adjustment for sun exposure, the relative risks (95% confidence interval) of melanoma associated with regular sunbed use were 8.1 (1.3-49.5), 2.2 (1.2-3.9) and 0.9 (0.4-2.2), respectively.

4. Four studies found some degree of increasing melanoma risk with increasing lifetime sunlamp/sunbed exposure (Table 9.1) [3,29-31].

Table 9.1 Duration of exposure to sunlamps or sunbeds and relative risk of cutaneous melanoma.[a]

Study place, year of publication [study years], numbers of cases/controls [reference]		Duration of exposure	Cases	Controls	Estimated melanoma relative risk	95% confidence interval
Scotland, 1988 [1979-84], 180/120 (Swerdlow et al., 1988) [29]		Never used	142	110	1.0[d]	–
		<3 months	6	3	0.7	0.10-3.80
		3 months – 1 year	24	5	3.1	1.00-9.90
		> 1 year	8	2	3.4	0.60-20.3
		Test for linear trend: P = 0.0029				
Ontario, 1990 [1984-86], 583/608 (Walter et al., 1990) [30]	Males	Never used	210	242	1.00[c]	–
		<180 minutes	25	20	1.44	0.75-2.82
		≥180 minutes	39	18	2.50	1.34-4.80
		Test for linear trend in males: P = 0.0012				
	Females	Never used	222	256	1.00[c]	–
		<180 minutes	39	39	1.17	0.70-1.95
		≥180 minutes	38	27	1.62	0.91-2.89
		Test for linear trend in females: P = 0.070				
Sweden, 1994 [1988-90], 400/640 (Westerdahl et al., 1994) [31]		Never used	282	479	1.0[d]	–
		1-3 sessions	44	67	1.1	0.70-1.90
		4-10 sessions	30	55	1.1	0.70-1.90
		>10 sessions	41	33	1.8	1.00-3.20
		Test for linear trend: P = 0.020				
Belgium, France, Germany, 1994[b] [1991-92], 420/447 (Autier et al., 1994) [3]	Exposure starts ≥1980	Never used	310	327	1.00[d]	–
		<10 hours	36	45	0.75	0.46-1.25
		≥10 hours	19	18	0.99	0.49-2.00
	Exposure starts <1980	<10 hours	16	15	1.00	0.47-2.13
		≥10 hours	18	7	2.12	0.84-2.12
		Test for linear trend: P = 0.033 when start < 1980; P = 0.89 when start ≥1980				
Connecticut, USA, 1998 [1987-89], 624/512 (Chen et al., 1998) [32]		Never used	483	417	1.00[d]	–
		<10 sunlamp uses	76	50	1.25	0.84-1.84
		≥10 sunlamp uses	63	40	1.15	0.60-2.20
		Test for linear trend: P = 0.068				
Sweden, 2000 [1995-97], 571//913[e] (Westerdahl et al., 2000) [7]		None	319[e]	538[e]	1.0[d]	–
		1-125 uses	22	32	2.8	1.00-7.80
		126-250 uses	34	31	3.1	1.30-7.10
		>250 uses	31	37	1.5	0.70-3.20
		Test for linear trend: P = 0.26				

[a]Duration of exposure, relative risk, and 95% confidences as in published reports. The Mantel χ2 for trend was calculated by us. [b]The 21 cases and 35 controls who were exposed to sunlamp or sunbed for non-tanning purpose are not reported in this Table. [c]Adjusted for age. [d]Adjusted for age, sex, natural sun sensitivity and recreational sun exposure. [e]Reported numbers of cases and controls could differ according to ways sunbed uses were computed.

Table 9.2 Earlier and recent exposure to sunlamp or sunbed and risk of cutaneous melanoma[a].

Study		Estimated Melanoma Risk (95% confidence interval)	
		First exposure earlier	First exposure more recent
Scotland, 1988[b] [29]		9.10 (2.00-40.6)*	1.90 (0.60-5.60)
Ontario, Canada, 1990[b] [30]	Males:	2.00 (1.21-3.34)*	1.52 (0.56-4.25)
	Females:	1.53 (0.96-2.46)	1.24 (0.67-2.31)
Belgium, France, Germany, 1994[c] [3]		2.12 (0.84-5.37)	0.99 (0.49-2.00)
Connecticut, USA, 1998[d] [32]		1.33 (0.84-2.12)	1.15 (0.64-2.07)

[a] These results were not reported in Swedish studies (Westerdahl *et al.*, 1994 [31]; Westerdahl *et al.*, 2000 [7]).
[b] Five years since last use, unadjusted odds ratio for ever exposed *vs* never exposed.
[c] First exposure took place before 1980, odds ratio for ten hours of exposure or more *vs* never exposed, adjusted for age, sex, natural sun sensitivity and recreational sun exposure.
[d] Exposures ≤ 1970 are earlier, and exposures after 1970 are more recent; adjusted for age, sex, natural sun sensitivity, and recreational sun exposure.
* $P \leq 0.05$

The following considerations must be taken into account for interpreting results from studies listed in Tables 9.1 and 9.2.

1. In the Ontario study [30], risk estimates were not adjusted for sun exposure.
2. In all studies, after adjustment for sun exposure and natural sun sensitivity, risks of melanoma associated with sunbed use were small and often statistically non significant.
3. Two studies did not find a consistent dose-effect trend [7,32]. The absence of clear dose-effect relationship in the Swedish study published in 2000 is troublesome as that study was performed in a population with a high level of sunbed use over at least fifteen years.
4. The data were obtained from retrospective questionnaires, and therefore, past sunlamp/sunbed exposure and sun exposure history were difficult to assess accurately. It is therefore not impossible that the moderate increase in melanoma risk still observed after adjustment for sun exposure was due to the residual confounding linked to inaccurate measurement of past sun exposure.
5. Associations found could be the consequence of "rumination" bias as melanoma patients might have been more likely to remember past exposures to artificial UV sources. However, the Ontario study performed a part of the interviews before patients were told they had a melanoma, and concluded that recall bias was not likely to explain their findings [30].

6. Time scales used in the six studies for expressing duration of sunlamp/sunbed exposure were quite variable. In the last Swedish study [7], the answer "regular use of sunbed" was not defined in more quantitative terms. Also, numbers of cases and controls reported in published tables varied quite considerably according to the way sunbed uses were reported, which renders difficult an unambiguous appraisal of results reported in that Swedish study [7].

7. The first five studies in Table 9.1 appraised sunlamp/sunbed exposure that took place in the seventies and eighties. It is very unlikely that a study could assess the eventual influence of sunlamp/sunbed exposure that took place in the ten years before the study.

Overall, while the six studies raise the possibility of a moderate positive association between sunlamp/sunbed use and melanoma, the results lack consistency. Furthermore, there is little chance that any epidemiological study has had the ability to measure the impact on melanoma of the indoor tanning fashion that became so common among young age groups after 1985. Hence, in June 2003, there is still no conclusive evidence on the influence of sunlamp/sunbed use on melanoma occurrence.

5.5   Results from epidemiological studies on non-melanoma skin cancers

Two studies examined past exposure to sunbeds in patients with non-melanoma skin cancer. One found no association [33], and another found positive associations between sunbed use and squamous cell (SCC) and basal cell skin cancers (BCC) [34]. In the latter study, the estimated relative risk associated with sunbed use was 2.5 (95% CI: 1.7 to 3.8) for squamous cell skin cancer (SCC) and 1.5 (95% CI: 1.1 to 2.1) for basal cell skin cancer (BCC). These findings are more in line with data on SCC in patients affected by severe psoriasis and treated with PUVA therapy (a combination of UVA irradiation and oral taking of psoralen – see below).

6.   PSORIASIS AND SKIN CANCERS

Patients suffering from severe psoriasis are often treated with UV radiation. UVB alone may be employed, but more frequently, treatments consist of UVA exposures in combination with oral psoralens (i.e., PUVA therapy). Psoriasitic patients have often recourse to sunbed exposure as a self-therapy for their lesions [35]. Also, high levels of sun exposure are common in psoriasis patients, and may represent a form of treatment for that skin condition (the "climatotherapy", usually on the Dead Sea in Israel [36]). All long-term follow-up of PUVA treated patients found a positive impact on non-melanoma skin cancers, mainly SCC [37-39]. Three prospective studies on psoriasis patients found no raised melanoma incidence with PUVA therapy, one study in a large cohort of PUVA treated patients in Sweden found a significantly deceased risk of melanoma [39], and one study in the USA found an increased melanoma risk associated with PUVA in patients with severe psoriasis [40,41]. In the US study, the increased risk was mainly apparent in psoriatic patients who had received 250 treatments or more. It was however impossible to ascertain which treatment component was implicated in the higher melanoma risk, since psoralens are potent photocarcinogens, and a proportion of patients received various other potentially carcinogenic treatments (e.g., coal tar). Also, sun exposure history of patients was not assessed.

Thus, in regard to considerable amounts of UVA exposure (through either PUVA or sunbed exposure), there is so far little support for a raised melanoma incidence among PUVA-treated psoriasitic patients.

7.   ARGUMENTS OFTEN EVOKED FOR THE DEFENSE OF INDOOR TANNING

The sunbed industry, tanning enthusiasts, and a fraction of the medical community exploit several lines of argument to defend the use of artificial tanning devices (e.g., *www.suntanning.com*). Many arguments have surfaced as a consequence of the lack of knowledge we have on the type of UV radiation causing melanoma, on the biological mechanisms involved in melanoma development, on which mechanisms would or would not be sun-induced, and on the relationship between tan acquisition and carcinogenic processes. The subtlest position is the recognition of good and bad effects of indoor tanning, but that finally, good effects would outweigh bad effects. Arguments put forward by indoor tanning advocates are often speculative and of questionable scientific validity, but they represent the justification that indoor tanning is not an unacceptable health threat. These arguments are often accepted as true science by many doctors, institutions active in cancer prevention, and decision makers. We review and briefly discuss the most important of them.

1. *"The UV spectrum emitted by sunbeds is safer than the solar spectrum."*
    This argument suggests that a tan acquired through sunbed use will be safer than a tan acquired through sunbathing on a beach. It is largely based on the fact that compared to the summer Mediterranean sun, the

UV spectrum of a modern sunbed contains more UVA and less UVB. However, recent studies suggest that tanning is a direct consequence of UV-induced DNA damage [42]. Substantial skin DNA damage is detectable after sunbed exposure, which is comparable to the DNA damage induced by exposure to natural sunlight: this would be chiefly due to the UVB fraction present in the output of most sunbeds [43,44]. Thus, at present, the available scientific data hardly support the idea that an artificially acquired tan is safer than a tan acquired through sun exposure.

2. "Acquisition of a tan with sunbed use would achieve the maximum protective effect through a combination of pigmentation and skin thickening." Recent data show that acquisition of a pre-vacation tan offers only little protection against sun-induced DNA damage [45,46], and the moderate skin thickening induced by sunbed use would afford even less photoprotection than tanning [47]. Also, recent studies have raised the possibility that the induction of melanin synthesis could be involved in skin carcinogenesis [48,49].

3. *"A pre-vacation tan confers protection against sunburns and other deleterious effects of the sun."* This argument is a corollary of the former one. Surveys in various fair skinned communities show that between 25 and 50% of sunbed users report that they want to "prepare the skin for holidays." However, because a pre-vacation tan offers some protection against sun-induced erythema, a pre-vacation tan may induce hazardous sun exposure behaviors such as the promotion of prolonged sun exposure. Hence, the risk of melanoma ultimately associated with indoor tanning would include not only the exposure to UV-radiation emitted by tanning devices, but also the possibility of increased sun exposure at the start of the holiday [45].

4. Currently, the main argument develops around the fact that the fashion of intentional sun exposure and tan acquisition will not change in the short term. The literature shows how ineffective are efforts deployed to convince adolescents and young adults to refrain from sunbathing. Typical sunbathing during sunny holidays entails heavy sun exposure every (or nearly every) day, with few interruptions, and often, the occurrence of sunburn. At least 48 hours are needed for repair of skin UV-induced DNA damage. Every day sunbathing leads to accumulation of DNA damage, which would favor skin cancer occurrence. Exposure to sunbeds equipped with lamps having an output resembling the solar spectrum allows tanning programs resembling sunbathing on a beach. For some authors, tan acquisition through sunbed exposure would be less dangerous than that acquired on beaches because sessions are spaced by 4-5 days, allowing full repair of UV-induced DNA damage [17].

Furthermore, because sunbed sessions are limited in time, sunburn occurrence should be rarer than when on the beach. Thus, tan acquisition through well-planned sunbed sessions would be safer than through sunbathing activities. These lines of arguments are often presented under the heading of "Sensible Sunbathing" [17,50]. These new types of arguments rest on apparently more solid scientific foundations. But available data suggest that the UVB would be the UV wavelength mainly involved in photocarcinogenesis [51]. Furthermore, no proven link exists between time allowed to repair UV-induced DNA, and melanoma occurrence, whereas, sufficient evidence exists of links between tan acquisition and melanoma occurrence.

8. RECOMMENDATIONS AND REGULATIONS

A number of reports from various scientific domains have triggered reactions intended to discourage exposure to sunbeds [52-55]. Standards for cosmetic use of UV emitting devices have been published by official organizations [56-59]. Since 1990, many countries (e.g., Sweden, United Kingdom, France, Belgium, United States of America, Canada) have issued specific rules for sunbed installation, with indications as to which of the different types of tanning device can be made available to the general public, commercial facilities, and health professionals. There is a wide variation in the content of these rules: some are regulations issued by governmental agencies, but others are just recommendations issued by non-governmental institutions. In Europe, there is no standardization of regulations on sunbed commercialization and use. In some countries (e.g., in the United Kingdom, Canada and The Netherlands), recommendations are formulated by, or in association with, the sunbed industry or organizations of professional sunbed operators.

In general, regulations also include recommendations on how tanning units must be operated, and the information that operators must deliver to consumers. Eyes should be protected with goggles. Consumers possibly taking photosensitizing medications or lotions should be identified. Many regulations discourage sunbed exposure for subjects having a poor or no ability to tan (e.g., red haired subjects with many freckles).

A frequently asked question is whether there is a limit below which indoor tanning would be safe. Several expert groups have suggested maximum numbers of tanning sessions, but these are best guesses not supported by human data. For instance, in 1990, the British Photodermatology Group recommended that exposures were not to exceed a cumulative amount of 10 hours of indoor tanning per year [60]. A document entitled "Outdoors and Indoors: Sun Wisely" produced under the auspices of the Dutch Cancer Society [50], argues that sunbed exposure not exceeding 50 minimal erythemal doses per year (MED) is acceptable (1 MED corresponds to the UV dose triggering minimal skin erythema in a moderately sun sensitive subject). A thirty minute sunbed session represents an exposure to 0.7 to 1 MED, and two weeks of summer holidays on the Mediterranean coast with daily sunbathing may represent a cumulative UV dose of 100 MED. Hence, the limits suggested for duration of sunbed exposure are well above the levels of sun exposure known to be associated with increased melanoma risk.

9.   IMPACT OF REGULATIONS

An important achievement of regulations is the requirement for better information for consumers. In some countries (e.g., in France), the need to have trained operators has prevented the multiplication of automated tanning parlors working without the surveillance of an operator. Also, these regulations are likely to protect consumers against the most dangerous UV devices. They can prevent consumers who are taking photosensitizing drugs from using sunbeds.

The impact of these regulations on potential health hazards associated with sunbed use is however difficult to estimate, because the bottom line is that each time a subject desires to acquire a tan, or to feel a sensation of well-being, either through sunbathing or through sunbed use, there is exposure to biologically effective, potentially carcinogenic doses of UV. Furthermore, regulations or recommendations rarely reflect the numerous uncertainties we have on the association between UV exposure and skin cancers, or other UV-induced lesions such as premature skin aging and eye lesions. In that respect, most existing regulations could just result in giving a false sense of security to both consumers and tanning parlor operators, and thus encourage indoor tanning. Hence, from a strict point of view of exposure to a hazardous health agent, the sunbed market remains largely unregulated.

Also, enforcement of regulations remains a challenge [4,21,61], and surveys repeatedly show the ignorance of both sunbed users and tanning facility operators about health hazards associated with indoor tanning [62]. Moreover, regulations do not apply to the private use of sunbeds.

10.   IS IT POSSIBLE TO REDUCE THE ATTRACTION OF SUNBED TANNING FOR YOUNG PEOPLE?

The studies done so far [8,10] show that people know about possible dangers associated with sunbed use, but that knowledge does not alter their tanning behaviors in general. Regulations restricting indoor tanning do not make sunbed users more cautious [63], and indoor tanning facilities continue to promote frequent tanning sessions [64].

11.   NEED FOR EPIDEMIOLOGICAL SURVEILLANCE

In the absence of a valid animal model for human melanoma, and given the ignorance we still have on the ultraviolet radiation implicated in melanoma development, the study of an eventual link between sunbed use and melanoma is left to epidemiological investigation. Epidemiological surveillance of the eventual influence of sunlamp/sunbed exposures on melanoma could be carried out in populations where the use of indoor tanning has been frequent since the early eighties (e.g., the Nordic countries). In order to maximize exposure rates to sunlamps/sunbeds, new studies should be performed in subjects less than 50 years old. Large numbers of subjects should be included, to yield sufficient data among subjects with both earlier and prolonged sunlamp/sunbed exposure. New studies should aim at reconstituting the individual's sunlamp/sunbed exposure history, giving attention to the types of tanning unit used over time. Data on sunburns incurred during tanning sessions, and any other symptoms, should be recorded. Unwarranted cosmetic effects of artificial tanning should also be studied more carefully, as such effects are more likely to dissuade young women from using tanning devices.

Realistic prospective epidemiological designs for investigating the issue are not easy to formulate and to fund. Prospective studies could only be performed in countries equipped with population cancer registers, and with high levels of exposure to sunlamps/sunbeds, e.g., the Nordic countries.

CONCLUSIONS

It is unlikely that public health control of indoor tanning will take place effectively in the absence of clear evidence of life-threatening conditions attributable to that fashion. With time, the melanoma risk conveyed by indoor tanning will become more apparent, mainly in the northern areas of America and Europe. As long as valid animal models for human melanoma are not available, epidemiological surveillance is needed to monitor the impact of sunbed use on the occurrence of skin and eye cancers, and to definitely establish whether an increased risk emerges, even after a long latency period.

The *precautionary principle* is frequently evoked in the shaping of health policies. In brief, that principle consists of regulating the general public use of a substance or a device whose safety remains open to question. In that respect, as long as the sunbed-melanoma association remains unsettled, health prevention programs should continue to discourage sunbed use.

SUMMARY POINTS

- Sunbed use has become a frequent behavior in most Caucasian populations. The highest levels of sunbed exposure are found in Nordic countries and in Canada, but sunbed use is becoming common in sunny areas.
- Sunbed use is tightly linked to the tanning fashion, and to unverified lines of argument suggesting that tan acquisition with sunbed use would be safer than with sunbathing.
- Examination of results from the six epidemiological studies that specifically explored the history of sunbed use among patients with cutaneous melanoma and unaffected controls raised the possibility of a moderate positive association between sunbed use and melanoma, but the results lack consistency, and in July 2002, there is still no conclusive evidence on the influence of sunbed use on melanoma occurrence.
- Limited epidemiological data, and long term follow up of patients with severe psoriasis treated with PUVA (a combination of UVA and psoralens) suggest the possibility of some increase in squamous cell and basal cell skin cancer incidence associated with high sunbed use.
- Future epidemiological studies on the sunbed-melanoma issue should adopt designs different from the classic case-control approach. However, the implementation of long-term prospective designs for examining the sunbed-melanoma issue poses numerous difficulties and will be possible only in areas equipped with population-based cancer registers and complete recording of melanoma cases.

IMPLICATIONS FOR PUBLIC HEALTH

- Epidemiological surveillance of the possible impact of sunbed use on skin cancer should be conducted in countries equipped with population-based cancer registers.
- As long as there is no clear scientific evidence on the real effects of sunbed use on skin cancers (and other health aspects), health prevention programs should continue to discourage sunbed use.
- Prevention messages should be targeted to adolescents and young adults, with the main objectives of providing correct information on the possible health hazards of indoor tanning, and combating unverified beliefs accompanying the marketing of that fashion.
- New regulations should be formulated independently from the sunbed industry or tanning parlor operators.
- Where regulations exist do, the main challenge remains their enforcement.

REFERENCES

1. International Agency for Research on Cancer Expert Group (1992) *Solar and Ultraviolet Radiation.* IARC Monographs on the Evaluation of Carcinogenic Risks to Humans, Vol. 55. Lyon, France: IARC Press.pp.217-228
2. International Agency for Research on Cancer Expert Group (2001) *Sunscreens.* IARC Handbooks of Cancer Prevention, Vol. 5. Lyon, France: IARC Press.
3. Autier P, Doré JF, Lejeune F, *et al* (1994) Cutaneous malignant melanoma and exposure to sunlamps or sunbeds: An EORTC multicenter case-control study in Belgium, France and Germany. *Int J Cancer* **58**: 809-813.
4. Oliphant JA, Forster JL, McBride CM (1994) the use of commercial tanning facilities by suburban Minnesota adolescents. *Am J Pub Health* **84**: 476-478.
5. Rhainds M, De Guire L, Claveau J (1999) A population-based survey on the use of artificial tanning devices in the province of Québec, Canada. *J Am Acad Dermatol* **40**: 572-576.
6. Boldeman C, Beitner H, Jansson B, Nilsson B, Ullen H (1996) Sunbed use in relation to phenotype, erythema, sunscreen use and skin disease: A questionnaire survey among Swedish adolescents. *Br J Dermatol* **135**: 712-716.
7. Westherdahl J, Ingvar C, Masback A, Olsson H (2000) Risk of cutaneous malignant melanoma in relation to use of sunbeds: further evidence for UVA carcinogenicity. *Br J Cancer* **82**: 1593-1599.
8. Boldeman C, Bränström R, Dal H, *et al.* (2001). Tanning habits and sunburn in a Swedish population age 13-50 years. *Eur J Cancer* **37**: 2441-2448.
9. Naldi L, Gallus S, Imberti GL, Cainelli T, Negri E, La Vecchia C (2000) Sunlamps and sunbeds and the risk of cutaneous melanoma. *Eur J Cancer Prev* **9**: 133-134.
10. Monfrecola G, Fabbrocini G, Posteraro G, Pini D (2000) What do young people think about the dangers of sunbathing, skin cancer and sunbeds? A questionnaire survey among Italians. *Photodermatol Photoimmunol Photomed* **16**: 15-18.

11. Chouela E, Pellerano G, Bessone A, Ducard M, Poggio N, Abeldano A (1999). Sunbed use in Buenos Aires, Argentina. *Photodermatol Photoimmunol Photomed* **15**: 100-103.

12. Dobbinson S, Borland R (1999) Reaction to the 1997/98 SunSmart Campaign: results from a representative household survey of Victorians. In: Anti-Cancer Council of Victoria, eds. *SunSmart Evaluation Studies No 6.* Melbourne: Anti-Cancer Council of Victoria, pp. 69-92.

13. McGintley J, Martin CJ, MacKie RM (1998). Sunbeds in current use in Scotland: a survey of their output and patterns of use. *Br J Dermatol* **139**: 428-438.

14. Diffey BL, Farr PM, Ferguson J (1990) Tanning with ultraviolet A sunbeds. *Br Med J* **301**: 773-774.

15. Wright AL, Hart GC, Kernohan E, Twentyman G (1996) Survey of the variation in ultraviolet outputs from ultraviolet A sunbeds in Bradford. *Photodermatol Photoimmunol Photomed* **12**: 12-16.

16. Wright AL, Hart GC, Kernohan EE (1997) Dangers of sunbeds are greater in the commercial sector. *Br Med J* **314**: 1280-1281.

17. de Winter S, Pavel S. Zonnebanken: onduidelijk effect on huidkankerrisico (2000) [Tanning beds: effect on skin cancer risk unclear]. *Ned Tijdschr Geneeskd* **144**:467-470. (in Dutch).

18. Arthey S, Clarke VA (1995) Suntanning and sun protection: a review of the psychological literature. *Soc Sci Med* **40**: 265-274.

19. Nissen JB, Avrach WW, Hansen ES, Stengaard-Pedersen K, Kragballe K (1998) Increased levels of enkephalin following natural sunlight (combined with salt water bathing at the Dead Sea) and ultraviolet A irradiation. *Br J Dermatol* **139**: 1012-1019.

20. Lam RW, Buchanan A, Mador JA, Corral MR, Remick RA (1992) The effects of ultraviolet-A wavelengths in light therapy for seasonal depression. *J Affect Disord* **24**: 237-243.

21. Spencer JM, Amonette EA (1995) Indoor tanning: risks, benefits, and future trends. *J Am Acad Dermatol* **33**: 288-298.

22. Daxecker F, Blumthaler M, Ambach W. Keratitis solaris and sunbeds (1995) *Ophthalmologica* **209**: 329-330.

23. Latarjet J, Tranchant P, Boucaud C, Robert A, Foyatier JL (1993) Les brûlures sévères dues aux psoralènes (severe skin burns due to psoralens). *La Lettre du Brûlologue* **15**:2-3. (In French)

24. Diffey BL (1986) Use of UVA sunbeds for cosmetic tanning. *Br J Dermatol* **115**: 67-76.

25. Roza L, Baan RA, Van Der Leun JC, Kligman L (1989) UVA hazards in skin associated with the use of tanning equipment. *J Photochem Photobiol B: Biology* **3**: 281-287.

26. Autier P, Joarlette M, Lejeune F, Lienard D, Andre J, Achten G (1991) Cutaneous malignant melanoma and exposure to sunlamps and sunbeds: a descriptive study in Belgium. *Melanoma Res* **1**: 69-74.

27. Moseley H, Davidson M, Ferguson J (1998) A hazard assessment of artificial tanning units. *Photodermatol Photoimmunol Photomed* **14**: 79-87.

28. Wester U, Boldemann C, Jansson B, Ullén H (1999) Population UV-dose and skin area - Do sunbeds rival the sun? *Health Physics* **77**: 436-440.

29. Swerdlow AJ, English JSC, MacKie RM (1988) Fluorescent lights, ultraviolet lamps, and risk of cutaneous melanoma. *Br Med J* **297**: 647-650.

30. Walter SD, Marrett LD, From L, Hertzman C, Shannon HS, Roy P (1990) The association of cutaneous malignant melanoma with the use of sunbeds and sunlamps. *Am J Epidemiol* **131**: 232-243.

31. Westerdahl J, Olsson H, Masbäck A *et al* (1994) Use of sunbeds or sunlamps and malignant melanoma in Southern Sweden. *Am J Epidemiol* **140**: 691-699.

32. Chen Y, Dubrow R, Zheng T, Barnhill RL, Fine J, Berwick M (1998) Sunlamp use and the risk of cutaneous malignant melanoma: a population-based case-control study in Connecticut, USA. *Int J Epidemiol* **27**: 758-765.

33. Bajdik CD, Gallagher RP, Astrakiankis G, Hill GB, Fincham S, McLean DI (1996) Non-solar ultraviolet radiation and the risk of basal and squamous cell skin cancer. *Br J Cancer* **73**: 1612-1614.

34. Karagas MR, Stannard VA, Mott LA, Slattery MJ, Spencer SK, Weinstok MA (2002) Use of tanning devices and risk of basal cell and squamous cell skin cancers. *J Natl Cancer Inst* **94**: 224-226.

35. Turner RJ, Walshaw D, Diffey BL, Farr PM (2000) A controlled study of ultraviolet A sunbed treatment of psoriasis. *Br J Dermatol* **143**: 957-963.

36. Frentz G, Olsen JH, Avrach WW (1999) Malignant tumours and psoriasis: climatotherapy at the Dead Sea. *Br J Dermatol* **141**: 1088-1091.

37. Stern RS, Lunder EJ. Risk of squamous cell carcinoma and methoxsalen (psoralen) and UV-A radiation (PUVA) (1998) A meta-analysis. *Arch Dermatol* **134**:1582-1585.

38. Morison WL, Baughman RD, Day RM, *et al* (1998) Consensus workshop on the toxic effects of long-term PUVA therapy. *Arch Dermatol* **134**; 595-598.

39. Boffetta P, Gridley G, Lindelöf B (2001) Cancer risk in population-based cohort of patients hospitalised for psoriasis in Sweden. *J Invest Dermatol* **117**: 1531-1537.

40. Stern RS, Nichols KT, Vakeva LH (1997) Malignant melanoma in patients treated for psoriasis with methoxsalen (psoralen) and ultraviolet A radiation (PUVA). The PUVA Follow-Up Study. *N Engl J Med* **336**: 1041-1045.

41. Stern RS, and the PUVA Follow-up Study (2001) The risk of melanoma in association with long-term exposure to PUVA. *J Am Acad Dermatol* **44**: 755-761.

42. Pedeux R, Al-Irani N, Marteau C, *et al* (1998) Thymidine dinucleotide induce S phase cell cycle arrest in addition to increased melanogenesis in human melanocytes. *J Invest Dermatol* **111**: 472-477.

43. Woollons A, Clingen PH, Price ML, Arlett CF, Green MH (1997) Induction of mutagenic damage in human fibroblasts after exposure to artificial tanning lamps. *Br J Dermatol* **137**: 687-692.

44. Woollons A, Kipp C, Young AR, *et al.* (1999) The 0.8% ultraviolet B content of an ultraviolet A sunlamp induces 75% of cyclobutane pyrimidine dimers in human keratinocytes in vitro. *Br J Dermatol* **140**: 1023-1030.

45. Hemminki K, Bykov VJ, Marcuson JA (1999) Re: Sunscreen use and duration of sun exposure: A double-blind, randomised trial. *J Nat Cancer Inst* **91**: 2016-2047.

46. Bykov VJ, Marcusson JA, Hemminki K (2001) Protective effects of tanning on cutaneous melanoma. *Dermatology* **202**: 22-26.

47. Sheehan JM, Potten CS, Young AR (1998) Tanning in human skin types II and III offers modest photoprotection against erythema. *Photochem Photobiol* **68**: 588-592.

48. Barker D, Dixon K, Medrano EE, *et al* (1995) Comparison of the responses of human melanocytes with different melanin contents to ultraviolet B irradiation. *Cancer Res* **55**: 4041-4046.

49. Kvam E, Tyrell RM (1999) The role of melanin in the induction of oxidative DNA base damage by ultraviolet A irradiation of DNA or melanoma cells. *J Invest Dermatol* **113**: 209-213.

50. Dutch Cancer Society (1995) *Outdoors and Indoors: Sun Wisely.* Report on the "Sensible Sunbathing" Consensus Meeting held under the auspices of the Dutch Cancer Society in Utrecht on October 6, 1995.

51. de Gruijl FR (2000) Photocarcinogenesis: UVA vs UVB. *Methods Enzymol* **319**: 359-366.

52. Council on Scientific Affairs (1989) Harmful effects of ultraviolet radiation. *JAMA* **262**: 380-384.
53. Cascinelli N, Krutmann J, MacKie R, *et al* (1994) European School of Oncology advisory report. Sun exposure, UVA lamps and risk of skin cancer. *Eur J Cancer* **30A**: 548-560.
54. World Health Organisation (1994) *Environmental Health Criteria 160: Ultraviolet Radiation.* An authoritative scientific review of environmental and health effects of U.V. with reference to global ozone layer depletion. Joint publication by WHO, UNEP, ICNIRP, Geneva.
55. Boyle P, Veronesi U, Tubiana M, *et al.* (1995) European Code Against Cancer *Eur J Cancer* **31A**: 1395-1405.
56. Food and Drug Administration (1985) Sunlamps products: performance standards: final rule (21 CFR 1040). *Federal Register* **50**: 36548-36552.
57. European Committee for Electrotechnical Standardization (1992). *Safety of household and similar electrical appliances: Part 2: Particular requirements for ultra-violet and infra-red skin treatment appliances for household and similar use.* International Electrotechnical Commission IEC 335-2-27: 1987 + amendement 1: 1989 modified, Brussels.
58. International Non-Ionizing Radiation Committee of the International Radiation Protection Association (1991) Health issues of ultraviolet "A" sunbeds used for cosmetic purpose. *Health Physics* **61**: 285-288.
59. International Commission on Non-Ionizing Radiation Protection (1995) *Global Solar UV Index.* Publication ICNIRP - 1/95, Oberschleibheim, Germany.
60. Diffey BL, Farr PM (1991) Tanning with UVA and UVB: an appraisal of risks. *J Photochem Photobiol B Biol* **8**: 219-223.
61. Culley CA, Mayer JA, Eckhardt L, *et al* (2001) Compliance with federal and state legislation by indoor tanning facilities in San Diego. *J Am Acad Dermatol* **44**: 53-60.
62. Ross RN, Phillips B (1994) Twenty questions for tanning facility operators: a survey of operator knowledge. *Can J Public Health* **85**: 393-396.
63. Beasley TM, Kittel BS (1997) Factors that influence health risk behaviors among tanning salon patrons. *Eval Health Prof* **20**: 371-388.
64. Kwon HT, Mayer JA, Walker KK, Yu H, Lewis EC, Belch GE (2002) Promotion of frequent tanning sessions by indoor tanning facilities: two studies. *J Am Acad Dermatol* **46**: 700-705.

Chapter 10

Animal models of ultraviolet radiation-induced skin cancer

Vivienne E. Reeve[1], Ph.D.; Ronald D. Ley[2], Ph.D.
[1]Faculty of Veterinary Science, University of Sydney, New South Wales, Australia; [2]Department of Cell Biology and Physiology, University of New Mexico, School of Medicine, Albuquerque, NM, USA

Key words: mouse, wavelength dependence, DNA damage, immune suppression, chemoprevention

INTRODUCTION

Solar ultraviolet (UV) radiation induces a number of pathologic conditions in mammals including erythema, edema, sunburn cell formation, immunosuppression, skin cancer and cataracts. Animal models have been invaluable in the study of the underlying mechanisms involved in the induction of these pathologies. Furthermore, animal-based studies have been very useful in determining efficacies of preventive and therapeutic modalities. As cancer formation is the result of an interactive series of events, the use of whole animals is essential to the study of this process. The following presents the results of animal studies that have provided significant understanding of photocarcinogenesis.

D. Hill et al. (eds.), Prevention of Skin Cancer, 177-194.
© 2004 Kluwer Academic Publishers. Printed in the Netherlands.

1.   ANIMAL MODELS OF ULTRAVIOLET RADIATION-INDUCED SKIN CANCER

Animal models of human disease have been of tremendous value in determining risk factors and underlying mechanisms of various diseases including skin cancer. The mouse model for skin cancer, particularly the albino hairless mouse, has been used extensively for over 25 years. Mice develop squamous cell carcinomas in response to chronic UV exposure. In contrast to humans, basal cell carcinomas and melanomas have not been described. Recently, techniques of engineering the murine genome have provided transgenic and gene knockout mice that have given insight into the role of various pathways in the formation of UV radiation-induced skin cancer.

One of the earlier transgenic mice used in UV radiation-induced skin cancer studies was a strain of mouse which carried the SV40 T antigen under control of the tyrosine promoter and expressed only in melanocytes [1]. The transgenic animals develop spontaneous cutaneous and ocular melanoma and short-term exposure to relatively low doses of UV radiation accelerates the appearance of melanotic tumors. Other transgenic mouse lines have been established with a mutated human Ha-ras gene also under control of the tyrosinase promoter [2]. These mice are susceptible to the induction of melanomas upon exposure to UV radiation alone. More recently, a further transgenic mouse in which the metallothionein gene promoter forces the overexpression of hepatocyte growth factor/scatter factor (HGF/SF), and in which sporadic melanomas develop spontaneously with aging, was found to respond to a single burning dose of UV radiation to neonates (but not adults) with subsequent accelerated melanoma development. In this mouse, the melanomas resembled human melanomas in their epidermal involvement [3].

A number of studies have been carried out using knockout mice that lack the TP53 tumor suppressor gene or the xeroderma pigmentosum group A (XPA) and group C (XPC) genes. Mice lacking one or both copies of the TP53 gene have increased susceptibility to UV-induced skin cancer with the homozygous knockout being the more susceptible [4,5]. The XPA and XPC knockout mice are deficient in nucleotide excision repair (NER) and express enhanced susceptibility to UV radiation-induced skin cancer [6,7]. Knockout mice also have been constructed that have defects in one of the two subpathways of NER, transcription-coupled repair (TCR) and global genomic repair (GGR) [8]. Deficiencies in these two pathways have different effects on susceptibility to UV radiation-induced pathologies of the skin. The absence of TCR results in higher susceptibility to sunburn than does the absence of GGR. Conversely, GGR-deficient mice are more susceptible to UV radiation-induced skin carcinogenesis than TCR-deficient mice. Both TCR- and GGR-deficient mice are more susceptible to sunburn and skin carcinogenesis than wildtype animals [8].

While a number of animal models have been used to study the induction of cutaneous melanoma, the majority of these models require treatment with chemical carcinogens with or without exposure to UV radiation for melanoma formation [9]. This includes a xenograft model with human skin on a RAG-1 mouse that is immunologically suppressed [10]. Induction of melanoma in the human skin grafts required treatment with 7,12-dimethyl(a)benzanthracene and UV radiation. In three non-murine species, however, melanoma has been induced upon exposure to UV radiation alone. These three species are the Angora goat [11], the South American opossum *Monodelphis domestica* [12], and hybrids or backcrosses of species of *Xiphophorus* (hybrid fish) [13]. Both the opossum and *Xiphophorus* species can remove UV radiation-induced pyrimidine dimers in DNA by enzymatic photoreactivation [9]. Photoreactivation is a light-dependent process whereby UV radiation-induced dimers between adjacent pyrimidines on the same DNA strand can be split *in situ* by the combined action of the photoreactivation enzyme and radiation in the region of 300-500 nm. In both models, photoreactivation has been used to identify pyrimidine dimers as initiating lesions for the formation of UV radiation-induced melanoma [12,13].

2.   WAVELENGTH DEPENDENCE FOR THE INDUCTION OF NON-MELANOMA SKIN CANCER IN ANIMAL MODELS

A wavelength dependency for the induction of non-melanoma skin cancer in mice has been constructed from the wealth of data that came from the Photobiology Unit of the former Skin and Cancer Hospital in Philadelphia and the Department of Dermatology of the University of Utrecht. Squamous cell carcinomas were induced in Skh hairless, albino mice with chronic exposure to 14 different broad-spectrum UV radiation sources. The tumor induction data from these studies were used to generate an action spectrum which transformed the various tumor responses obtained with different wavelength spectra into a common dose-response relationship [14]. The general shape of the skin cancer action spectrum in mice is similar to the action spectrum for the induction of erythema in humans [15]. It is also interesting to note that the peaks of both the action spectrum for the induction of skin cancer in mice [14] and for the induction of pyrimidine dimers in mouse epidermal DNA [16] are at 293 nm. This similarity of action spectra supports the notion that pyrimidine dimers are the initiating lesion for UV-induced skin cancer in the mouse.

3.   WAVELENGTH DEPENDENCE FOR THE INDUCTION OF MELANOMA IN ANIMAL MODELS

Xiphophorus and *M. domestica* have been used to investigate wavelength dependency for the induction of melanoma. Studies to date with the fish model indicate that wavelengths in the UVA (320-400 nm) and visible range are orders of magnitude more effective at inducing melanoma than would be predicted from the action spectra for erythema induction in humans or non-melanoma skin cancer in mice [17]. Contrary to what was observed with the fish model, the ability of UVA to induce melanoma (or melanoma precursors) in the opossum [18] is not substantially greater than would be predicted from its capacity to induce non-melanoma skin cancer in mice [14] or erythema in humans [15]. Thus, the action spectrum for melanoma induction in the fish model would *not* be expected to predict susceptibility to melanoma in mammals. This conclusion is supported by neonatal exposure of *M. domestica* to UVB, which resulted in widespread melanoma formation [19] but extremely low melanoma susceptibility upon exposure to UVA [20].

4.   MOLECULAR EVENTS

4.1   DNA damage induction and repair

The relative abundance of various classes of DNA damage changes as a function of wavelength of UV radiation exposure [21]. Exposure to shorter wavelengths of UV radiation in the UVB regions induces predominantly *cyclobutane pyrimidine dimers*. Two adjacent pyrimidines can be photodimerized with the loss of the 5,6 double bonds and formation of a four-carbon cyclobutane ring. In addition to the cyclobutane pyrimidine dimers, the *pyrimidine-pyrimidone 6-4 photoproduct* is also formed at the shorter wavelengths. This 6-4 adduct results from a single covalent linkage between the 6 carbon of one pyrimidine and the 4 carbon of an adjacent pyrimidine. The 6-4 photoproducts are less frequent than the cyclobutane pyrimidine dimers. Both photoproducts are formed upon direct absorption of UVB by DNA.

At the longer wavelengths in the UVA portion of the wavelength spectrum, the low energy photons are weakly absorbed by DNA but are capable of generating reactive oxygen species (ROS) through interaction with cellular photosensitizers. The oxidative DNA base damage, *7,8-dihydro-8-oxoguanine*, is induced in DNA upon exposure to UVA and the sensitized generation of singlet oxygen [22]. It has been estimated that exposure of the skin to solar radiation, which provides a proportion of UVB to UVA of approximately 1 to 20, could oxidize an amount of guanine equal to or greater than the number of cyclobutane dimers induced by direct absorption [22]. This could make oxidative damage in the form of 7,8-dihydro-8-oxoguanine a significant factor in the induction of skin cancer by sunlight [22], and would suggest that antioxidants may provide an effective means of preventing skin cancer in humans.

The rates of induction of DNA damage in skin exposed chronically to UV radiation are altered by UV radiation-induced changes in the optical properties of the skin [23-25]. Attenuation of levels of photoproducts in the skin can be attributed to melanogenesis, epidermal hyperplasia and increased thickness of the stratum corneum. These changes have the potential of confounding quantitative dose-response relationships in photocarcinogenesis.

A number of pathways are present in skin to repair UV radiation-induced DNA damage. *Monodelphis domestica* (see above) possesses a light-activated repair pathway that specifically repairs UV radiation-induced pyrimidine dimers in DNA. Photoreactivation repair does not appear to be active in mice and its presence in human skin is controversial [26]. Nucleotide excision repair (NER) is present in human, murine and marsupial skin [21,27]. This repair process is active on both UV radiation- and chemically-induced DNA damage. NER requires numerous gene products to: 1) recognize the DNA damage; 2) incise the damaged strand on both sides of the lesion; 3) remove the damaged nucleotide and adjacent nucleotides; 4) fill in the gap with DNA repair synthesis; and, 5) ligate the newly synthesized region to the existing strand. The importance of this process in preventing skin cancer is obvious from the high risk of skin cancer in individuals who suffer from the xeroderma pigmentosum syndrome (XP) [28].

4.2   Mutations in critical genes

The TP53 gene product is a multifunctional protein involved in transcription, cell cycle regulation, apoptosis and DNA repair (for review see reference [29]). Mutations in the TP53 gene are found in over 50% of all human cancers. In UV radiation-induced non-melanoma skin cancer, TP53 mutations have been found in 90% of all squamous cell carcinomas and ~50% of all basal cell carcinomas [30]. The majority of these mutations were cytosine-to-thymine (C→T) or CC→TT transitions, the signature mutations of UV radiation exposure [30]. Alterations in the TP53 gene or in p53 expression are also involved in melanoma formation, but to a lesser extent than in non-melanoma skin cancer [31]. Mutations in the TP53 gene and the p16 gene similar to those found in human skin cancers have also been described in UV radiation-induced skin cancers in mice (see Chapter 7).

5.   IMMUNOSUPPRESSION

5.1   Photoimmunosuppression and skin cancer

Some decades ago, it became apparent that UV radiation-induced murine skin cancers differed from cancers induced in mice by chemical carcinogens, being particularly resistant to successful transplantation to syngeneic mice. It was observed however that the transplanted tumors would survive and grow in the host, if the mouse was pretreated with immunosuppressive drugs or X-radiation, or interestingly, if the mouse was pretreated with a sub-carcinogenic dose of UV radiation. Thus, the observations that UV radiation-induced tumors were relatively highly antigenic, and that pre-transplantation irradiation of the host mouse with UV radiation could supply the necessary immune suppression to support their ongrowth, formed the founding basis of the science of photoimmunology. It was soon demonstrated in mice receiving chronic UV irradiations in order to induce skin cancer, that the injection of T lymphocytes purified from other UV-irradiated donor mice accelerated the production of the skin tumors [32], confirming that suppressive immune cells were generated in the spleen by even sub-carcinogenic UV doses, and were regulators of tumor development. Therefore, in addition to the primary initiation of the skin tumor by the DNA-damaging effect of UV radiation, a secondary activity could also be assigned to UV radiation, that of suppression of the immune system preventing tumor recognition and rejection.

5.2   Characteristics of immunosuppression

Studies then proceeded to identify the characteristics of this photoimmunosuppression, and to reveal the pathways by which it was induced. The early studies found that UV irradiated skin became depleted of Langerhans cells, and was thus defective in normal antigen presentation

[33]. They also found that T cell mediated immune functions specifically were impaired, whereas B cell activity and humoral immunity remained normal. The contact hypersensitivity and delayed type hypersensitivity reactions, being typical T cell mediated responses, became ideal assay methods for measuring the relevant immune function, and were shown to be readily suppressed by UV radiation exposure, even at moderate doses. It was shown that photoimmunosuppression could be revealed by contact sensitization of the mouse, both through the locally irradiated (and Langerhans cell-depleted) skin and through distant unirradiated skin [34]; in other words, that the immune suppression was a systemic defect.

In addition to suppression of the contact and delayed type hypersensitivity reactions, evidence is accumulating to show that other T cell regulated immune responses are sensitive to UV radiation. There is accumulating evidence of exacerbated severity of several microbiological and parasitic infections, e.g., *Herpes simplex*, *Mycobacteria*, *Candida*, *Leishmania*, *Listeria*, *Trichinella* [35-37]. Vaccination responses have also been found to be decreased by UV irradiation [38]. It is likely that the T cell immune defects that have been identified in response to UV irradiation may represent only a minor proportion of the real effect of this ubiquitous environmental immunosuppressant on human and animal health.

5.3   Photoimmunosuppression in humans

In humans, the association between skin cancer risk and immunosuppression was first observed in renal transplant patients, who were surviving for extended periods as improved immunosuppressive drugs were developed [39]. However, the onset of multiple and aggressive skin cancers after some years of successful transplant function was unexpected and difficult to control without terminating the immunosuppressive therapy. Apart from the transplant patients, it has been reported that skin cancer patients can invariably be categorized as "UV-sensitive" for their susceptibility to immunosuppression by UV radiation [40]. Other observations have revealed that sun-exposed skin sites on humans are less able to respond immunologically to sensitizers in the delayed type hypersensitivity reaction [41], and in patients with the hereditary disease, xeroderma pigmentosum, in which there is an inability to repair UV radiation-induced DNA damage, and a great susceptibility to skin cancers at an early age, there is a concomitant defective T cell immunity [42]. Experimentally, UV irradiation has been shown to result in Langerhans depletion and depressed delayed type hypersensitivity in human subjects [38].

5.4   Cutaneous photoreceptors for immunosuppression

Action spectrum studies in mice found that photoimmunosuppression was a property of the shortest UVB waveband occurring in terrestrial sunlight, the peak response being at 260-280 nm [43]. Therefore, a photoreceptor was sought which would possess the relevant UV radiation absorption characteristics, and be localized in the epidermal layer, since UVB radiation does not penetrate deeper into the skin, and two contenders were identified. Firstly the epidermal DNA itself, and secondly an epidermal molecule localized particularly in the stratum corneum, *trans*-urocanic acid (deaminated histidine), which photoisomerizes to *cis*-urocanic acid upon UVB exposure. The most abundant UVB-induced DNA lesion was known to be the cyclobutane pyrimidine dimer; enhanced repair of these dimers in the skin of the mouse [44] or the opossum, *M. domestica* [45], was shown to prevent photoimmunosuppression. At the same time, *cis*-urocanic acid was found to have immunosuppressive properties that simulated the UVB effects on contact hypersensitivity [46], and together with the pyrimidine dimer, accounted for the mediators of two apparently independent pathways leading to the UVB-induced immune defect.

5.5   Urocanic acid photoimmunology

Mice can be readily immunosuppressed by exogenous *cis*-urocanic acid administered topically or parenterally whereas the *trans* isomer is inactive [47,48]. Examination of the immune altering properties of a series of structural analogues of *cis*-urocanic acid revealed that histamine was similarly immunosuppressive, and subsequently it was shown that histamine receptor antagonists like cimetidine were protective against photoimmunosuppression, and therefore that histamine played a key role in the immunosuppression. While keratinocytes do release some histamine after UV radiation exposure, the major source of histamine seems to be the dermal mast cells, which infiltrate the dermis shortly after UV radiation exposure. Dermal mast cell prevalence was shown to correlate with *cis*-urocanic acid-induced immunosuppression, implying a synergy between histamine and *cis*-urocanic acid resulting in immunosuppression [49].

5.6   Other immunosuppressive mediators

Other molecules responding to UVB irradiation have been identified as photoimumune modulators. Prostaglandins, particularly prostaglandin-E2, appear to be a prerequisite for immunosuppression by both UVB radiation [50] and *cis*-urocanic acid, and their synthesis to be a histamine-dependent response following UV irradiation [51]. In fact, the synergy between histamine and *cis*-urocanic acid resulted in increased prostaglandin-E2 formation [52], and furthermore, the inhibition of prostaglandin-E2 synthesis by the cyclooxygenase inhibitor, the non-steroidal anti-inflammatory drug indomethacin, was shown to be photoimmunoprotective [52]. It remains unclear just how these molecules activate the immune suppression.

In addition, the cytokine response to UV radiation is robust, a large array of these immune-mediating protein messengers being released from the irradiated keratinocytes. Identification of the key cytokines that might result in photoimmunosuppression has been difficult; however, it is now apparent that the creation of a preponderance of cytokines functionally associated with the class of T helper-2 cells over the T helper-1 cytokines like interferon-gamma and interleukin-12 is critical to photoimmunosuppression [53]. The use of cytokine gene knockout mice has been important in assigning the major immunosuppressive function to the over-expression of the T helper-2 interleukins-4 and -10. There also appears to be a role for the pleiotropic cytokines, tumor necrosis factor-alpha and interleukin-6 [54,55], which can display either T helper-1 or -2 characteristics under different conditions, although this is less well understood. Further, the apoptosis pathway plays a role in photoimmunosuppression, and the expression of the apoptotic ligand known as FasL is intimately involved with at least local photoimmunosuppression [56]. Co-stimulatory factors like the intercellular adhesion molecules also seem to be involved [57].

Recently it has become apparent that oxidative processes are also related to photoimmunosuppression, and to the actions of *cis*-urocanic acid. A variety of antioxidants, both endogenous – such as vitamin C [58], vitamin E [59], carnosine [60], metallothionein [61], glutathione and N-acetylcysteine [62] – and exogenous plant derived compounds, usually of flavonoid structure – such as green tea polyphenols [63] or fruit and vegetable-derived phenolic flavonoids [64], or sulfydryl-rich garlic [65] – effectively prevent the immunosuppression in mice. Upregulation of enzymatic antioxidant defenses, for example of the oxidative stress-responsive enzyme haem oxygenase by UVA irradiation, also provides immunoprotection from UVB radiation and *cis*-urocanic acid [66].

The exact oxidative reactions associated with photoimmunosuppression are unclear at present. Since several of the immune-protective antioxidants have been shown to antagonize *cis*-urocanic acid, and since the immunosuppressive action of *cis*-urocanic acid does not appear to function by the induction of cytokine derangements [67], perhaps the cyclooxygenase pathway accounts for the oxidant requirement for photoimmunosuppression downstream from both *cis*-urocanic acid formation and cytokine activity.

6. PREVENTION OF PHOTOCARCINOGENESIS
(see also Chapter 8)

6.1 Sunscreens

Since sunscreens contain UVB-absorbers to protect from sunburn, and the action spectrum for photoimmunosuppression peaks also in the UVB waveband, it is reasonable to predict that sunscreens will also protect from immunosuppression. However, there is great controversy on this issue, and the outcomes from the many murine studies that have used a variety of UV radiation sources, UV radiation dosages, UV radiation-absorbing sunscreen ingredients, and different assays of immune function, have been confusing. It seems that sunscreens protect less well from photoimmunosuppression than from sunburn, but experiments comparing different UV radiation-absorbers have not been technically comparable or informative, nor have the studies been extended to chronic irradiation regimes in order to demonstrate the effect on photocarcinogenesis. There is a pressing need for good controlled studies in this area, since protection from photoimmunosuppression in humans should result in protection from the secondary promotion phase of skin tumor development for tumors initiated by either inadvertent unprotected sunlight exposure or the breakthrough UVB radiation penetrating a sunscreen. The latest epidemiological data indicate that sunscreen usage in humans may provide protection from squamous cell carcinoma, but there is inadequate evidence for protection from the commonest human skin cancer, basal cell carcinoma, or from melanoma [68].

6.2 Dietary fat

The promotion phase of chemical carcinogenesis has long been recognized to be modulated by dietary lipids, being enhanced by both increased lipid content of the diet, and by increased polyunsaturated fatty acid content. More recently, skin cancer outgrowth has been observed to follow the same trend, and high polyunsaturated corn or sunflower oil content accelerated the appearance of tumors induced in mice by UV radiation, whereas hydrogenated corn or sunflower oil retarded them [69]. The dietary fat effects, both qualitative and quantitative, are significant even if applied after the UV-initiation of the tumors, and are related to their modulation of the immune response to UV radiation [70]. Thus, feeding a polyunsaturated sunflower oil-based diet resulted in exacerbated suppression of contact hypersensitivity by both UVB radiation and *cis*-urocanic acid, in comparison with feeding predominantly saturated butterfat [71]. In chronically UV-irradiated mice, a low corn oil diet (0.75% oil) significantly protected the delayed type hypersensitivity response, the production of suppressor T lymphocytes, and the ability to reject a transplanted UV radiation-induced tumor, in comparison with a high corn oil diet (12% oil) [72]. In a study feeding mixed fat diets to mice, it was shown that the greater the proportion of polyunsaturated fat, the greater was both the photoimmunosuppression and the photocarcinogenic response [70].

Studies have also compared the effect of feeding increased omega-3 fatty acids such as are found in fish oils, with the plant-derived omega-6 fats in corn oil, and have reported a marked reduction in UV radiation-induced tumor development by omega-3-containing menhaden (from mackerel) oil [73]. The omega-3 fats compete with omega-6-derived arachidonic acid for the production of pro-inflammatory prostaglandins like prostaglandin-E2, and menhaden oil diets have been found to suppress dramatically the increase in plasma and cutaneous prostaglandin-E2 levels in response to UV irradiation. The importance of prostaglandin-E2 for the photoimmunosuppression that is associated with the enhancement of photocarcinogenesis becomes evident again in these studies, and is consistent with the observations that indomethacin inhibits both UVB- and *cis*-urocanic acid-induced suppression of contact hypersensitivity [52] and the expression of photocarcinogenesis in the mouse [74]. Very recently, additional studies in the mouse [75] have shown that the selective inhibition by the drug celecoxib of the inducible form of cyclooxygenase (cyclooxygenase-2), the prostaglandin synthesizing enzyme, also has dramatic protective effects against photocarcinogenesis. The advantage of inhibiting only cyclooxygenase-2 is the avoidance of the gastrointestinal damaging effects incurred by inhibition of constitutive cyclooxygenase-1. Human actinic keratoses, squamous cell carcinoma and keratoacanthomas (but not basal cell carcinoma) all expressed high amounts of cyclooxygenase-2, suggesting that these lesions could be targeted effectively by selective cyclooxygenase-2 inhibitors.

6.3 Phytochemicals

Flavonoids are polyphenolic ring compounds occurring naturally in a wide variety of plants and vegetables. They have been found to have anti-carcinogenic properties in numerous experimental models of chemically induced cancers. They are also antioxidants, and are effective free radical scavengers, consistent with their having been shown to inhibit both chemical carcinogen tumor initiation, which requires oxidative metabolism of the environmental pre-carcinogen, and tumor promotion by phorbol esters, which is also oxidant-dependent. Their antioxidant role has been demonstrated by their ability to upregulate the endogenous cellular antioxidants such as glutathione, glutathione peroxidase, catalase, systems that become depleted with chronic UV irradiation, and it has been suggested that therapy with endogenous antioxidants, either administered or stimulated, might offer superior UV radiation photoprotection [76]. Flavonoids also act as inhibitors of the tyrosine kinases that activate certain oncogenes and growth factors like epidermal growth factor, and can thus affect cell proliferative responses. Flavonoids also can induce apoptosis. The isoflavones comprise a subclass of flavonoids and have a molecular structure enabling them to display oestrogenic activity. The prototype isoflavone, genistein, has been most intensely studied, and is known for its occurrence, together with daidzein, in the soyabean. Other leguminous plants, such as red clover, are claimed to have a higher and more varied isoflavone content.

A hallmark premutagenic lesion induced by many oxidatively active reactants in the DNA, including UV radiation, is 7,8-dihydro-8-oxoguanine, but its significance to photocarcinogenesis is not yet clear. However, genistein has protected from 7,8-dihydro-8-oxoguanine formation by UVC radiation *in vitro* [77], and from tumor promoter-induced expression of the oncogenes c-*fos* and c-*jun* in mouse skin [78]. Genistein has been found to inhibit the UVB-induced production of prostaglandin-E2 in human epidermal cultures and in human skin [79], the inhibition of UVB-induction of cyclooxygenase-2 perhaps being mediated via its tyrosine kinase suppression. It is therefore predictable that flavonoids will inhibit UV radiation-induced immunosuppression, as has been reported for a diet of fruits and vegetables extract, and for the flavonoids quercetin and chrysin, when fed to hairless mice undergoing chronic UV irradiation. Unexpectedly, quercetin was not found to inhibit photocarcinogenesis [64,80], whereas the flavonoid apigenin, also widespread through the edible plants and vegetables, significantly inhibited photocarcinogenesis in mice when applied topically [81]. Apigenin induces cell cycle arrest in keratinocytes and fibroblasts, suggesting that it may check uncontrolled mitosis of tumor cells via a mechanism inducing the cyclin dependent kinase inhibitor p21, an effector of the p53 tumor suppressor protein [82]. A study in mice with an isoflavone, equol (a daidzein metabolite that has been identified in human urine), has provided dose-responsive data for protection from UV radiation-induced suppression of contact hypersensitivity when applied topically. The equol was remarkably efficacious, at lotion concentrations of 5-20 uM [83]. Silymarin is yet another flavonoid, isolated from the milk thistle, that has been found to protect from photocarcinogenesis and co-carcinogenesis of 7,12-dimethylbenz(a)anthracene plus chronic UV irradiation, when applied topically to mouse skin. In addition, the silymarin inhibited sunburn and sunburn cell formation in the epidermis, edema, the depletion of catalase, and the induction of cyclooxygenase activity [84].

The polyphenolic catechins found in tea are also flavonoids, and have been extensively studied as anti-carcinogenic agents, especially towards photocarcinogenesis in mice. Green tea polyphenols in the drinking water or applied topically, have inhibited photoimmunosuppression [63], photocarcinogenesis, the "sunburn" reaction, co-carcinogenesis induced by 7,12-dimethylbenz(a)anthracene and chronic UV irradiation, and the progression of skin tumors towards malignancy [85,86]. It is consistent that the green tea polyphenols also enhance the endogenous antioxidant enzymes in various tissues, including the skin [87].

CONCLUSIONS

Models of UV radiation-induced skin carcinogenesis in normal, mutant or transgenic mouse strains have provided valuable information on the genetic damage critical to skin tumor production, the importance of damage repair capacity, the UV wavelength dependency, and the regulatory influence of the immune system. The clarification of the photocarcinogenic and photoimmunosuppressive UV waveband in mice has been the basis for the design of UV-blocking sunscreening products for humans. The murine models have also been used extensively to identify chemopreventive strategies that can be applied orally or topically for the inhibition of tumor growth.

SUMMARY POINTS

- Mouse models for the UV induction of squamous cell carcinoma and melanoma have been developed.
- The DNA-damaging lesions and the genetic location of the important mutations have been identified.
- The role of the UV-immunosuppressed state in regulating skin tumor growth is partially clarified in mouse skin.
- Protection by sunscreens and chemoprevention by antioxidants, reduced dietary fat and various phytochemicals has been demonstrated in mice.

IMPLICATIONS FOR PUBLIC HEALTH

The similarity of the action spectra for non-melanoma skin cancer induction in mice, DNA damage in mice, and erythema induction in human skin, indicates that strategies that have been found to protect mice from photocarcinogenesis may also inhibit at least squamous cell carcinoma development in humans. Thus UVB-blocking sunscreens, primarily developed to prevent sunburn, can be expected also to protect from non-melanocytic skin cancer. There is, however, uncertainty about the wavelength dependency for melanoma induction as the animal models for this cancer are less effective models of human melanoma. Photoimmunosuppression in mice has a strong pro-photocarcinogenic effect that has human parallels, and therefore methods found in mice to protect the immune system from UV radiation are also likely to be immunoprotective in humans. Mouse studies have indicated that there is a significant contribution of UV-induced oxidative damage to both photoimmunosuppression and photocarcinogenesis, and the future development of the use of exogenous antioxidants, topically or as dietary supplements, is anticipated to have a chemopreventive effect against human skin cancers.

REFERENCES

1. Klein-Szanto AJ, Silvers WK, Mintz B (1994) Ultraviolet radiation-induced malignant skin melanoma in melanoma-susceptible transgenic mice. *Cancer Res* **17:** 4569-4572.
2. Broome Powell M, Gause PR, Hyman P, *et al.* (1999) Induction of melanoma in Tpras transgenic mice. *Carcinogenesis* **20:** 1747-1753.
3. Noonan FP, Recio JA, Takayama H, *et al.* (2001) Neonatal sunburn and melanoma in mice. *Nature* **413:** 271-272.
4. Li G, Ho VC, Berean K, Tron VA (1995) Ultraviolet radiation induction of squamous cell carcinomas in p53 transgenic mice. *Cancer Res* **55:** 2070-2074.
5. Jiang W, Ananthaswamy HN, Muller HK, Kripke ML (1999) p53 protects against skin cancer induction by UV-B radiation. *Oncogene* **18:** 4247-4253.
6. De Vries A, Berg RJ, Wijnhoven S, *et al.* (1998) XPA-deficiency in hairless mice causes a shift in skin tumor types and mutational target genes after exposure to low doses of U.V.B. *Oncogene* **16:** 2205-2212.
7. Van Steeg H, Mullenders LH, Vijg J (2000) Mutagenesis and carcinogenesis in nucleotide excision repair-deficient XPA knock out mice. *Mutat Res* **450:**167-180.
8. Berg RJ, Rebel H, van der Horst GT, *et al.* (2000) Impact of global genome repair versus transcription-coupled repair on ultraviolet carcinogenesis in hairless mice. *Cancer Res* **60:** 2858-2863.
9. Kusewitt DF, Ley RD (1996) Animal models of melanoma. *Cancer Surveys* **26:** 35-70.
10. Atillasoy ES, Seykora JT, Soballe PW, *et al.* (1998) UVB induces atypical melanocytic lesions and melanoma in human skin. *Amer J Path* **152:** 1179-1186.

11. Green A, Neale R, Kelly R, *et al.* (1996) An animal model for human melanoma. *Photochem Photobiol* **64:** 577-580.
12. Ley RD, Applegate LA, Padilla RS, Stuart TD (1989) Ultraviolet radiation-induced malignant melanoma in *Monodelphis domestica. Photochem Photobiol* **50:** 105.
13. Setlow RB, Woodhead AD, Grist E (1989) Animal model for ultraviolet radiation-induced melanoma: platyfish-swordtail hybrid. *Proc Natl Acad Sci USA* **86:** 8922-8926.
14. De Gruijl FR, Henricus JCM, Sterenborg P, *et al.* (1993) Wavelength dependence of skin cancer induction by ultraviolet irradiation of albino hairless mice. *Cancer Res* **53:** 53-60.
15. Parrish JA, Jaenicke KF, Anderson RR (1982) Erythema and melanogenesis action spectra of normal human skin. *Photochem Photobiol* **36:** 187-191.
16. Ley RD, Peak MJ, Lyon L (1983) Induction of pyrimidine dimers in epidermal DNA of hairless mice by UV-B: An action spectrum. *J Invest Dermatol* **80:** 188-189.
17. Setlow RB, Grist E, Thompson K, Woodhead AD (1993) Wavelengths effective in induction of malignant melanoma. *Proc Natl Acad Sci USA* **90:** 6666-6670.
18. Ley RD (2001) Dose Response for Ultraviolet Radiation A-Induced Focal Melanocytic Hyperplasia and Non-melanoma Skin Tumors in *Monodelphis domestica. Photochem Photobiol* **73:** 20-23.
19. Robinson ES, Hubbard GB, Colon G, Vandeberg JL (1998) Low-dose ultraviolet exposure early in development can lead to widespread melanoma in the opossum model. *Int J Exp Path* **79:** 235-244.
20. Robinson ES, Hill RH, Kripke ML, Setlow RB (2000) The *Monodelphis* melanoma model: Initial report on large ultraviolet A exposures of suckling young. *Photochem Photobiol* **71:** 743-746.
21. Black HS, de Gruijl FR, Forbes PD, *et al.* (1997) Photocarcinogenesis: an overview. *J Photochem Photobiol B.* **40:**29-47.
22. Kvam E, Tyrrell RM (1997) Induction of oxidative DNA base damage in human skin cells by UV and near visible radiation. *Carcinogenesis* **18:** 2379-2384.
23. de Gruijl FR, Berg RJ (1998) In situ molecular dosimetry and tumor risk: UV-induced DNA damage and tumor latency time. *Photochem Photobiol* **68:** 555-560.
24. Mitchell DL, Greinert R, De Gruijl FR, *et al.* (1999) Effects of chronic low-dose ultraviolet B radiation on DNA damage and repair in mouse skin. *Cancer Res* **59:** 2875-2884.
25. Mitchell DL, Byrom M, Chiarello S, Lowery MG (2001) Attenuation of DNA damage in the dermis and epidermis of the albino hairless mouse by chronic exposure to ultraviolet-A and –B radiation. *Photochem Photobiol* **73:** 83-89.
26. Ley RD (1993) Photoreactivation in humans (Commentary). *Proc Natl Acad Sci USA* **90:** 4337.
27. Applegate LA, Ley RD (1987) Excision repair of pyrimidine dimers in marsupial cells. *Photochem Photobiol* **45:** 241-245.
28. van Steeg H, Kraemer KH (1999) Xeroderma pigmentosum and the role of UV-induced DNA damage in skin cancer. *Molec Med Today* **5:** 86-94.
29. Selivanova G, Wiman KG (1995) p53: A cell cycle regulator activated by DNA damage. *Adv Cancer Res* **66:** 143-180.
30. Ziegler A, Leffell DJ, Kunala S, *et al.* (1993) Mutation hotspots due to sunlight in the p53 gene of nonmelanoma skin cancers. *Proc Natl Acad Sci USA* **90:** 4216-4220.
31. Weiss J, Schwechheimer K, Cavenee WK, *et al.* (1993) Mutation and expression of the p53 gene in malignant melanoma cell lines. *Int J Cancer* **54:** 693-699.
32. Fisher MS, Kripke ML (1982) Suppressor T lymphocytes control the development of primary skin cancers in UV-irradiated mice. *Science* **216:** 1133-1134.

33. Aberer W, Schuler G, Stingl G, Honigsman H, Wolff K (1981) UV light depletes surface markers of Langerhans cells. *J Invest Dermatol* **76**: 202-210.

34. Noonan FP, De Fabo EC (1990) Ultraviolet B dose response curves for local and systemic immunosuppression are identical. *Photochem Photobiol* **52**: 801-810.

35. Goettsch W, Garssen J, Deijns A, De Gruijl FR, Van Loveren H (1994) UVB exposure impairs resistance to infection by *Trichinella spiralis*. *Environ Health Perspect* **102**: 298-301.

36. Yasumoto S., Hayashi Y, Aurelian L (1987) Immunity to Herpes simplex virus Type 2: Suppression of virus induced immune responses in ultraviolet B-irradiated mice. *J Immunol* **139**: 2788-2793.

37. Jeevan A, Brown E, Kripke ML (1995) UV and infectious diseases. In: Krutmann J, Elmets CA, eds. *Photoimmunology*. Oxford: Blackwell Sci., pp. 153-163.

38. Cooper KD, Oberhelman L, Hamilton TA, *et al.* (1992) UV exposure reduces immunization rates and promotes tolerance to epicutaneous antigens in humans: relationship to dose, CD1a-DR+ epidermal macrophage induction, and Langerhans cell depletion. *Proc Natl Acad Sci USA* **89**: 8497-8501.

39. Sheil AGR, Mahoney JF, Horvath JS, *et al.* (1981) Cancer following successful cadaveric donor renal transplant. *Transplantation Proc* **XII**: 733-735.

40. Yoshikawa T, Rae V, Bruins-Slot W, Van den Berg JW, Taylor JR, Streilein JW (1990) Susceptibility to effects of UV radiation on induction of contact hypersensitivity as a risk factor for skin cancer. *J Invest Dermatol* **95**: 530-536.

41. O'Dell BL, Jessen RT, Becker LE, Jackson RT, Smith EB (1980) Diminished immune response in sun-damaged skin. *Arch Dermatol* **116**: 559-561.

42. Morison WL, Bucana C, Hashem N, Kripke ML, Cleaver JE, German JL (1985) Impaired immune function in patients with xeroderma pigmentosum. *Cancer Res* **45**: 3929-3931.

43. De Fabo EC, Kripke ML (1980) Wavelength dependence and dose-rate independence of UV radiation-induced immunologic unresponsiveness of mice to a UV-induced fibrosarcoma. *Photochem Photobiol* **32**: 183-188.

44. Vink AA, Yarosh DB, Kripke ML (1995) Chromophore for UV-induced immunosuppression: DNA. *Photochem Photobiol* **63**: 383-386.

45. Applegate LA, Ley RD, Alcalay J, Kripke ML (1989) Identification of the molecular target for the suppression of contact hypersensitivity by ultraviolet radiation. *J Exp Med* **170**: 1117-1131.

46. De Fabo EC, Noonan FP (1983) Mechanism of immune suppression by UV radiation in vivo. 1. Evidence for the existence of a unique photoreceptor in skin and its role in photoimmunology. *J Exp Med* **157**: 84-98.

47. Norval M, Simpson TJ, Ross JA (1989) Urocanic acid and immunosuppression. *Photochem Photobiol* **50**: 267-271.

48. Norval M, Gibbs NK, Gilmour J (1995) The role of urocanic acid in UV-induced immunosuppression: Recent Advances (1992-1994). *Photochem Photobiol* **62**: 209-217.

49. Hart PH, Grimbaldeston MA, Swift GJ, Hosszu EK, Finlay-Jones JJ (1999) A critical role for dermal mast cells in cis-urocanic acid-induced systemic suppression of contact hypersensitivity responses in mice. *Photochem Photobiol* **70**: 807-812.

50. Chung H, Burnham DK, Robertson B, Roberts LK, Daynes RD (1986) Involvement of prostaglandins in the immune alteration caused by the exposure of mice to ultraviolet radiation. *J Immunol* **137**: 2478-2484.

51. Pentland AP, Mahoney M, Jacobs C, Holtzman J (1990) Enhanced prostaglandin synthesis after ultraviolet injury is mediated by endogenous histamine stimulation. A mechanism for irradiation erythema. *J Clin Invest* **86**: 556-574.

52. Jaksic A, Finlay-Jones J, Watson CJ, Spencer LK, Santucci I, Hart PH (1995) *Cis*-urocanic acid synergizes with histamine for increased PGE_2 production by human keratinocytes: Link to indomethacin-inhibitable UVB-induced immunosuppression. *Photochem Photobiol* **61**:303-309.

53. Ullrich S (1996) Does exposure to UV radiation induce a shift to a Th-2-like immune reaction? (Review) *Photochem Photobiol* **64**:254-258.

54. Nishimura N, Tohyama C, Satoh M, Nishimura H, Reeve VE (1999) Defective immune response and severe skin damage following UVB irradiation in interleukin-6-deficient mice. *Immunology* **97**: 77-83.

55. Moodycliffe AM, Kimber I, Norval M (1994) Role or tumour necrosis factor-alpha in ultraviolet B light-induced dendritic cell migration and suppression of contact hypersensitivity. *Immunology* **81**: 79-84.

56. Schwarz A, Grabbe S, Grosse-Heitmeyer K, *et al.* (1998) Ultraviolet light-induced immune tolerance is mediated via the Fas/Fas-ligand system. *J Immunol* **160**: 4262-4270.

57. Krutmann J, Grewe M (1995) Involvement of cytokines, DNA damage, and reactive oxygen intermediates in ultraviolet radiation-induced modulation of intercellular adhesion molecule-1 expression. *J Invest Dermatol* **105**(S): 67-70.

58. Nakamura T, Pinnell SR, Darr D *et al.* (1997) Vitamin C abrogates the deleterious effects of UVB radiation on cutaneous immunity by a mechanism that does not depend on TNF-α. *J Invest Dermatol* **109**: 20-24.

59. Yuen KS, Halliday GM (1997) Alpha-tocopherol, an inhibitor of epidermal lipid peroxidation, prevents ultraviolet radiation from suppressing the skin immune system. *Photochem Photobiol* **65**: 587-592.

60. Reeve VE, Bosnic M, Rozinova E (1993) Carnosine (β-alanylhistidine) protects from the suppression of contact hypersensitivity by ultraviolet B (280-320 nm) radiation or by *cis*-urocanic acid. *Immunology* **78**: 99-104.

61. Reeve VE, Nishimura N, Bosnic M, Michalska AE, Khoo KHA (2000) Lack of metallothionein-I and –II exacerbates the immunosuppressive effects of UVB. *Immunology* **100**: 399-404.

62. Steenvoorden D, Vanhenegouwen G (1998a) Glutathione synthesis is not involved in protection by N-acetylcysteine against UVB-induced systemic immunosuppression in mice. *Photochem Photobiol* **68**: 97-100.

63. Katiyar SK, Elmets CA, Agarwal R, Mukhtar H (1995) Protection against ultraviolet-B radiation-induced local and systemic suppression of contact hypersensitivity and edema responses in C3H/HeN mice by green tea polyphenols. *Photochem Photobiol* **62**: 855- 861.

64. Steerenberg PA, Garssen J, Dortant P, *et al.* (1998) Protection of UV-induced suppression of skin contact hypersensitivity – a common feature of flavonoids after oral administration. *Photochem Photobiol* **67**: 456-461.

65. Reeve VE, Bosnic M, Rozinova E, Boehm-Wilcox C, (1993a) A garlic extract protects from ultraviolet B (280-320 nm) radiation-induced suppression of contact hypersensitivity. *Photochem Photobiol* **58**: 813-817.

66. Reeve VE, Tyrrell RM, (1999) Heme oxygenase induction mediates the photoimmunoprotective effect of UVA radiation in the mouse. *Proc Natl Acad Sci USA* **96**: 9317-9321.

67. Zak-Prelich M, Norval M, Venner TJ, *et al.* (2001) *cis*-Urocanic acid does not induce the expression of immunosuppressive cytokines in murine keratinocytes. *Photochem Photobiol* **73**: 238-244

68. International Agency for Research on Cancer Expert Group (2001) *Sunscreens*. IARC Handbooks of Cancer Prevention, Vol. 5. Lyon, France: IARC Press, p.149.

69. Black HS, Lenger W, Phelps AW, Thornby JI (1983) Influence of dietary lipid upon ultraviolet light carcinogenesis. *Nutr Cancer* **5**: 59-68.
70. Reeve VE, Bosnic M, Boehm-Wilcox C (1996) Dependence of photocarcinogenesis and photoimmunosuppression in the hairless mouse on dietary polyunsaturated fat. *Cancer Letts* **108**: 271-279.
71. Cope RB, Bosnic M, Boehm-Wilcox C, Mohr D, Reeve VE (1996) Dietary butter protects against ultraviolet radiation-induced suppression of contact hypersensitivity in Skh:HR-1 hairless mice. *J Nutr* **126**: 681-692.
72. Black HS, Okotie-Eboh G, Gerguis J, Urban JI, Thornby JI (1995a) Dietary fat modulates immunoresponsiveness in UV-irradiated mice. *Photochem Photobiol* **62**: 964-969.
73. Orengo IF, Black HS, Kettler AH, Wolf JE Jr. (1989) Influence of dietary menhaden oil upon carcinogenesis and various cutaneous responses to ultraviolet radiation. *Photochem Photobiol* **49**: 71-77.
74. Reeve VE, Matheson MJ, Bosnic M, Boehm-Wilcox C (1995) The protective effect of indomethacin on photocarcinogenesis in the hairless mouse. *Cancer Letts* **95**: 213-219.
75. Fischer SM, Lo HH, Gordon GB, *et al.* (1999) Chemopreventive activity of celecoxib, a specific cyclooxygenase-1 inhibitor, and indomethacin against ultraviolet light-induced skin carcinogenesis. *Mol Carcinogenesis* **25**: 231-240.
76. Steenvoorden DPT, van Henegouwen GMJB (1997) The use of endogenous antioxidants to improve photoprotection (Review). *J Photochem Photobiol B* **41**(1-2): 1-10.
77. Wei HC, Cai QY, Rahn RO (1996) Inhibition of UV light- and Fenton reaction-induced oxidative DNA damage by the soybean isoflavone genistein. *Carcinogenesis* **17**: 73-77.
78. Wei H., Barnes S, Wang Y (1996a) The inhibitory effect of genistein on a tumour promoter c-*fos* and c-*jun* expression in mouse skin. *Oncol Rep* **3**: 125-128.
79. Isoherranen K, Punnonen K, Jansen C, Uotila P (1999) Ultraviolet irradiation induced cyclooxygenase-2 expression in keratinocytes. *Br J Dermatol* **140**: 1017-1022.
80. Steerenberg PA, Garssen J, Dortant P *et al* (1997) Quercetin prevents UV-induced local immunosuppression, but does not affect UV-induced tumor growth in SKH-1 hairless mice. *Photochem Photobiol* **65**: 736-744.
81. Birt DF, Mitchell D, Gold B, Pour P, Pinch HC (1997) Inhibition of ultraviolet light induced skin carcinogenesis in Skh-1 mice by apigenin, a plant flavonoid. *Anticancer Res* **17**: 85-91.
82. Lepley DM, Pelling JC (1997) Induction of p21/WAF1 and G(1) cell-cycle arrest by the chemopreventive agent apigenin. *Mol Carcinogenesis* **19**: 74-82.
83. Widyarini S, Spinks N, Husband AJ, Reeve VE (2001) Isoflavone derivatives from red clover (*Trifolium pratense*) protect from inflammation and immune suppression induced by UV radiation. *Photochem Photobiol* **74**: 465-470.
84. Katiyar SK, Korman NJ, Mukhtar H, Agarwal R (1997) Protective effects of silymarin against photocarcinogenesis in a mouse skin model. *J Natl Cancer Inst* **89**: 556-565.
85. Wang ZY, Agarwal R, Bickers DR, Mukhtar H (1991) Protection against ultraviolet B radiation-induced photocarcinogenesis in hairless mice by green tea polyphenols. *Carcinogenesis* **12**: 1527-1530.
86. Wang ZY, Huang M, Ferraro T, *et al* (1992) Inhibitory effect of green tea in the drinking water on tumorigenesis by ultraviolet light and 12-*O*-tetradecanoylphorbol-13-acetate in the skin of Skh-1 mice. *Cancer Res* **52**: 1162-1170.
87. Khan SG, Katiyar SH, Agarwal R, Mukhtar H (1992) Enhancement of antioxidant and phase II enzymes by oral feeding of green tea polyphenols in drinking water to Skh-1 hairless mice: possible role in cancer chemoprevention. *Cancer Res* **52**: 4050-4052.

Chapter 11

Skin cancer induction by UV radiation: molecular UV targets and quantitative risk models

Frank R. de Gruijl[1], Ph.D.; Harry Slaper[2], Ph.D.
[1]*Dermatology, Leiden University Medical Center, Leiden, The Netherlands;* [2]*Lab. For Radiation Research, National Institute for Public Health and Environment, Bilthoven, The Netherlands*

Key words: skin cancer, UV radiation, signaling pathways, oncogenes, tumor suppressor genes

INTRODUCTION

Cancer research is making great strides in the fundamental understanding of how a normal cell can turn malignant, i.e., proliferate and spread uncontrollably. The relevant changes (carcinogenic "events") that lead to cancer can be detected or even quantified in terms of frequency of occurrence. In animal experiments on UV-induced skin cancers, the relation between such early carcinogenic events and wavelength, exposure and lapse of time can be studied in great detail. Epidemiology revealed the importance of solar (UV) exposure in the etiology of human skin cancer (see Chapters 5, 6) and early carcinogenic events can, in principle, also be detected in humans. Quantitative risk models can be refined and improved by integrating these experimental and epidemiological data. Such refined and detailed quantitative models are, however, in their infancy.

In this chapter we provide an overview that attempts to identify cross-linkages between molecular, animal and epidemiological studies on UV-induced skin cancers. Referring to this body of data, we discuss current risk

D. Hill et al. (eds.), Prevention of Skin Cancer, 195-209.

models of UV-induced skin cancers. These models are used in the scenario studies of the stratospheric ozone layer thickness (see Chapter 4).

1. UV RADIATION AND ONCOGENIC PATHWAYS

In general, a cancer cell arises from corrupted biochemical signaling pathways that control the cell cycle, differentiation and cell death (a special form of cell death dubbed "apoptosis"). The most permanent disruption stems from mutated or lost genes that code for proteins that are used in these signaling pathways. Such defects in genes will be passed along to daughter cells, thus propagating potential oncogenic changes. As there is a redundancy in the control mechanisms in the cell, several genes/proteins need to be affected in order for a tumor to arise. Carcinogenesis is understood to be a multi-step (multi-mutation) process, and it appears that at least two types of changes need to occur: a) the activation of a mitogenic (proliferative) pathway, and b) de-activation of a growth controlling pathway. The first can be related to the conversion of a "proto-oncogene" to an activated "oncogene" (genetically dominant), and the latter to de-activation of a "tumor suppressor gene" (genetically recessive).

1.1 Tumor suppressor genes

The p53 protein plays a central role in a cell's protective responses to damage to its DNA. This protein is involved in arresting the cell cycle (proliferation) to allow for time to repair the damage or to force the cell into a well-orchestrated suicide (apoptosis) if the DNA is overly damaged. Replication of damaged DNA may lead to errors in DNA of a daughter cell (i.e., mutations) and the interventions controlled by p53 aim to prevent this. Dysfunctional p53 protein will, therefore, clearly jeopardize the integrity of the genetic code. The TP53 tumor suppressor gene that codes for the p53 protein was found to be mutated in a majority of squamous cell carcinomas (SCC), (about 90%), in basal cell carcinomas (BCC), (>50%), from White Caucasians in the USA [1,2]. Strikingly, the point mutations found in these genes were very characteristic for the action of UVB radiation: the mutations occur mainly at typical UVB target sites, i.e., sites with adjacent pyrimidine bases (di-pyrimidine sites) in the DNA, and in a majority of cases cytosine was substituted by thymine (C→T transitions) and sometimes two neighboring cytosines were replaced by two thymines (CC→TT tandem mutations). Similar point mutations in the TP53 gene have been found in tumors in extensive mouse experiments [3-6]. Experiments with hairless mice show that clusters of epidermal cells with mutant p53 occur long before

SCC become visible [7]; such clusters of mutant p53 have also been found in normal human skin [8,9]. The early occurrence of TP53 mutations may facilitate mutations in other genes and thus cause further carcinogenic progression. The dose-time dependency of these early p53-mutant cell clusters in the skin showed a close parallel to that of the ultimate tumors. Hence, the frequency of these p53-mutant cell clusters may be a direct indicator of skin cancer risk [10].

In cutaneous melanomas (CM), a defect in the tumor suppressive function of the p16 protein appears to play a role. Like p53, the p16 protein is involved in cell cycle arrest, and inhibiting proliferation from oncogenic signaling. In familial melanoma the gene coding for p16, the INK4a/CDKN2A, is often found mutated [11] (for an in-depth review see [12]). Partial or complete loss of a parental INK4a allele (loss of heterozygosity, LOH) is observed in a majority (about 60%) of cell lines derived from sporadic (non-familial) CM, and most of the remaining cell lines (e.g., 8 out of 11) bear point mutations that are typical of UV radiation, i.e., C→T transitions at dipyrimidine sites [13]. Although 60-70% of sporadic melanomas (n = 62) show a lack of p16^{INK4a} expression, and all (n = 5) of the metastases do [14], the high number of homozygous losses and mutations of INK4a found in cell lines is not reproduced in primary CM. Homozygous deletions are found in approximately 10% of primary CM, and reported mutation rates range from 0 to 25 % [12]. The reason for this discrepancy is not entirely clear but it could be due to a high selection for a loss or mutation of INK4a in generating the cell lines [15].

1.2   Oncogenes

A mutation in either the TP53 or the INK4a gene is clearly not enough to start a skin cancer. A "mitogenic" pathway, switching on cell proliferation, needs to be activated. In a majority of BCC the "Sonic Hedgehog" pathway appears to be activated, as can be detected by the expression of the transcription factor, GLI1, in the nucleus of the cells in BCC [16]. Activation of this pathway induces epidermal hyperplasia [17,18]. This pathway is normally activated by binding of the Sonic Hedgehog protein to the PTCH membrane receptor of the cell. Dysfunctional PTCH can activate the pathway without binding Sonic Hedgehog. Next to frequent LOH at the PTCH locus, many sporadic BCC show mutations in the (remaining) PTCH allele [19]: 12 out of 37 tumors in single stranded conformational polymorphism (SSCP) screening, and additionally, 9 of these tumors showed LOH of PTCH. (The SSCP technique was apparently not sensitive enough as two tumors without variant SSCP or LOH were both found to have mutations when analyzed by direct sequencing.) Seven of 15 mutations occurred at di-pyrimidinic sites and were C→T transitions (among which 2 were CC→TT tandem mutations), and could, therefore, have been caused by UVB radiation. Heterozygous Ptc knockout mice (Ptc is the murine homologue of human PTCH) develop more BCC faster when exposed to ionizing or UVB radiation [20]. These BCC show frequent loss of the wildtype Ptc allele, and all those tested (n = 12) showed expression of Gli1, whereas both SCC that were tested did not. Two of 5 UV-induced BCC-like tumors carried TP53 mutations (3 in total: 2 C→T and 1 C→G). These experimental data show that UV radiation can play an important role in causing or enhancing the development of BCC. Next to the induction of TP53 mutations, UV radiation could exert a more direct effect on the Sonic Hedgehog pathway by enhanced loss of the wildtype PTCH gene and/or possible mutation of this gene.

The mitogenic pathways involving proteins of the (proto-) oncogenes of the RAS family also appear to be involved in some skin cancers. Such pathways are normally triggered by binding of a growth factor to a receptor for tyrosine kinase (RTK) on the cell membrane. The RTK subsequently oligomerizes and thus activates a signaling cascade in which RAS proteins transfer the signal. Specific mutations in a RAS gene can lead constitutive activation of the downstream part of the pathway without any receptor binding. Activating mutations in H-RAS have been reported in a minority of SCC and BCC [21,22]. These activating mutations are restricted to the codons 12, 13 and 61, and are not specific to UV radiation. Increased expression of RAS without any mutation in the corresponding gene [21] indicates that the pathway may be activated by alterations upstream of RAS. RAS may also play a role in CM: 10-70% of CM from regularly sun-exposed sites have been reported to carry activating point mutations in N-RAS, whereas none of the CM from irregularly exposed sites carried such mutations [23,24]. In a comparative study the percentage of N-RAS mutated CM from sun-exposed sites was higher in an Australian population (24%) than in a European population (12%) [24]. These mutations occur in the vicinity of dipyrimidine sites, the typical UV targets, but they are not dominated by C→T transitions. Recently, a majority (70%) of melanomas was found to bear mutations in the gene coding for BRAF downstream of RAS [25]. These mutations were not characteristic of UV radiation. Proliferation of melanocytes can be stimulated through various RTKs (receptors for fibroblast growth factor, FGF-R, for hepatocyte growth factor, c-MET, and for mast cell growth factor, c-KIT) [26], and this stimulation can involve activation of RAS/BRAF. Melanoma cells constitutively express several activated proteins involved in mitogenic pathways.

1.2.1 Interaction between oncogenic and tumor suppressive proteins

As mentioned earlier, the RAS proteins function in mitogenic pathways that start by activation of RTK at the cell membrane, e.g., the receptor for epidermal growth factor, EGF-R. It is well known that oncogenic RAS will transform most immortal cell lines and make them tumorigenic upon transplantation into nude mice. Surprisingly, Serrano *et al.* [27] found that expression of oncogenic RAS (producing an activated H-RAS^{G12V}) in primary human or rodent cells results in a state that is phenotypically characterized as "senescence": the cells are viable and metabolically active but remain in the G1-phase of the cell cycle (the phase preceding DNA replication for cell division). This oncogenic RAS-induced arrest in G1 is accompanied by an accumulation of both p16 and p53. Inactivation of either p16 or p53 prevented this G1 arrest. Thus, cells immortalized by dysfunctional p16 or p53 will not go into senescence upon RAS activation, but may progress to a tumorigenic state.

In a fish model (with hybrids of *Xiphophorus maculatis* and *helleri*) an RTK gene (Xmrk) of the EGF-R family and an Ink4a homologue (CdknX or DIFF) appear to be important for hereditary CM [28,29]. This provides experimental evidence for the cooperation of an RTK mitogenic pathway and dysfunctional Ink4a in melanomagenesis. In further evidence, Chin *et al.* [30] demonstrated that Ink4a-null mice, in which expression of a human mutant H-RAS^{G12V} transgene was restricted to melanocytes, developed melanomas.

1.3 Combinations of oncogenes and tumor suppressor genes in skin cancer and UVB radiation

From the data stated above, it appears that at least a combination of an activated oncogenic pathway and an inactivated tumor suppressor gene is needed in order for a skin cancer to arise: in SCC it is possibly an activated RTK/RAS pathway in combination with dysfunctional p53 tumor suppression; in BCC, mostly the Hedgehog pathway with possibly dysfunctional p53; and in CM, possibly an activated RTK/RAS/BRAF in combination with inactivation of the INK4a locus. These combinations may be required, but not necessarily sufficient for the development of a tumor. Additional oncogenic events may be necessary.

Although skin cancers appear to be related to UV radiation, the effect of UV radiation is only unambiguously clear in point mutations of TP53 in SCC and BCC. The mutations found in the other relevant genes are of a wider variety, which may (in part) be caused by solar UV radiation.

Experiments are needed to clarify if and how UVB or UVA radiation can affect other relevant genes.

2.   DEPENDENCE OF TUMOR RATE ON WAVELENGTH, DOSE AND TIME

Tumor formation is a multi-step dynamic process in which one or more steps (mutations) may be driven by external carcinogens (e.g., UV radiation). A risk assessment needs to take the "quality" and "quantity" of the exogenous carcinogen properly into the equation. In UV carcinogenesis the *wavelength* of the irradiation determines its "quality" (its effectiveness), and *dose* (exposure regimen) and *time* (tumor latency) are the important quantities. The wavelength dependency of UV carcinogenesis is represented in an action spectrum (the inverse of daily exposure at each wavelength required to achieve a certain median induction time of a first tumor on an individual). Spectral weighting of the UV exposure can subsequently assess a carcinogenic dose. Only after a proper definition of carcinogenic UV dose, can a meaningful assessment be made of the relationship between (solar) exposures of different spectral compositions and tumor induction rates.

2.1   Action spectra

Shortwave UV radiation is directly absorbed by DNA and causes the formation of dimers at di-pyrimidine sites. Above 300 nm the efficiency of induction of these DNA adducts drops off steeply, and correspondingly, the mutation rate per J/m^2 drops off. A series of skin carcinogenesis experiments on hairless SKH-1 mice with various broadband UV sources has provided the data to establish the wavelength dependency of UV carcinogenesis: the result was dubbed the SCUP-m action spectrum (*S*kin *C*ancer *U*trecht-*P*hiladelphia-*m*urine) [31]. By correcting for differences in transmission of murine and human epidermis the carcinogenic action spectrum for humans was estimated and dubbed the SCUP-h action spectrum (h stands for human) [32]; this correction shifted the maximum from 293 to 299 nm. The SCUP-h action spectrum is depicted in Figure 11.1, together with the measured action spectrum for the induction of pyrimidine dimers in human skin by Freeman *et al.* [33]. The two action spectra resemble each other remarkably well, especially in the UVB, which confirms that UV-induced genotoxicity is indeed the major driving force behind UV carcinogenesis. The point mutations found in the TP53 gene from SCC and BCC confirm the important contribution of UVB radiation to the formation of these skin cancers.

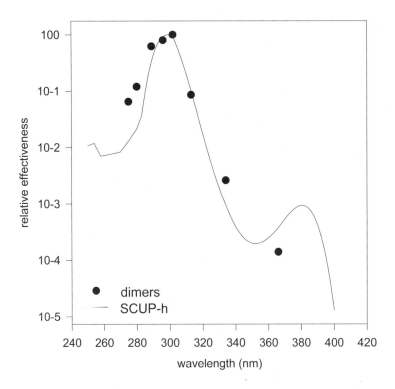

Figure 11.1 Comparison of the SCUP-h action spectrum [32] and the action spectrum for the induction of pyrimidine dimers in human skin [33].

It has recently been found that neonatal broadband UV irradiation causes CM in transgenic mice that over-express the hepatocyte growth factor (HGF, ligand to c-Met) [34], whereas chronic irradiation of adult mice does not induce CM. It should be feasible in the near future to determine the wavelength dependence of CM induction in this mouse model. UV irradiation of hybrid *Xiphophorus* fish was found to significantly increase the number of CM over the number that developed spontaneously [35]. UVA radiation was surprisingly effective in this model, only about 10 fold less effective than UVB radiation per unit radiant energy (J/m^2). This may, however, correspond more to the promotional activity of UV radiation on outgrowth of latent tumor foci than on the *de novo* induction (initiation) of CM. It is as yet unknown how UV radiation affected CdknX/Ink4a or the Xmrk/RTK mitogenic pathway in these fish. In the opossum *Monodelphis domestica* UVB radiation appears to induce CM [36], particularly when applied neonatally [37]. However, UVA radiation did not induce malignant CM in this model [38], and only benign melanocytic precursor lesions upon chronic exposure [39]. In a very recent study it was found that the UVB-induced CM from these opossums carried UVB-like mutations in the CDKN2A homologue, and that only the mutant allele was present and expressed in a metastatic cell line [40].

Overall, the data presently weigh most heavily toward the carcinogenic effect of UVB radiation: the latest data on experimental induction of malignant CM in the opossum *Monodelphis domestica* are not indicative of any contribution of UVA radiation comparable to the paramount carcinogenicity of UVB radiation.

2.2   Dose-time relationship

Among the multiple rate-limiting steps (mutations in oncogenes and tumor suppressor genes) in UV carcinogenesis some steps will be UV-driven and some will be independent of the UV exposure (the latter may be caused by endogenous metabolic processes which generate reactive oxygen species, ROS). The likelihood of the occurrence of a UV-dependent step will increase with the accumulated UV dose, whereas the likelihood of a UV-independent step will simply increase with the lapse of time. Clearly, the UV-independent steps will render the whole process of carcinogenesis less dependent on the UV dose: if the daily dose in mouse experiments was increased by a factor of 2, the tumor induction time was found to be shortened by less than a factor of 2, i.e., there was no direct reciprocity between daily dose and tumor induction time. Besides UV independent steps, adaptive processes that lessen the impact of higher daily doses may cause a failure in reciprocity between daily dose and tumor induction time; e.g., the UV-induced epidermal hyperplasia, which diminishes the penetration to the germinative basal cells, may have this effect [41].

From experiments in hairless mice it was found that the average number of tumors (SCC or precursors) per mouse, the yield Y (or tumor multiplicity), can be written as:

$$Y = (H/H_o)^{p1} (t/t_o)^p \qquad (1)$$

Equation 11.1

Where H is the daily UV exposure (in $J/m^2/d$), t is time (in days), and H_o, t_o, p1 and p are constants (when $H = H_o$ and $t = t_o$ then $Y = 1$, i.e., an average of 1 tumor per mouse; note that if $H = 2H_o$ then $t = t_o/2^{p1/p}$ for $Y = 1$) [42]. In a straightforward interpretation, the power of time, p, is likely to be proportional (not necessarily equal) to the total number of rate limiting steps that occur in the course of time (including those steps that depend on the daily UV exposure). The power of the daily UV exposure, p1, is likely to be proportional to the number of UV driven steps; which implies that $p1 \leq p$.

If all mice in a group are comparable (in sensitivity and treatment), the probability, P, for a mouse contracting a first tumor becomes:

$$P = 1 - \exp(-Y) \qquad (2)$$

Equation 11.2

Which, in the absence of any intervening deaths, equals the prevalence of tumor bearing animals in a (large) group. These relationships hold rather well in the experiments with albino hairless mice, where $p = 7.2 \pm 0.8$ and $p1 = 4.3 \pm 0.5$ for early tumors of 1 mm in diameter [42,43], with pigmented hairless mice $p1 = 2.1 \pm 0.2$ ($p1/p = 0.3$ computed from data in [44]; this lower dependency on the daily UV exposure is probably due to a better adaptation by pigmentation of the animals). When the daily exposure of the albino mice is discontinued after a couple of weeks, long before the appearance of tumors, then Y increases with t to the power 2.8 ± 0.2, which power equals $p-p1$ ($= 2.9 \pm 0.3$), the power related to the UV-independent steps [42].

In human populations, the age-specific incidence rates of cancers are measured, which equal the increase in Y per unit time (e.g., per year) if the fraction of patients with multiple tumors is small. The probability (calculated according to Equation 11.2) of SCC in the Dutch population follows a time-dependence which is quite comparable to that of albino hairless mice: $p = 6.6 \pm 0.4$ for males and 8.9 ± 0.7 for females [45]. Under a level of daily exposure comparable to the estimated average among Dutch males, the tumors in the mice occur about 250 times faster. This appears to indicate that the tumor kinetics in mouse and man are very similar, but that the developmental rate of SCC (the mutation rate) is much higher in the mice. By combining measurements of ambient UV loads and epidemiological data from USA it can be inferred that $p1 = 2.6 \pm 0.8$ for human SCC [46], a value of p1 that is very similar to the one for pigmented hairless mice. For BCC, p ranges between 4.5 and 5.5 and $p1 = 1.4 \pm 0.5$ [46].

3.   SCENARIO STUDIES

3.1   Skin cancer incidences and altered ambient UV radiation

As discussed in Chapter 4, comparison of two stable situations, one with a life-long low UV exposure and the other with a life-long high UV exposure, is the easiest way to quantify the effect of an increased UV exposure such as that caused by a depletion of the ozone layer. Assuming that the behavior and genetic composition of white Caucasian populations in various locations in the USA are sufficiently comparable and that the populations are in a stationary condition in relation to UV exposure and skin tumor incidences, the relationship between ambient UV loads and incidence rates can be used for the assessment. SCC would increase by 3% for each percent of ozone depletion, BCC by 1.7%, and CM by 0.5-1%, if the SCUP-h action spectrum is also applicable to CM [46-48]. The complication here is that the incidence rates of BCC and CM in particular are not stationary in the USA [46].

It is much harder to estimate transitional changes in incidence due to changes in UV exposure. More detailed knowledge is required, for example on whether UV acts early, late or continuously in the process of skin carcinogenesis. From current data it appears that UV acts throughout the genesis of SCC, but mainly in an early stage of BCC and CM development. For scenario studies on dynamic changes the tumor yield, Y, the right-hand side of Equation 11.1 may be factorized in a contribution from events driven by the *total* UV exposure, written as $(TH/H_o.t_o)^{p1}$, and a contribution from events purely dependent on time, taken as $(t/t_o)^{p-p1}$, where TH ($= H.t$) is the total UV exposure. For SCC these two factors are simply multiplied to calculate the yield, but for BCC and CM the two factors need to be convoluted in time because the UV-dependent events can be assumed to precede the purely time-dependent events, according to epidemiological data on the importance of childhood exposure. Thus, scenario studies of changes in ozone can be made [49] (see Chapter 4): without restrictions the skin cancer incidence could quadruple by the end of this century, and even initial restrictions under the Montreal Protocol would still yield a two-fold increase.

CONCLUSIONS

Basic research on the molecular-genetic mechanisms involved in skin cancer formation is shedding more light on the possible role of (solar) UV radiation. The mutations found in the TP53 gene from SCC and BCC are now classical examples of how a carcinogen can be recognized by the precise nature of changes in the cell's genetic material, DNA: the carcinogen, solar UVB radiation, has clearly left its signature. However, UV radiation also introduces other types of damage in the DNA, which leads to non-specific mutations that may be caused by other carcinogens as well. Proper experimental (animal) models may serve to elucidate the role of UV radiation in these ambiguous genetic changes. In particular, the precise role of solar UV radiation in the etiology of the most fatal skin cancer, CM, needs to be established more firmly (e.g., UVB versus UVA, childhood exposure versus intermittent exposure), but currently recent results from experiments with the opossum *Monodelphis domestica* appear to re-affirm the importance of UVB exposure for *malignant* CM and the importance of neonatal exposures.

By combining the epidemiological and animal-experimental data we have derived quantitative tumor-response models for SCC, BCC and CM (see Chapter 4). Knowledge on the (sequence of) molecular events leading up to skin cancer already contributes to a deeper understanding of these models (e.g., the early UVB-induced TP53 mutations). Integration of these molecular events into the quantitative models will refine and improve future modeling, and may lead to quantification of personal risk based on measurements of certain biological markers related to early carcinogenic changes.

SUMMARY POINTS

- (Skin) cancers arise from a combination of defects (gene mutations) in stimulating and inhibiting signaling pathways that control cell proliferation.
- UVB-related mutations are most clearly present in the TP53 tumor suppressor gene in skin carcinomas. UV radiation may (in part) be the cause of other gene mutations found in skin cancers, such as mutations in PTCH and RAS genes.
- Transgenic mouse models are instrumental in elucidating the fundamental mechanisms by which UV radiation causes various types of skin cancer, specifically basal cell carcinomas and cutaneous melanomas.
- Quantitative risk models can be refined by mouse experiments, particularly by results on early (onco-) genetic changes.

IMPLICATIONS FOR PUBLIC HEALTH

- Fundamental knowledge on the pathogenesis of skin cancers attained from mouse experiments is of direct importance in prevention. For example, the knowledge that UVB is far more carcinogenic than UVA radiation, including for cutaneous melanoma (as indicated by the Marsupial model), and the confirmation of the importance of neonatal exposure on the formation of cutaneous malignant melanoma later in life (as found in the Marsupial and the HGF-transgenic mouse models).
- Identification of early (UV-induced) oncogenic changes in human skin (e.g., TP53 mutations) may serve to assess a subsequent tumor risk, and measuring such changes in a population may serve as a surrogate for tumor incidences. Such data on UV-induced early oncogenic changes can obviously greatly refine current quantitative models on UV-related skin cancer risks, and make these models more reliable.

ACKNOWLEDGEMENTS

The authors wish to thank the Ministry of the Environment ("VROM") and the European Commission and the Dutch Cancer Society ("NKB/KWF") for the financial support of their research.

REFERENCES

1   Brash DE, Rudolph JA, Simon JA, *et al.* (1991) A role for sunlight in skin cancer: UV-induced *p53* mutations in squamous cell carcinomas. *Proc Natl Acad Sci USA* **88**: 10124-10128.
2. Ziegler AD, Leffel DJ, Kunala S, *et al.* (1993) Mutation hotspots due to sunlight in the *p53* gene of skin cancers. *Proc Natl Acad Sci USA* **90**: 4216-4220.
3. Kress S, Sutter SC, Strickland PT, Mukhtar H, Schweizer J, Schwarz M (1992) Carcinogen-specific mutational pattern in the *p53* gene in ultraviolet B radiation-induced squamous cell carcinomas of mouse skin. *Cancer Res* **52**: 6400-6403.
4. Kanjilal S, Pierceall WF, Cummings KK, Kripke ML, Ananthaswamy HN (1993) High frequency of *p53* mutations in ultraviolet radiation-induced skin tumors: evidence for strand bias and tumor heterogeneity. *Cancer Res* **53**: 2961-2964.
5. Van Kranen HJ, de Gruijl FR, de Vries A, *et al.* (1995) Frequent p53 alterations but low incidences of ras mutations in UV-B induced skin tumors of hairless mice. *Carcinogenesis* **16**: 1141-1147.
6. Dumaz N, Van Kranen HJ, de Vries A, *et al.* (1997) The role of UVB light in skin carcinomas through the analysis of *p53* mutations in squamous cell carcinomas of hairless mice. *Carcinogenesis* **18**: 897-904.

7. Berg RJW, van Kranen HJ, Rebel HG, *et al.* (1997) Early p53 alterations in mouse skin carcinogenesis by UVB radiation: immunohistochemical detection of mutant p53 protein in clusters of preneoplastic epidermal cells. *Proc Natl Acad Sci.USA* **93**: 274-278.

8. Jonason AS, Kunala S, Price GJ, *et al.* (1996) Frequent clones of *p53*-mutated keratinocytes in normal human skin. *Proc Natl Acad Sci USA* **93**: 14025-14029.

9. Ren ZP, Ponten F, Nister M, Ponten J (1996) Two distinct p53 immunohistochemical patterns in human squamous cell skin cancer, precursors and normal epidermis. *Int J Cancer* **69**: 174-179.

10. Rebel H, Mosnier LO, Berg RJ, *et al.* (2001) Early p53-positive foci as indicators of tumor risk in ultraviolet-exposed hairless mice: kinetics of induction, effects of DNA repair deficiency, and p53 heterozygozity. *Cancer Res* **61**:977-983.

11. Kamb A, Gruis NA, Weaver-Feldhaus J, *et al.* (1994) A cell cycle regulator potentially involved in geneisis of many tumor types. *Science* **264**: 436-440.

12. Ruas M., Peters G (1998) The p16^{INK4a}/CDKN2A tumor suppressor and its relatives. *Biochim Biophys Acta* **1378**: F115-F177.

13. Pollock PM, Yu F, Qui L, Parsons PG, Hayward NK (1995) Evidence for u.v. induction of CDKN2 mutations in melanoma cell lines. *Oncogene* **11**: 663-668.

14. Funk JO, Schiller PI, Barrett MT, Wong DJ, Kind P, Sander CA (1998) p16INK4a expression is frequently decreased and associated with 9p21 loss of heterozygosity in sporadic melanoma. *J Cutan Pathol* **25**: 291-296.

15. Flores JF, Walker GJ, Glendening JM, *et al.* (1996) Loss of the p16INK4a and p15INK4b genes as well as neighboring 9p21 markers, in sporadic melanoma. *Cancer Res* **56**: 5023-5032.

16. Dahmane N, Lee J, Robins P, Heller P, Ruiz i Alteba, A (1997) Activation of the transcription factor Gli1 and the hedgehog signalling pathway in skin tumors. *Nature* **389**: 876-881.

17. Fan H, Oro AE, Scott MP, Khavari PA (1997) Induction of basal cell carinoma features in transgenic human keratinocytes expressing Sonic Hedgehog. *Nat Med* **3**: 788-792.

18. Fan H, Khavari PA (1999) Sonic hedgehog opposes epithelial cell cycle arrest. *J Cell Biol* **147**: 71-76.

19. Gialini MR, Stahle-Bäckdahl M, Leffell DJ, *et al.* (1996) The role of the human homologue of *Drosophila* Patched in sporadic basal cell carcinomas. *Nature Gen* **14**: 78-81.

20. Aszterbaum M, Epstein J, Oro A, *et al.* (1999) Ultraviolet and ionizing radiation enhance the growth of BCCs and trichoblastomas in patched heterozygous knockout mice. *Nature Med* . **5**: 1285-1291.

21. Pierceall WE, Goldberg LH, Tainsky MA, Mukhopadhyay T, Ananthaswamy HN (1991) *Ras* gene mutation and amplification in human nonmelanoma skin cancers. *Mol Carcinog* **4**: 196-202.

22. Cambell C, Quinn AG, Rees JL (1993) Codon 12 Harvey-ras mutations are rare events in non-melanoma human skin cancer. *Br J Dermatol* **128**: 111-114.

23. Van 't Veer LJ, Burgering BMT, Versteeg R, *et al.* (1989) N-*ras* mutations in human cutaneous melanoma from sun-exposed body sites. *Mol Cell Biol* **9**: 3114-3116.

24. Van Elsas A, Zerp SF, van der Flier S, *et al.* (1996) Relevance of ultraviolet-induced N-ras oncogene point mutations in development of primary human cutaneous melanoma. *Am J Path* **143**: 883-893.

25. Davies H, Bignell GR, Cox C, *et al.* (2002) Mutations of the BRAF gene in human cancer. *Nature* **417**: 949-954.

26. Halaban R, Fan B, Ahn J, Funasaka Y, Gitay-Goren H, Neufeld G (1992) Growth factors, receptor kinases, and protein tyrosine phosphatases in normal and malignant melanocytes. *J Immunother* **12**: 154-161.

27. Serrano M, Lin WA, McCurrach ME, Beach D, Lowe SW (1997) Oncogenic *ras* provokes premature cell senescence associated with accumulation of p53 and p16[INK4a]. *Cell* **88**: 593-602.

28. Wittbrodt J, Adam D, Malitschek B, *et al.* (1989) Novel putative receptor tyrosine kinase encoded by melanoma-inducing *Tu* locus in *Xiphophorus. Nature* **341**: 415-421.

29. Kazianis S, Gutbrod H, Nairn RS, *et al.* (1998) Localization of a *CDKN2* gene in linkage group V of Xiphophorus fishes defines it as a candidate for the *DIFF* tumor suppressor. *Genes Chromosomes Cancer* **22**: 210-220.

30. Chin L, Pomerantz J, Polsky D, *et al.* (1997) Cooperative effects of *INK4a* and *ras* in melanoma susceptibility in vivo. *Genes Dev* **1**: 2822-2834.

31. De Gruijl FR, Sterenborg HJCM, Forbes PD, *et al.* (1993) Wavelength dependence of skin cancer induction by ultraviolet irradiation of albino hairless mice. *Cancer Res* **53**: 53-60.

32. De Gruijl FR, Van der Leun JC (1994) Estimate of the wavelength dependency of ultraviolet carcinogenesis in humans and its relevance to the risk assessment of a stratospheric ozone depletion. *Health Phys* **67**: 314-325.

33. Freeman SE, Hachan H, Gange RW, Maytum DJ, Sutherland JC, Sutherland BM (1989) Wavelength Dependence of pyrimidine dimer formation in DNA of human skin irradiated in situ with ultraviolet light. *Proc Natl Acad Sci USA* **86**: 5605-5609.

34. Noonan FP, Recio JA, Takayama H, *et al.* (2001) Neonatal sunburn and melanoma in mice. *Nature* **413**: 271-272.

35. Setlow RB, Woodhead AD, Grist E (1989) Animal model for ultraviolet radiation-induced melanoma: platyfish-swortail hybrid. *Proc Natl Acad Sci USA* **86**: 8922-8926.

36. Ley RD, Applegate LA, Padilla RS, Stuart TD (1989) Ultraviolet radiation-induced malignant melanoma in Monodelphis domestica. *Photochem Photobiol* **50**:1-5.

37. Robinson ES, Hubbard GB, Colon G, Vandeberg JL (1998) Low-dose ultraviolet exposure early in the development can lead to widespread melanoma in the opossum model. *Int J Exp Path* **79**:235-244.

38. Robinson ES, Hill RH Jr, Kripke ML, Setlow RB (2000) The Monodelphis melanoma model: initial report on large ultraviolet A exposures of suckling young. *Photochem Photobiol* **71**:743-746.

39. Ley RD (2001) Dose response for ultraviolet radiation A-induced focal melanocytic hyperplasia and nonmelanoma skin tumors in Monodelphis domestica. *Photochem Photobiol* **73**:20-23.

40. Chan J, Robinson ES, Atencio J, *et al.* (2001) Characterization of the CDKN2A and ARF genes in UV-induced melanocytic hyperplasias and melanomas of an opossum (Monodelphis domestica). *Mol Carcinog* **31**: 16-26.

41. De Gruijl FR, Van der Leun JC (1983) Effect of chronic UV exposure on epidermal transmission in mice. *Photochem Photobiol* **36**: 433-441.

42. De Gruijl, FR, Van der Leun JC (1991) Development of skin tumors in hairless mice after discontinuation of ultraviolet irradiation. *Cancer Res* **51**: 979-984.

43. De Gruijl FR, Van der Meer JB, Van der Leun JC (1983) Dose-time dependency of tumor formation by chronic UV exposure, *Photochem Photobiol* **37**: 53-62.

44. Davies RE, Forbes PD (1988) Retinoids and photocarcinogenesis: a review. *J Toxicol Cut Ocul Toxicol* **7**: 241-253.

45. De Gruijl FR (1997) Health effects from solar UV radiation. *Rad Protect Dosimetry* **72**: 177-196.

46. De Gruijl FR, Van der Leun JC (1993) Influence of ozone depletion on the incidence of skin cancer. In: Young AR, Björn LO, Moan J, Nultsch W, eds. *Environmental UV Photobiology*. New York: Plenum Press, pp. 89-112.

47. Longstreth JD, De Gruijl FR, Kripke ML, Takizawa Y, Van der Leun JC (1995) Effects of increased solar ultraviolet radiation on human health. *Ambio* **24**: 153-165.

48. Scotto J, Fears TR (1987) The association of solar ultraviolet and skin melanoma incidence among Caucasians in the Unites States. *Cancer Invest* **5**: 275-283.

49. Slaper H, Velders GJM, Daniel JS, De Gruijl FR Van der Leun JC (1996) Estimates of ozone depletion and skin cancer incidence to examine the Vienna Convention achievements. *Nature* **384**: 256-258.

Chapter 12

Patterns and causes of sun exposing and sun protecting behavior

Suzanne Dobbinson, M.Sc., Ph.D.; David J. Hill, Ph.D.
Centre for Behavioural Research in Cancer, The Cancer Council Victoria, Melbourne, Victoria, Australia

Key words: sun exposure, sun protection, sunburn, skin cancer, sun related behavior

INTRODUCTION

Sun-related behavior increases or decreases exposure of the skin or eyes to solar ultraviolet radiation and may significantly alter skin cancer risk. Sun exposing behavior may be intentional or incidental. Intentional sun-exposing behavior is exposure to the sun with the primary purpose of achieving a biological response, such as a tan [1] usually with limited attention to sun protection and maximal concern for extended exposure. Wearing brief clothing and use of sunscreens with a low sun protection factor (SPF), or no sunscreen, when outdoors characterizes intentional exposure. Incidental sun-exposure occurs as a result of being outdoors without adequate protection whilst pursuing activities not directed exclusively at obtaining a suntan, such as in occupational sun exposure. In contrast, "sun protective behavior" (SPB) minimizes the skin's exposure to ultraviolet radiation. It includes employing personal protective aids to minimize skin exposure when outdoors using covering clothing, a sunscreen of SPF ≥15, sunglasses, or umbrellas; and, or, seeking shade. People may also reduce exposure through minimizing outdoor activity when UV levels are raised, such as around solar noon, at high altitudes, or latitudes near the equator.

D. Hill et al. (eds.), Prevention of Skin Cancer, 211-240.

1.   INFLUENCES

To a large extent a person's sun-related behavior will depend on the physical environment, opportunities for outdoor activity, personal disposition, and sun-related attitudes and beliefs. These determinants have complex, direct and indirect effects on behavior. The patterns of human outdoor activity vary and much of this behavior is a response to specific contexts. Reinforcement contingencies may operate both in favor of and against sun protective behavior. A brief overview of some of the key influences is considered here and the reader is referred to Hill and Boulter [2] and Arthey and Clarke [3] for other reviews. Much of the evidence is correlational and reported from cross-sectional descriptive studies. A few studies report the successful application of theoretical psychosocial models to sun protective behavior, including Azjen's Theory of Planned Behavior [4] and Rosenstock's Health Belief Model [5-7].

Awareness of skin cancer risk, for example through media messages and health education, has variable influence on sun-related behaviors. Clarke *et al.* [8] posit that for most adolescents a degree of optimistic bias in assessing personal risk counters knowledge about skin cancer in influencing suntanning and sun protection. Nevertheless, in an early study of sunbathing, knowledge of skin cancer was a predictor of not sunbathing. Social contact with people who had skin cancer was associated with sunscreen use [9]. Moreover, experiencing anxiety during sunbathing was associated with perceived susceptibility and use of sunscreen [9]. Thus beliefs about personal susceptibility to skin cancer may develop from knowledge of skin cancer. Other studies also report knowledge and perceived susceptibility to be associated with sunscreen use [10,11]. In contrast, experience of "relaxation" during sunbathing has predicted frequent sunbathers [12].

Attitudes and beliefs about sun protection and sun exposure arise from personal dispositions and interactions with the social and physical environments. For example, pro-tan beliefs may stem from social influences including the media portrayal of wealthy, healthy and attractive people with deep suntans [9,13,14]. Beliefs about the attractiveness of a tan are a strong correlate of sunbathing [9-11,15,16]. Sunbathers seeking a tan are shown to place a high value on appearance [9,15] and tend to have a high opinion of their physical appearance [11]. Sunbathing is also a social activity and often correlated with friends' sunbathing [9,11]. Similarly, for sun protection behavior the influence of the social environment is important. Children's sun protection has been found to be consistently linked with parent's sun protection [17-20].

Beliefs about specific sun protective aids may be a deterrent to use. For example, Hill *et al.* describe the following barriers to use among a community sample: that hats are "uncomfortable", "hot" and "spoil hairstyle", sunscreens are "greasy" or "a nuisance" to apply, and shirts are "uncomfortable in heat" and are "overdressed" for the beach, while the main benefits of use were protection from sunburn and skin cancer [7]. Jackson and Aiken's psychosocial model of sun protection finds such perceived barriers to influence young women's sun protection intentions both directly and through altering self-efficacy for sun protection [6].

Enabling factors such as availability and cost of suitable summer attire can have a significant influence on sun protective and sun exposing behavior. The fashion industry has considerable influence on popular styles and availability of clothing, hats and sunglasses. Only recently has suitable protective summer attire such as covering lycra suits for swimming and UV protection labeling for clothing become available. In addition, sunscreens are now included in a much wider range of cosmetic products as the industry embraces the anti-aging benefits of reducing daily UV exposure.

It is posited that experience of painful sunburn provides a strong negative reinforcement for sun protection behavior [8,21]; while ease of tanning may act to reward sunbathing efforts and decrease concern with sun protection [8]. Age and gender also influence these behaviors, both through life-stage activity needs as well as social influences.

2.   BEHAVIORAL PATTERNS OF EXPOSURE

Few countries have conducted regular population-wide surveys of sun-related behaviors. In addition, in countries with different climates and UV environments, behavior associated with increased risk of skin cancer varies. In countries with high UV environments, such as Australia, incidental exposure during daily activities may increase risk. In cooler climates with low UV environments, such as the United Kingdom, Norway and Sweden, high risk may be associated with taking holidays in warmer countries with high UV or using artificial UV sources to promote tanning (see Chapter 9). Only three European studies reported the prevalence of holidays in warmer climates [11,22,23]. Throughout this chapter much of the detailed analysis of sun protection behavior is sourced largely from studies from the United States, Canada, Australia and New Zealand where there has been most commitment to skin cancer control.

2.1   Sun exposure and sunburn

We use tables to summarize key findings from recent studies that purport to provide population estimates of sun exposure for adults (Table 12.1), adolescents (Table 12.2) and children (Table 12.3) in several countries. Sun exposure is defined as being outdoors in the sun, regardless of deliberate protection used at that time. Different ways of measuring and reporting the data make it hard to generalize. In the Australian and New Zealand studies of adults, people reported on how long they had been outdoors between 11 and 3 (summer time) on the preceding two weekend days and the average was greater than half that period. The United States and Canadian studies asked people to indicate how much time during the whole summer day they spent outside, and in the United States nearly half spent over 5 hours compared to one quarter spending more than 2 hours in Canada.

The results for adolescents suffer from lack of comparability among studies, but the levels in Table 12.2 support quite strongly that, compared with adults (Table 12.1), adolescents are more exposed than adults in the same country. It also appears from the available data (Table 12.3) that young children spend long periods outdoors, possibly due to having greater activity needs or more available recreational time during the day than adults.

Sunburn reflects behavior only to some extent, as it is also a result of susceptibility (skin type) and environmental conditions (UVR levels). Nevertheless, sunburn can be taken as a marker of exposure levels likely to indicate increased risk of skin cancer [24].

Cumulative self-reported "summer sunburn" has been the most common measure of sunburn used in population studies (see Tables 12.1-3). This measure suffers from poor recall. Reports of sunburn on specific days, such as immediate-past weekends, provide a more accurate measure but do not represent the occurrence of sunburn over a whole season. Estimates of weekend sunburn over summer can be obtained from weekly data collection but this method is not widely used in population studies except in Australia and New Zealand. The measurement of sunburn related to outdoor activities on specific days has allowed examination of the behavioral components of trends in sunburn by adjusting for UV and temperature data for the relevant dates. Only in Victoria, Australia, has this method been used to monitor trends in sunburn related to behavioral change and health promotion activities [25,26].

Table 12.1 Sunburn and sun exposure representative population surveys: Adults

Country	Year	Study	Population	n	Sun exposure – usual (hours)	Sun exposure – specific occasion (hours)	Summer sunburn[a]	Weekend sunburn[b]
Australia	1988	[24]	14-69 yrs	1655	-	=2.08 (t2 w)	-	16%
	1990	[25]	14-69 yrs	1376	-	72% >15min (t2 w)	-	-
	1992	[27]	14-69 yrs	2317	-	=1.87 (t2 w)	-	20%
	1998	[28]	14+ yrs	601	-	-	41%	-
New Zealand	1994	[29]	15-65 yrs	1243	-	=2-3 (t4 w)	-	12%
Canada	1996	[30]	25+ yrs	3449	26% >2h	-	50%	-
United States	1996	[31]	18+ yrs	1010	43% >5h	-	39%	-

Note: Year is publication year if the year of data collection is not reported.

Reports of exposure:
( ) the mean "daily" exposure; or (% >x hours/minutes) the proportion of people who spent a minimum number of hours outside.
In addition, some studies' measures *restricted times* to between:
   t1 = daylight hours; t2 = 11am & 3pm; t3 = 10am & 4pm; t4 = 11am & 4pm; w = days on weekend

Reports of sunburn:
(a) Individuals report retrospectively on whether sunburned in the *past summer*.
(b) Individuals report on whether they experienced at least mild erythema on the *previous weekend*.

Table 12.2 Sunburn and sun exposure representative population surveys: Adolescents

Country	Year	Study	Population	n	Sun exposure – usual (hours)		
					M	F	P
Australia	1990	[32]	12-17 yrs	4721	-	-	-
	1990	[33]	13-15 yrs	972	-	-	-
New Zealand	1997	[34]	12-17 yrs	203	-	-	-
	1994	[35]	21 yrs cohort	909	-	-	-
Canada	1996	[36]	15-24 yrs	574	-	-	36%>2hr
United States	1998	[37]	11-18 yrs	1192	=3.5-4	-	- (t3 w)
	1994	[38]	11-19 yrs	658	=5.7	=5.1	=5.4 (t1 w)
					=5.3	=3.9	=5.1 (t1 WD)
	1992	[10]	Gr. 9 & 10	1703	=5.2	=4.5	- (t1)
	1993	[16]	17-23 yrs	266	-	-	72% >1hr
Norway	1992	[11]	School students	15169	=2.4	=3.3 /when sunbathing	-

M= Males; F= Females; P= People

Reports of exposure:
( ) the mean "daily" exposure; or (% >x hours/minutes) the proportion of people who spent a minimum number of hours outside.
In addition, some studies' measures *restricted times* to between:
    t1 = daylight hours; t2 = 11am & 3pm; t3 = 10am & 4pm; t4 = 11am & 4pm; t5 = peak UV;
    w = days on weekend; WD = week days
    and some are reported "of those people outdoors" = /of

Reports of sunburn:
(a) Individuals report retrospectively on whether sunburned in the *past summer.*
(b) Individuals report on whether they experienced at least mild erythema on the *previous weekend.*

Sun exposure – specific occasion (hours)			Summer sunburn[a]	Weekend sunburn[b]
M	F	P	P	P
-			66%	-
~80% >2hr	~60% >2hr	- [(t5)]	-	-
/during both Sat & Sun				
-	-	43% >2hr [(t4w)]	-	31% [(t4 w)]
		/of		/of
-	-	-	35% blistered sunburn in past 6 yrs	-
-	-	-	68%	-
-	-	-	-	-
-	-	-	-	-
-	-	-	-	-
-	-	-	-	-
-	-	-	-	-

Table 12.3 Sunburn and sun exposure representative population surveys: Children

Country	Year	Study	Population	n	Sun exposure – usual (hours)	Sun exposure – specific occasion (hours)	Summer sunburn[a]	Weekend sunburn[b]
Australia	1996	[39]	5-13 yrs	735**	-	-	56%[c]	15%[d]
New Zealand	1996	[40]	2-12 yrs	887	-	-	29% (Jan)	-
	1994	[17]	≤10 yrs	285	-	-	-	7% (w) /of
Canada	1996	[41]	≤12 yrs	1051	51% >2h	-	45% (June-Aug)	-
United States	1997	[42]	≤12 yrs	503	=5.1 (t3) =7.5 (t1 w)	-	-	13% (past weekend/ week day)
Germany	1996	[23]	5-8 yrs	287	-	-	50% (ever)	-
South France	1992	[43]	3-15 yrs	573	50% >6h	-	89% (ever)	-

** *Select sample of primary school students*

Reports of exposure:
( ) the mean "daily" exposure or (% >x hours/minutes) the proportion of people who spent a minimum number of hours outside
In addition, some studies' measures *restricted times* to between:
    t1 = daylight hours; t2 = 11am & 3pm; t3 = 10am & 4pm; t4 = 11am & 4pm; w = days on weekend
    and some are reported "of those people outdoors" =/of

Reports of sunburn:
(a) Individuals report retrospectively on whether sunburned in the *past summer*
(b) Individuals report on whether they experienced at least mild erythema on the *previous weekend.*
(c) Cumulative over 8 weeks in *spring*
(d) Point prevalence average over 8 weeks

Returning to the commonly reported incidence of summer sunburn, it is important to note that while estimates of sunburn in different countries varied, to a large extent these differences might be attributed to populations of varied skin type and different UV environments. The data on the incidence of "summer sunburn" among adults in three countries was comparable, ranging from 39% in the United States [31], 41% in Australia [28], and 50% in Canada [30]. In a study in Britain, the majority of burns in the last 12 months occurred in the spring and summer months and 46% were the result of sun exposure abroad [44].

There is some evidence that incidence of summer sunburn varies with age in a pattern closely reflecting the groups less likely to report regular sun protection. In the 1996 national surveys conducted in Canada, summer sunburn was lowest among children (45%) compared to youth (68%) and adults (50%) [30,36,41]. Sunburn on specific summer weekends also appears to be less prevalent among children. In New Zealand, 7% of children [17] and 12% of adults [29] were sunburned on summer weekends.

A number of studies reported sunburn by gender. For adults, sunburn was consistently more common among males than females [24,25,28-31]. Sunburn among male and female adolescents was more variable, with two studies reporting more sunburn among females [35,36] and one study reporting more sunburn among males [38]. Sunburn was equally likely among girls and boys in one study [39] and slightly higher among girls in the other study [40].

In some studies, people with sensitive skin types experienced the most sunburn [10,24,38,39,41,42,45]. In others, people with moderately sensitive skin (burn then tan) experienced more sunburn than those with very sensitive skin (burn only), while those with less sensitive skin (tan only) suffered the least sunburn [8,28,30,46].

2.2　Sun protection

Tables 12.4-6, summarizing data from 29 studies, provide an overview of the use of specific sun protection strategies by people in the United States, Canada, Australia and New Zealand. The data on sun protection in other countries was excluded from the tables on sun protection, as they were often limited to certain age groups and smaller non-representative samples. The excluded studies were from northern European countries focusing on protection used during sunbed use and holidays to warmer climates [11,46,47], or from southern European countries with warmer climates reporting children's sun protection during recreational activities outdoors [18,23,43], and one study in Japan reporting on sunscreen use of adults [48].

Table12.4 Regular summer sun protection population surveys: Adults

Country	Year	Study	Population	n	Seek shade			Wear hats		
					M	F	P	M	F	P
Australia	1998	[28]	14+ yrs	601	57% (T2 i)	73%	65% [a]	62% (T2 i)	41%	51% [a]
	1992†	[27]	14-69 yrs	2317	- (T2 i)	-	36% [b]	- (T2 i)	-	56% [b]
	1990†	[25]	14-69 yrs	1376	-	-	-	32% (T2 i)	26%	29% [b]
	1988	[24]	14-69 yrs	1655	-	-	-	23% (T2 i)	14%	18% [b]
New Zealand	1994	[29]	15-65 yrs	1243	-	-	-	- (T3 i)	-	38% [b]
Canada	1996	[30]	25+ yrs	3449	36% (ii)	48%	44% [a]	54% (ii) cover head	34%	45% [a]
	1987	[49]	35-64 yrs	3843	-	-	-	43% (T4)	26%	- [a]
United States	1996†	[31]	18+ yrs	1010	- (iii)	-	39% [c]	- (iii)	-	32% [c]
	1992	[50]	17+ yrs	10048	22% (iii)	37%	30% [c]	-	-	-
	1994	[51]	18-65 yrs	864 San Diego residents	-	-	-	- (iv)	-	13% [a]

* Publication year (time of data collection not reported).
** Select sample - Birth Cohort
† Trend study most recent year's data reported
     M = Males; F = Females; P = People
     wb = wide-brimmed; l/sleeved = long-sleeved; (p) = wear protective clothing

(a) Use reported when outside as either in the *highest category* (if a 4-point scale used) or in the *highest two categories* (if a 5-point scale used eg. "often" and "always"), is reported.
(b) Use reported when outside for *a specific occasion or time* of high sun exposure.
(c) Likely use reported when out more than 1 hour on a sunny day.

Use covering clothing			Use sunscreen			Avoid sun			Composite sun protection behavior		
M	F	P	M	F	P	M	F	P	M	F	P
-	-	47% [a]	30%	55%	43% [a]	46%	68%	56%	-	-	-
(T2 i) wear covering clothes (gender n.s.)			(T2 i) SPF 15+			(T2) ever in last summer					
-	-	-	28% (T2 i)	43%	33% [b]	-	-	-	-	-	0.61 [b]
									mean body cover		
-	-	-	15% (T2 i)	28%	21% [b]	-	-	-	0.72	0.69	0.71 [b]
									mean clothing cover		
-	-	-	16% (T2 i)	25%	21% [b]	-	-	-	0.67	0.67	- [b]
									mean clothing cover		
-	-	-	- (T3 i)	-	32% [b]	-	-	-	-	-	-
50% (ii) (p)	40%	45% [a]	22% on face (ii)	57%	38% [a]	31% (T3)	45%	38% [a]	-	-	-
			- on body	-	32% [a]						
27% (T4) cover-up arms & legs	18%	- [a]	15% (T4) SPF 8+	35%	- [a]	14% (T4)	35%	- [a]	-	-	-
-	-	-	- (iii)	-	42% [c]	-	-	-	-	-	-
27% (iii) (p) eg, wb hats or l/sleeved shirts	29%	28% [c]	22% (iii)	41%	32% [c]	-	-	-	-	-	53%
									use of 1 or more sun protection behaviors		
- (iv) a shirt with sleeves	-	26% [a]	- on face (iv)	-	20% [a]	-	-	-			
			- on body	-	11% [a]						

When in sun/outside:
   (i)   >15 minutes
   (ii) > 30 minutes
   (iii) > 1 hour
   (iv) during recreation

In addition, some studies assessed behaviors restricted to certain times of the day
   T1 = daylight hours; T2 = 11am-3pm; T3 = 11am-4pm; T4 = 10am-2pm

Table12.5 Regular summer sun protection population surveys: Adolescents

Country	Year	Study	Population	n	Seek shade			Wear hats		
					M	F	P	M	F	P
Australia	1996	[52]	12-17 yrs	49373	28% (T2) (iii)	34%	31% [a]	64% (T2) (iii)	38%	50% [a]
	1993	[53]	Yr 7-12	23915	23% (T2) (iii)	30%	- [a]	62% (T2) (iii)	38%	- [a]
	1990	[33]	13-15 yrs	972	-	-	-	-	-	10% [b]
	1990	[32]	12-17 yrs	4721	-	-	-	- (T2)	-	12% [a]
New Zealand	1997	[34]	12-17 yrs	203	-	-	-	33% (T3) hat	21%	28% [b]
	1994	[35]	21 yrs**	909	-	-	-	-	-	-
	1991	[54]	13-15 yrs	345	-	-	-	43% sunhat	20%	31% [a]
Canada	1996	[36]	15-24 yrs	574	22% (ii)	29%	26% [a]	55% (ii) hat/cover head	19%	38% [a]
United States	1998	[37]	11-18 yrs	1192	22% (iii) stay in shade	22%	22% [a]	4% (iii) wb hat	4%	4% [a]
	1994	[38]	11-19 yrs	658	-	-	-	56% cap	20%	- [c]
	1996*	[45]	11 yrs	509	-	-	-	45%	19%	32% [b]
	1992*	[10]	High school	1703	-	-	-	-	-	-
	1993*	[16]	17-23 yrs	266	-	-	-	-	-	-

*   Publication year (time of data collection not reported).
** Select sample - Birth Cohort
     M = Males; F = Females; P = People; SPB = Sun Protection Behaviors
     wb = wide-brimmed; l/sleeved = long-sleeved; (q) = clothes covering most of the body

(a) Use reported when outside as either in the *highest category* (if a 4-point scale used) or in the *highest two categories* (if a 5-point scale used eg. "often" and "always"), is reported.
(b) Use reported when outside *for a specific occasion or time* of high sun exposure.
(c) Likely use reported when out more than 1 hour on a sunny day.

Use covering clothing			Use sunscreen			Avoid sun			Composite sun protection behavior		
M	F	P	M	F	P	M	F	P	M	F	P
28% (T2)(iii)(q)	21%	24% [a]	51% (T2)(iii)	72%	61% [a]	19% (T2) stay inside	19%	19% [a]	-	-	-
27% (T2)(iii)(q)	22%	25% [a]	54% (T2)(iii) max SPF	73%	- [a]	- (T2/T4) stay inside	-	<20% [a]	-	-	-
- shirts to elbows or wrists	-	46% [b]	-	-	13% [b]	-	-	-	-	-	-
-	-	-	- (T2) SPF 15+	-	27% [a]	-	-	-	-	-	-
-	-	-	30% (T3)	51%	39% [b]	45% (T3) chose out of sun /of those outdoors	61%	51% [b]	-	-	-
-	-	-	-	-	42% [a]	-	-	-	-	-	-
58%	46%	52% [a]	49%	59%	54% [a]	-	-	-	-	-	-
35% (ii) protect with clothing	27%	31% [a]	25% (ii) on face	47%	35% [a]	20% (T3)	32%	26% [a]	-	-	-
23% (iii) wear long pants (4% l/sleeved shirt)	18%	20% [a]	25% (iii)	38%	31% [a]	-	-	-	54% use 1-2 SPB	64%	59% [a]
-	-	-	-	-	-	-	-	-	- use 3-6 SPB	-	10%
- l/sleeved shirt	-	4% [c]	17%	35%	26% [a]	-	-	-	-	-	-
45% shirts with sleeves	55%	50% [b]	11% [b]	21% [b]	-	-	-	-	-	-	-
-	-	-	-	-	23% [a]	-	-	-	-	-	-
-	-	-	8%	17%	- [a]	-	-	-	-	-	-
-	-	-	-	-	7% [a]	-	-	-	-	-	-

When in sun/outside:
- (i)   >15 minutes
- (ii) >30 minutes
- (iii) >1 hour
- (iv) during recreation

In addition, some studies assessed behaviors restricted to certain times of the day
  T1 = daylight hours; T2 = 11am-3pm; T3 = 11am-4pm; T4 = 10am-2pm

Table12.6 Regular summer sun protection population surveys: Children

Country	Year	Study	Population	n	Seek shade	Wear hats
Australia	1996	[39]	5-13 yrs	735[†]	53% [a]	86% [a]
New Zealand	1996/97	[40]	2-12 yrs	887	22% [a] (T3)	64% [a] (T3) legionnaires cap
	1994	[17]	≤10 yrs	285	-	59% [b] (T3) hat/cap
Canada	1996	[41]	≤12 yrs	1051	38% [a] (ii)	71% [a] (ii)
	1993	[19]	age not specified	925[‡]	20% [c] (ii) have child play in shade	70% [c] (ii) insist child wears a hat
United States	1997	[42]	≤12 yrs	503	30% [c] stay in shade	27% [c] hat with 4-inch brim

†   Sample of 5 Melbourne primary schools
‡   Sample of parents with children attending emergency dept of pediatric hospital
          wb = wide-brimmed; l/sleeved = long-sleeved

(a) Use reported when outside as either in the *highest category* (if a 4-point scale used) or in the *highest two categories* (if a 5-point scale used eg. "often" and "always"), is reported.
(b) Use reported when outside for a *specific occasion or time* of high sun exposure.
(c) Likely use reported when out more than 1 hour on a sunny day.

Use covering clothing	Use sunscreen	Avoid sun	Composite sun protection behavior
70% [a] cover-up with clothes	72% [a]	46% [a] (T2) stay inside	-
15% [a] (T3) l/sleeved shirts 12% [a] (T3) cover legs	86% [a] (T3) SPF 15+	-	-
-	52% [b] (T3)	-	53% [b] (T3) a hat & sunscreen
58% [a] when in sun >2 hrs wear clothing	76% [a] (ii) use on both face/body	36% (T3) avoid sun	-
50% [c] (ii) favor protective clothing	66% [c] (ii) apply sunscreen to all exposed skin	-	35% [c] (ii) hat & shirts & sunscreen
8% [c] l/sleeved shirt	53% [c] SPF 15+ 50% [b]	-	-

When in sun/outside:
  (i)   >15 minutes
  (ii)   >30 minutes
  (iii) >1 hour
  (iv)   during recreation

In addition, some studies assessed behaviors restricted to certain times of the day:
  T1 = daylight hours; T2 = 11am-3pm; T3 = 11am-4pm; T4 = 10am-2pm

As with the measures of sun exposure, measures of sun protection varied widely. Most of these studies specified sun protection "when in the sun" or "outdoors on sunny days", often during the middle of the day for at least 15 minutes or more. The type of activity was generally not specified; however, the data mainly apply to sun protection during incidental exposure, including activities such as play, gardening, passive and active recreation, socializing and doing chores. Data for children were generally by parents' proxy report.

2.2.1   Sun protection by country

Overall, the prevalence patterns showed little consistency between countries but some of these differences might be attributed to the different timing of the surveys. Despite this, there appears to be a trend for increased prevalence of a range of sun protection behaviors in countries where skin cancer control efforts have been sustained for several years.

In Australia and New Zealand, sunscreen was widely used by all age groups [28,29,39,40,52,54] and was most prevalent among children at 72% [39] and 86% [40] respectively. Sunscreen use was less common among adolescents and adults in Canada [30,36] but the large majority of Canadian children (76%) [41] regularly used sunscreen when outdoors. In the United States sunscreen use was less common overall, including a lower prevalence of use among children (53%) [42].

In Australia, regular use of shade was also common among adults (65%) [28] compared to use in the other countries, for example to 39% of adults in the United States [31]. Although regular hat use was reasonably common in all four countries, there were little data on protective styles of hats used. Recent prevalence estimates of hat use ranged from 59% to 86% for children, 32% to 51% for adults and 28% to 50% of adolescents.

Use of clothing as a means of sun protection was generally low in all four countries. Nonetheless, measures of use of clothing cover varied widely and prevalence estimates appear to be influenced by subtle differences in the context of measures. Reporting whether "clothing cover" was worn by adults was nearly double the prevalence (at 47% and 45% of adults respectively) [28,30] as those studies where the measure was "long-sleeve shirts or wide-brimmed hats" (26% and 28%) [50,51]. Prevalence estimates in studies of adolescents also appear to vary according to the specificity of the measures. A study in Australia reported only 24% of adolescents wore clothing "covering most of" the body [52]. A study in New Zealand reported the highest use of clothing by adolescents with 52% reporting they "protect themselves" with clothing [54]. Children's regular use of clothing showed similar variability by type of clothing specified. Children's use of covering clothing ranged from 8% of children in the United States who regularly used "long-sleeved shirts" [42], to 70% of children in an Australian study who wore "covering clothing" on sunny days [39].

Few studies report on one of the most efficient means of minimizing UV exposure, that is "limiting time outside during the middle of the day." Recent studies report 56% of adults [28], 19% of adolescents [52] and 46% of children in Australia [39]; and 38% of adults [30], 20% of male youth, 32% of female youth [36] and 36% of children [41] in Canada choose to stay inside or avoid the sun.

2.2.2   Composite measures of sun protection

Given that to some extent one form of sun protection may be substituted for another, assessing the total combined protection of all the precautions a person has taken is better than counting them separately. Few authors report on protection achieved by the combined effects of clothing, sunscreen, and hat use. In one Australian study an algorithm was developed to provide a "total body exposure index" which was shown to vary by age, sex and skin-type [24]. A limitation of this type of index is that it is only applicable for a particular point in time and therefore is limited to use in point-prevalence studies of sun protection behavior. Another study reported "adequate sun protection" defined by use of either "a hat and shirt" or "sunscreen" or "in the shade" for each opportunity. As recorded in sun protection diaries, 40% of students in the study were adequately protected when outdoors for two hours or more [55,56].

A few studies report the proportion of people who usually use at least one form of sun protection. A national study of children in the United States found the majority of children (74%) used at least one form of sun protection [57]. Similarly, the majority of parents (91%) attending a Canadian pediatric hospital indicated they would ensure their children used at least one form of sun protection, including hats, sunscreen or clothing, when playing outdoors in the sun for more than 30 minutes [19]. Over two-thirds (69%) reported they would use two forms of sun protection and 35% would use all three for their children at every opportunity. The overall proportion of adults who usually use at least one form of sun protection was somewhat lower. A study of adults in the United States report just over half usually would use one form of sun protection when they were outdoors [50].

2.2.3   Sun protection by age

Despite the varied adoption of sun protection in different countries, with few exceptions, consistent patterns in sun protection can be noted for different age groups and genders. Children were generally best protected:

use of hats, clothing, and sunscreen was on average 20% to 30% higher than for adolescents and adults. This is encouraging, as adults largely control children's sun protection [58]. It suggests that parents and caregivers have at least recognized that children, if not themselves, need to be protected from the sun. Children's use of shade during lengthy time outside was one exception and was generally less commonly used than other sun protection strategies. For example, in Australia 53% of children [39], compared to 65% of adults [28], regularly sought shade. Compared to other strategies regularly used by children for sun protection, avoidance of midday sun was also limited. Some indication of the practicalities of avoiding the midday sun was given by parents in the national survey in the United States, with more parents agreeing that outdoor activities were usually easier to plan after 4 pm (68%) than before 10 am (46%) [42].

Studies of adolescents' sun protection behavior were often not directly comparable to population data on adults. Nonetheless, available data using standard measures suggests adolescents generally perform sun protective strategies less frequently than adults. Data from a national survey in Canada showed young people, compared to adults, less frequently used shade (26% cf. 44%), clothing (31% cf. 45%), and sunscreen (35% cf. 38%); hats were also worn less frequently by female youth (19% cf. 34%) but male adults and adolescents commonly wore hats (55% cf. 54%) [30,36].

It is disappointing that the gains in sun protection during childhood do not translate into habitual sun protection during adolescence. The decline in sun protection during adolescence is often attributed to increased concern about appearance, development of pro-tan attitudes and more independence from parents [8,32]. Many adolescents spend lengthy periods outdoors during leisure activities [43,59], along with higher activity needs and more opportunity for outdoor leisure than adults, and their apparent neglect of sun protection is cause for concern.

2.2.4   Gender differences

Regular use of hats was more common among males than females during both adolescence and adulthood. Hats in particular appear to be widely used by men in many countries, particularly among adolescents, with estimates of frequent use between 43% to 64% of males in Canada, the United States, New Zealand and Australia. A few studies reporting the type of hat worn find few people wear protective broad-brimmed or legionnaire styles [53,60]. While children more commonly wear the legionnaire style of hat [39,40], caps appear to be more popular for adolescents and adults [61] and may be worn more for fashion or in preference to sunglasses to reduce glare when participating in sports.

In contrast, females more frequently used sunscreen [10,24,25,27,28, 30,32,34-37,45,49,50,52-54]. This may result from heavy marketing of sunscreen to women and women's habitual use of other skin care products, which more recently are likely to contain sunscreens to retard skin ageing. Females were also generally more likely to report they regularly utilized shade for sun protection [28,30,36,50,52,53]. There was, however, little consistent difference among men and women in the use of covering clothing for sun protection.

2.3   Prevalence of sunbathing and intentional tanning

Exposing skin to sunlight for the *purpose of getting a tan* may be a secondary (and intended) reason to engage in a range of outdoor activities. Sunbathing is for some people the clearest example of intentional sun exposure and is thereby given separate treatment here. Use of artificial UV sources in intentional tanning, as mentioned previously, is covered in Chapter 9. Thirteen large studies reported on the prevalence of sunbathing and intentional tanning for specific populations. Unfortunately, most of the data in these studies were relatively dated or among unrepresentative samples [4,10,12,16,33,47,54]. Recent data on the prevalence of intentional tanning found 25% of adults in the United States [31], 28% in New Zealand [29], and 33% in Britain [44] "work on" or "attempt" a suntan over summer or in the past year. Intentional tanning was slightly more common among Canadian youth, at 44% reporting active seeking of a suntan over the last summer [36]. Twenty-six percent of male and 30% of female Swedish university students reported regular sunbathing with the intention of getting a tan [62].

There is little reported on the prevalence of sunbathing or tanning in children. One study in New Zealand reported that 40% of parents surveyed at the beginning of summer intended to let their child get a suntan over summer, while 60% did not. They found parental intentions predicted children with a suntan in mid-summer, but by the end of summer the vast majority of children had gained a suntan and parental intentions were no longer correlated with suntan outcome [40].

In all studies reporting gender differences, tanning and sunbathing was more prevalent among females than males.

2.4   Populations at the beach or sunbathing

Specific studies of sunbathers, beachgoers and sunbed users reveal the degree of risk and factors associated with people's tanning and sunbathing. Studies reviewed include 16 studies, 13 at beaches [21,63-74] and one of

sunbathers at parks and a beach [75,76]. Two studies provide details on
sunbathers' sun exposure over a whole holiday period rather than at a
specific time [77,78]. Thirteen of the studies at beaches had data on sun
exposing or sun protective behavior. Three other studies not included in this
section reported more on psychosocial correlates of suntanning and not on
the prevalence of sun-related behaviors [9,79,80]. Detail on "usual"
exposure during suntanning or when at the beach is available from larger
population studies [12,51,81,82].

It appears that tanning motivates the majority of beachgoers. This was
the case for each of the studies mentioning reasons for beach attendance. In
1988/89, 57% of beachgoers in Puerto Rico [70], and in 1995 70% of
beachgoers in Connecticut [68] were at the beach to get or maintain a suntan.
Similarly, a study on a surf beach in Australia in 1990/91 reports a high
prevalence of "sunbaking" motivation among adolescents [63]. More
females than males reported suntanning motivation at these Connecticut and
Australian beaches [63,68].

2.4.1   Time outside

With surprising consistency in these settings, intended sunbathing
exposures were on average three to four hours (see Table 12.7) [63,64,67-
69,75]. A recent randomized trial of sunscreen use by French and Swiss
university students on summer vacations suggests that use of higher SPF
sunscreen while sunbathing was likely to extend time spent sunbathing [77].

Four of these studies reported the frequency of sunbathing. New Jersey
beachgoers reported they spent 2.3 days per week sunbathing [69];
adolescent beachgoers in Victoria (Australia) spent an average of 19 days
over summer at the beach [63]; and study participants in the sunscreen trial
spent 19 to 20 days sunbathing on their summer vacations [77]. The majority
of white beachgoers at a Cape Peninsula beach in South Africa reported
being at the beach during peak UV periods and spending more than 10 days
sunbathing over the summer [72].

Estimates of total exposure annually and over summer have also been
reported. Thirty-five percent of children and 45% of adolescents in a city in
southern France spend more than 15 hours per week outside in their
swimsuit over July [78]. Of beachgoers at Puerto Rico, residents spent an
average of 80 hours per year and tourists 55 hours per year in intense leisure
exposure [70].

Exposure times of specific groups were assessed in three of these studies:
Pratt *et al.* found that more male than female adolescents were frequent
beachgoers (21 versus 16 days) and stayed longer when at the beach (142
versus 103 minutes) [63]. Similarly, Nguyen *et al.* found males spent longer

at the beach. In addition, young adults and people who tanned easily and were sunburned rarely spent longer at the beach [69]. In one study of Danish sunbathers there was no difference in sun exposure by skin type [75].

Table 12.7 Average length of exposure at the beach.

Country each setting	Studies	Population	Average time at beach/ sunbathing	Comment
United States				
3 New Jersey beaches	[69]	13-87 yrs	3.7 hours	
3 Connecticut beaches	[68]	12+ yrs	4 hours	
Galveston Island Beach	[67]	15-69 yrs	3 hours	
Denmark				
4 parks & 1 beach	[75]	av 28 yrs	3.4 hours	Of sunbathers had applied sunscreen
			3.3 hours	Of sunbathers not using sunscreen
South Africa				
3 Cape Peninsula beaches	[72]	18+ yrs	12-3pm (65%)	
Australia				
1 Victoria surf beach	[63]	15-20 yrs		
			2 hours	Spent at the beach between 11-3pm
			1 hour	Spent at the beach at other times of the day
2 Victoria beaches	[64]	8-12 yrs	>2 hours (75%)	Parent proxy report
France/Switzerland				
Sunbathers on holiday	[77]	18-24 yrs		(Daily over holiday)
			3.1 hours	SPF 30 group
			2.6 hours	SPF10 group

In contrast, other population studies reporting on "usual exposure" times found more frequent sunbathing and longer exposure times among females, but confirm more frequent sunbathing among younger adults. In a national survey of adults in the United States, 27% of women compared to 23% of men reported frequent sunbathing of at least 11 or more days in the past year [81]. Likewise, a survey of high school students in Norway reports, on average, females spent more time sunbathing than males (at 3.3 and 2.4 hours respectively) [11]. A survey of San Diego residents found that, of the 54% of residents who spent at least 10% of their time in the sun trying to get a tan, on average, younger people were more frequent tanners. Those aged 18 to 24 years spent nearly one-third of their time in the sun "tanning" while those aged 45 to 54 years spent one-fifth of their time in the sun "tanning" [51]. Similarly, Koh *et al.* [81] report more frequent sunbathing among people aged less than 40 years.

2.4.2   Sunburn

Sunburn specific to a sunbathing episode is rarely reported, as it requires follow-up at the end of the sunbathing period. Stender *et al.* surveyed sunbathers' sunburn the following day. Twenty-nine percent of sunbathers who had not used sunscreen and 22% of sunscreen users got sunburn as a result of the previous day's sunbathing [75]. Seasonal sunburn, over summer months or on a recent holiday, is more frequently reported. In this case the incidence may not relate specifically to the intentional exposure. For example, Autier *et al.* report 45% of sunbathers were sunburned at least once on their summer holiday. Frequent sunbathing was a common activity for this group but they may also have been sunburned during other outdoor activities [77]. Paradoxically, duration or extent of exposure is not a strong predictor of sunburn. However, perceived susceptibility strongly predicts sunburn occurrence. A study of San Diego tanners reported, in fact, that those who spent the most time sunbathing experienced the least sunburn [51].

2.4.3   Use of sunscreen

Measurement of sun protection used during sunbathing and at the beach in these studies was generally limited to sunscreen use. The mean prevalence of use of sunscreens was 69% in 14 studies of beachgoers and sunbathers. On average more females than males had applied sunscreen (an average of 72% cf. 58% in five studies) [66,68,69,72,75]. Sunscreen was also more commonly used by children (75% of children in five studies [21,64,65, 73,74] cf. 67% of adolescents in three studies [63,65,71] and 64% of adults in eight studies [65,67-70,72,73,75] were using sunscreens). Nevertheless, while the majority used sunscreens, there was considerable variation and some studies reported high proportions of beachgoers and sunbathers not using any sunscreen. In 1988/89 half of residents compared to 23% of tourists visiting Puerto Rican beaches [70], and on Connecticut beaches in 1995, 52% of males and 40% of females were not using sunscreen [68].

Only five of these studies report use of sunscreens with a sun protection factor of at least SPF 15. This may be due to a number of factors, including historically a limited availability and marketing of maximum protection sunscreens in many countries and hence limited reporting of their use. The average proportion of beachgoers using a maximum protection sunscreen in these five studies was 77%, ranging from 63% to 100% of sunscreen users [64-66,69,73]. Use of more protective sunscreens appears to be more common among beachgoers with sensitive skins and among children. Reported use of SPF 15 sunscreen by New South Wales beachgoers was as high as 85% among children and somewhat lower for other age groups [65]. Moreover, children under 10 years of age were more likely to be wearing higher SPF sunscreens in a study of Danish sunbathers [76]. Puerto Rican beachgoers with fairer skin types more commonly used a sunscreen of at least SPF 4 [70].

2.4.4 How sunscreen is used

A few studies also provide some insight into how people use sunscreens when at the beach. There appears to be considerable variation in use/ application. In Australia, two studies report the majority of beachgoers had applied sunscreen on arrival or within 10 minutes of arrival at the beach [64,65]. In a more detailed observational study of sunscreen use, Robinson *et al.* reported the delay in commencing applying sunscreen by families arriving at a Lake Michigan beach was usually 9 minutes. In addition, families took up to 42 minutes to finish applying sunscreen to all family members [73]. Application at the start of exposure was less common on San Juan beaches, only 40% of sunscreen users having applied sunscreen on arrival at this beach [71]. In contrast, the majority of sunbathers had applied sunscreen prior to arriving at their sunbathing location in Denmark [76].

It is recommended that, even when using waterproof sunscreens, reapplication is required after swimming to ensure maximum protection (see Chapter 13). Reapplication of sunscreen after swimming varied widely. Of those using sunscreens, 61% at Queensland beaches [66], 30% at San Juan beaches [71] and 42% of Danish sunbathers over 10 years of age [75] reapplied sunscreen after leaving the water. Only one study reported on use of water-resistant sunscreens. On Queensland beaches in 1989, as many as 88% of sunscreen users chose to wear a water-resistant formula [66].

Another common misuse of sunscreens is that people do not apply them to all exposed skin. There is little consistency in body areas left exposed, but it would appear that the legs, in particular, are frequently left unprotected [66,74]. In addition, at least in one beach study the face was better protected than the body [72], with similar reports among tanners in population studies [36,51]. Three studies report a body cover index, with mean protection from clothing or sunscreen ranging from approximately one-third to one-half of the body [63,64,74]. Two of these studies report on children's composite protection, with a fair proportion inadequately protected. At one lake beach in the United States children had better cover than mothers or fathers, but almost one-third of girls at the beach had no protection other than a bathing suit and only 10% had protected their legs [74]. Similarly, at a beach in Victoria, Australia, one-fifth of children had no head cover from either sunscreen or a hat [64]. The other study reported on sunscreen use on exposed skin over all ages, with up to three-quarters of sunscreen users having applied sunscreen to their whole body when sunbathing and 10% or less having used a lower sun protection factor on some body areas [76].

Table 12.8 Sunscreen use at the beach.

Country Beach setting	Year	Studies	Population	Point prevalence of sunscreen use		
				Total	Males	Females
United States						
3 New Jersey beaches	1993*	[69]	13-87 yrs	78%	71%	84%
3 Connecticut beaches	1995	[68]	12+ yrs	56%	48%	60%
Galveston Island Beach	1991	[21]	Children < 12 yrs‡	51%	-	-
Galveston Island Beach	1997	[67]	15-69 yrs	75%	-	-
Lake Michigan beach	1996	[73]				
			Children 1-10 yrs ‡	76%		
			Parents	-	46%	71%
New Hampshire lake beach	1995	[74]	Children 2-9 yrs‡	79%	-	-
Puerto Rico						
Puerto Rico beach	1988/89	[70]				
			Residents	50%	-	-
			Tourists	70%	-	-
Puerto Rico	1991/92	[71]	Adolescents 13-18 yrs	68%†	-	-
Denmark						
4 parks & 1 beach	1994	[75]	av 28 yrs	67%	52%	73%
South Africa						
3 Cape Peninsula beaches	1991/92*	[72]	18+ yrs	50%	49%	74%
Australia						
Queensland beaches	1989	[66]	2-78 yrs	70%	68%	71%
2 Victoria beaches	1989	[64]	Children 8-12 yrs‡	75%	-	-
1 Victoria surf beach	1990/91	[63]	15-20 yrs	74%	-	-
6 NSW beaches	1993*	[65]	Adults 15+ yrs & Children ‡	82%	-	-

Note:
* Publication year (time of data collection not reported)
‡ Proxy = Parent report
† "always use" unclear if this is a point prevalence or not

CONCLUSION

The studies described in this chapter highlight the variable nature of people's sun protective and sun exposing behaviors. These sun-related behaviors varied widely by country and by setting. Comparisons internationally are problematic because of a limited use of standard measures for sun-related behaviors and a lack of representative population studies in many European countries. Moreover, reporting of sun-related behaviors is strongly influenced by context and by recall bias. In recent years more studies have adopted the prevalence methods that minimize recall bias as the data often relates to the previous weekend. However, many of the studies reported behaviors over summer using various measure of frequency. Nevertheless, these studies reveal consistent prevalence patterns identifying risk groups to target in skin cancer control.

In general, average time spent exposed to the sun was much greater than that of the minimum erythemal dose. Average times spent at the beach were commonly over three hours. The prevalence of intentional exposure was variable but commonly less than one third in most countries. Nevertheless, sunbathing and tanning was more common among women than men, and relatively high among adolescents. Increased risk is also associated with incidental exposure when limited attention is paid to sun protection. The data suggests men in particular are at risk here, due to their extended time spent outdoors without the use of sunscreens or other adequate sun protection. Although limited data were available on children's sun exposure, there is some evidence that children spend more time outdoors than other age groups.

Most studies did not report in a way that permits evaluation of overall protection afforded by the various sun-protective behaviors people adopted. Studies of children's sun protection suggest that the majority uses at least one form of sun protection and, in general, children were best protected and suffer less sunburn than adults. Some sun protection strategies were more widely used than others, although these varied by age and gender. Overall, hats and sunscreens appear to be used widely, while people less frequently wore long-sleeved or covering clothing or minimized time outside during peak UV periods. Use of shade was variable. The underlying principle of adequate sun protection is to take an integrated approach to protect all skin. Options for sun protection are varied: some require forethought, preparation and cost; while others such as sun avoidance and seeking shade are more readily achieved.

Some concern has been expressed that skin cancer among sunscreen users may be relatively high. In this chapter there was little data to suggest that sunscreen use was any more favored as a form of sun protection during incidental exposure for any age group. Nonetheless, the studies of beachgoers' and sunbathers' sun protection suggest sunscreen is more widely used than other forms of protection in these contexts. Although sunscreen is a product intended to reduce UV exposure, paradoxically, it is posited that, through higher use among people of susceptible skin type, problems with application and its ability to allow extended exposure by prevention of sunburn, there is evidence of increased risk associated with use (see Chapter 8) [1]. The studies of beachgoers described earlier highlight some other important behavioral considerations in use of sunscreen. These included failing to apply sunscreen prior to exposure, failing to apply to all skin exposed to the sun, and failing to reapply sunscreen. In Chapter 13 strong arguments are also made for the benefits of applying sunscreen twice, due to problems in obtaining reasonable coverage of the skin in one application.

SUMMARY POINTS

- Modifying people's sun exposing and sun protective behaviors has the potential to be of significant benefit to skin cancer prevention efforts.
- Both incidental and intentional sun exposures contribute to an individual's risk of skin cancer with the average exposure times, as reviewed here, being well over that of the minimal erythemal dose.
- The population and beach studies reviewed here highlight the contingent nature of people's sun protective behaviors and wide variability in patterns of use. Children appear to be best protected and adolescent sun protection is often lacking, while both spend long periods of time outdoors. Males more often wear hats, while females more often wear sunscreen, stay indoors or seek shade but report more sunbathing.
- Inadequate application and reliance on sunscreen during time at the beach or sunbathing is cause for concern, suggesting continued monitoring and focus for public health promotion efforts is needed in this area.
- The review was limited in its ability to distinguish differences between countries given issues with comparability in measures and timing of surveys. In addition, it should be noted that many of the earlier studies reviewed are not relevant in light of current prevention efforts. Nonetheless, there was some data to suggest a trend for increased prevalence of a range of sun protection behaviors in countries where skin cancer control efforts have been sustained for several years.

IMPLICATIONS FOR PUBLIC HEALTH

Public health efforts need to address over-reliance on sunscreen use and work towards providing adequate alternatives. Prevention messages might promote selection of more protective styles of clothing for swimming and other water sports (rather than brief styles), provision of and use of shade, and avoidance of peak UV periods of the day. Equally, adequate sun protection during incidental sun exposure is important for skin cancer control efforts. This is especially so for children and adolescents, as early exposure is posited to increase risk later in life and because, as noted in this chapter, they also appear to be most likely to spend extended periods outside. Here research into barriers to regular use may prove valuable. The chapter also highlights some of the key influences in sun-related behavior that might be targeted in skin cancer control programs. Skin-type, personal dispositions to tanning and sun protection, social norms, enabling factors and the physical environment each play a role. In Chapter 14 recent skin cancer control initiatives are reviewed, providing an assessment of the efficacy of specific intervention strategies.

REFERENCES

1. International Agency for Research on Cancer Expert Group (2001) *Sunscreens.* IARC Handbooks of Cancer Prevention, Vol. 5. Lyon, France: IARC Press.
2. Hill J, Boulter J (1996) Sun protection behaviour – Determinants and trends. *Cancer Forum* **20(3):** 204-211.
3. Arthey S, Clarke VA (1995) Suntanning and sun protection: a review of the psychological literature. *Soc Sci Med* **40:** 265-274.
4. Hillhouse JJ, Adler CM, Drinnon J, Turrisi R (1997) Application of Azjen's theory of planned behavior to predict sunbathing, tanning salon use, and sunscreen use intentions and behaviors. *J Behav Med* **20:** 365-378.
5. Carmel S, Shani E, Rosenberg L (1994) The role of age and an expanded Health Belief Model in predicting skin cancer protective behavior. *Health Educ Res* **9:** 433-447.
6. Jackson K, Aiken L (2000) A psychosocial model of sun protection and sunbathing in young women: The impact of health beliefs, attitudes, norms and self-efficacy for sun protection. *Health Psychol* **19:** 469-478.
7. Hill D, Rassaby J, Gardner G (1984) Determinants of intentions to take precautions against skin cancer. *Community Health Stud* **VIII (1):** 33-43.
8. Clarke VA, Williams T, Arthey S (1997) Skin type and optimistic bias in relation to the sun protection and suntanning behaviors of young adults. *J Behav Med* **20:** 207-222.
9. Keesling B, Friedman HS (1987) Psychosocial factors in sunbathing and sunscreen use. *Health Psychol* **6:** 477-493.
10. Mermelstein RJ, Riesenberg LA (1992) Changing knowledge and attitudes about skin cancer risk factors in adolescents. *Health Psychol* **11:** 371-376.
11. Wichstrom L (1994) Predictors of Norwegian adolescents' sunbathing and use of sunscreen. *Health Psychol* **13:** 412-420.
12. Hillhouse JJ, Stair A, Adler CA (1996) Predictors of sunbathing and sunscreen use in college undergraduates. *J Behav Med* **19:** 544-561.
13. George PM, Kuskowski M, Schmidt C (1996) Trends in photoprotection in American fashion magazines, 1983-1993 will fashion make you look old and ugly? *J Am Acad Dermatol* **34:** 424-428.
14. Broadstock M, Borland R, Gason R (1992) Effects of suntan on judgements of healthiness and attractiveness by adolescents. *J Appl Soc Psychol* **22:** 157-172.
15. Miller AG, Ashton WA, McHoskey JW, Gimbel J (1990) What price attractiveness? Stereotype and risk factors in suntanning behaviour. *J Appl Soc Psychol* **20(15):** 1272-1300.
16. Leary MR, Jones JL (1993) The social psychology of tanning and sunscreen use: Self – presentational motives as a predictor of health risk. *J Appl Soc Psychol* **23:** 1390-1406.

17. McGee R, Williams S, Glasgow H (1997) Sunburn and sun protection among young children. *J Paediatr Child Health* **33**: 234-237.
18. Kakourou T, Kavadias G, Gatos A, Bilalis L, Krikos X, Matsniotis MD (1995) Mothers' knowledge and practices related to sun protection in Greece. *Pediatr Dermatol* **12(3)**: 207-210.
19. Zinman R, Schwartz S, Gordon K, Fitzpatrick E, Camfield C (1995) Predictors of sunscreen use in childhood. *Arch Pediatr Adolesc Med* **149**: 804-807.
20. Foltz AT (1993) Parental knowledge and practices of skin cancer prevention: a pilot study. *J Pediatr Health Care* **7**: 220-225.
21. Maducdoc L, Wagner J, R F, Wagner KD (1992) Parents' use of sunscreen on beach-going children: The burnt child dreads the fire. *Arch Derrmatol* **128**: 628-629.
22. Bourke JF, Healsmith MF, Graham-Brown RAC (1995) Melanoma awareness and sun exposure in Leicester. *Br J Dermatol* **132**: 251-256.
23. Abeck D, Feucht J, Schafer T, Behrendt H, Kramer U, Ring J (2000) Parental sun protection management in preschool children. *Photodermatology Photoimmunology & Photomedicine* **16**: 139-143.
24. Hill D, White V, Marks R, Theobald T, Borland R, Roy C (1992) Melanoma prevention: Behavioural and nonbehavioural factors in sunburn among an Australian urban population. *Prev Med* **21**: 654-669.
25. Hill D, White V, Marks R, Borland R (1993) Changes in sun-related attitudes and behaviours, and reduced sunburn prevalence in a population at high risk of melanoma. *Eur J Cancer Prev* **2**: 447-456.
26. Centre for Behavioural Research in Cancer (2000) Unpublished data. In: *SunSmart Campaign 2000-2003*. Melbourne, Victoria: Anti- Cancer Council of Victoria p32.
27. Baade PD, Balanda KP, Lowe JB (1996) Changes in skin protection behaviours, attitudes and sunburn: In a population with the highest incidence of skin cancer in the world. *Cancer Detect Prev* **20(6)**: 566-575.
28. Dobbinson S, Borland R (1999) Reaction to the 1997/98 SunSmart Campaign: Results from a representative household survey of Victorians. In: *SunSmart Evaluation Studies No. 6. The Anti-Cancer Council of Victoria's skin cancer control program and related research and evaluation.* Melbourne, Victoria: Anti-Cancer Council of Victoria, Chapter 7, p69-92.
29. McGee R, Williams S, Cox B, Elwood M, Bulliard J (1995) A community survey of sun exposure, sunburn and sun protection. *NZ Med J* **108**: 508-510.
30. Shoveller JA, Lovato CY, Peters L, Rivers JK (1998) Canadian national survey on sun exposure & protective behaviours: adults at leisure. *Cancer Prev Control* **2**: 111-116.
31. Robinson JK, Rigel DS, Amonette RA (1997) Trends in sun exposure knowledge, attitudes, and behaviors: 1986 to 1996. *J Am Acad Dermatol* **37**: 179-186.
32. Broadstock M, Borland, Hill D (1996) Knowledge, attitudes and reported behaviours relevant to sun protection and suntanning in adolescents. *Psychol Health* **11**: 527-539.
33. Fritschi L, Green A, Solomon PJ (1992) Sun exposure in Australian adolescents. *J Am Acad Dermatol* **27**: 25-28.
34. Richards R, McGee R, Knight RG (2001) Sunburn and sun protection among New Zealand adolescents over a summer weekend. *Aust NZ J Public Health* **25**: 352-354.
35. Douglass H, McGee R, Williams S (1997) Sun behaviour and perceptions of risk for melanoma among 21-year-old New Zealanders. *Aust NZ J Public Health* **21**: 329-334.
36. Lovato C, Shoveller J, Peters L, Rivers JK (1998) Canadian national survey on sun exposure & protective behaviours: youth at leisure. *Cancer Prev Control* **2**: 117-122.
37. Cokkinides VE, Johnston-Davis K, Weinstock M, *et al.* (2001) Sun exposure and sun-protection and attitudes among U.S. youth, 11 to 18 years of age. *Prev Med* **33**: 141-151.

38. Robinson JK, Rademaker AW, Sylvester JA, Cook B (1997) Summer sun exposure: knowledge, attitudes, and behaviors of Midwest adolescents. *Prev Med* **26:** 364-372.
39. Dixon H, Borland R, Hill D (1999) Sun protection and sunburn in primary school children: The influence of age, gender, and coloring. *Prev Med* **28:** 119-130.
40. Morris J, McGee R, Bandaranayake M (1998) Sun protection behaviours and the predictors of sunburn in young children. *Paediatr Child Health* **34:** 557-562.
41. Lovato CY, Shoveller JA, Peters L, Rivers JK (1998) Canadian national survey on sun exposure and protective behaviours: Parents' reports on children. *Cancer Prev Control* **2(3):** 123-128.
42. Robinson J, Rigel D, Amonette R (2000) Summertime sun protection used by adults for their children. *J Am Acad Dermatol* **42:** 746-53.
43. Vergnes C, Daures J, Sancho-Garnier H, *et al.* (1999) Patterns of sun exposure and sun protection of children in the south of France. *Ann Dermatol Venereol* **126:** 505-511.
44. Melia J, Bulman A (1995) Sunburn and tanning in a British population. *J Public Health Med* **17:** 223-229.
45. Reynolds KD, Blaum JM, Jester PM, Weiss, Soong SJ, Diclemente RJ (1996) Predictors of sun exposure in adolescents in a southeastern US population. *J Adolesc Health* **19(6):** 409-415.
46. Boldeman C, Beitner H, Jansson B, Nilsson B (1996) Sunbed use in relation to phenotype, erythema, sunscreen use and skin diseases A questionnaire survey among Swedish adolescents. *Br J Dermatol* **135:** 712-716.
47. Hughes BR, Altman DG, Newton JA (1993) Melanoma and skin cancer: evaluation of a health education programme for secondary schools. *Br J Dermatol* **128:** 412-417.
48. Kawada A, Hiruma M, Noda T, Kukita A (1989) Skin typing, sun exposure, and sunscreen use in a population of Japanese. *J Dermatol* **16:** 187-190.
49. Campbell HS, Birdsell JM (1994) Knowledge, beliefs, and sun protection behaviours of Alberta adults. *Prev Med* **23:** 160-166.
50. Hall HI, May DS, Lew RA, Koh HK, Nadel M (1997) Sun protection behaviors of the US white population. *Prev Med* **26:** 401-407.
51. Newman WG, Agro AD, Woodruff SI, Mayer JA (1996) A survey of recreational sun exposure of residents of San Diego, California. *Am J Prev Med* **12:** 186-194.
52. Livingston PM, White VM, Ugoni AM, Borland R (2001) Knowledge, attitudes and self-care practices related to sun protection among secondary students in Australia. *Health Educ Res* **16:** 269-278.
53. Lowe JB, Borland R, Stanton WR, Baade P, White V, Balanda KP (2000) Sun-safe behaviour among secondary school students in Australia. *Health Educ Res* **15:** 271-281.
54. McGee R, Williams S (1992) Adolescence and sun protection. *NZ Med J* **105:** 401-403.
55. Cockburn J, Hennrikus D, Scott R, Sanson-Fisher R (1989) Adolescent use of sun-protection measures. *Med J Aust* **151:** 136-140.
56. Sanson-Fisher R (1992) Re: "Adolescent use of sun-protection measures" by Jill Cockburn, Deborah Hennrikus, Robert Scott, Robert Sanson-Fisher (Med J Aust 1989; 151: 136-140). *Med J Aust* **157:** 216.
57. Robinson J, Rigel D, Amonette R (1998) Sun-protection behaviors used by adults for their children: United States, 1997. *MMWR* **June 19, 1998:** 480-482.
58. Hill D, Dixon H (1999) Promoting sun protection in children: rationale and challenges. *Health Educ Behav* **26:** 409-417.
59. Fritschi L, Green A (1995) Sun damage in teenagers' skin. *Aust J Public Health* **19:** 383-386.
60. Centre for Behavioural Research in Cancer (2000) Unpublished data. In: *SunSmart Campaign 2000-2003*. Melbourne, Victoria: Anti- Cancer Council of Victoria, p30.

61. SunSmart Schools Program (1999) *Secondary schools become SunSmart: some case studies.* Melbourne, Victoria: Anti-Cancer Council of Victoria.
62. Jerkegren E, Sandrieser L, Brandberg Y, Rosdahl I (1999) Sun-related behaviour and melanoma awareness among Swedish university students. *Eur J Cancer Prev* **8:** 27-34.
63. Pratt K, Borland R (1994) Predictors of sun protection among adolescents at the beach. *Aust Psychol* **29(2):** 135-139.
64. Bennetts K, Borland R, Swerissen H (1991) Sun protection behaviour of children and their parents at the beach. *Psychol Health* **5:** 279-287.
65. Foot G, Girgis A, Boyle CA, Sanson-Fisher RW (1993) Solar protection behaviours: a study of beachgoers. *Aust J Public Health* **17:** 209-214.
66. Pincus MW, Rollings PK, Craft AB, Green A (1991) Sunscreen use on Queensland beaches. *Australas J Dermatol* **32:** 21-25.
67. McCarthy EM, Ethridge KP, Wagner RF, Jr (1999) Beach holiday sunburn: the sunscreen paradox and gender differences. *Cutis* **64(1):** 37-42.
68. Zitser BS, Shah AN, Adams ML, St -Clair J (1996) A survey of sunbathing practices on three Connecticut State beaches. *Conn Med* **60:** 591-594.
69. Nguyen GT, Topilow AA, Frank E (1994) Protection from the sun: a survey of area beachgoers. *NJ Med* **91:** 321-324.
70. Ross SA, Sanchez JL (1990) Recreational sun exposure in Puerto Rico: trends and cancer risk awareness. *J Am Acad Dermatol* **23:** 1090-1092.
71. Rodriguez G, Ortiz R, Suarez R (1993) Patterns in sun exposure and sunscreen use among Puertorrican adolescents. *Bol Asoc Med P R* **85:** 21-23.
72. von-Schirnding Y, Strauss N, Mathee A, Robertson P, Blignaut R (1991) Sunscreen use and environmental awareness among beach-goers in Cape Town, South Africa. *Public Health Rev* **19:** 209-217.
73. Robinson JK, Rademaker AW (1998) Sun protection by families at the beach. *Arch Pediatr Adolesc Med* **152:** 466-470.
74. Olson A, Dietrich A, Sox C, Stevens M, Winchell C, Ahles T (1997) Solar protection of children at the beach. *Pediatrics* **99:** 1-5.
75. Stender IM, Lock-Andersen J, Wulf HC (1996) Sun-protection behaviour and self-assessed burning tendency among sunbathers. *Photodermatol Photoimmunol Photomed* **12:** 162-165.
76. Stender IM, Andersen JL, Wulf HC (1996) Sun exposure and sunscreen use among sunbathers in Denmark. *Acta Derm Venereol* **76:** 31-33.
77. Autier P, Dore JF, Negrier S, *et al.* (1999) Sunscreen use and duration of sun exposure: a double-blind, randomized trial. *J Nat Cancer Inst* **91:** 1304-1309.
78. Grob JJ, Guglielmina C, Gouvernet J, Zarour H, Noe C, Bonerandi JJ (1993) Study of sunbathing habits in children and adolescents: Application to the prevention of melanoma. *Dermatology* **186:** 94-98.
79. Eiser JR, Eiser C, Sani F, Sell L, Casas RM (1995) Skin cancer attitudes: a cross-national comparison. *Br J Soc Psychol* **34:** 23-30.
80. Rossi JS, Blais LM, Weinstock MA (1994) The Rhode Island sun smart project: Skin cancer prevention reaches the beaches. *Am J Public Health* **84(4):** 672-674.
81. Koh HK, Bak SM, Geller AC, *et al.* (1997) Sunbathing habits and sunscreen use among white adults: results of a national survey. *Am J Public Health* **87:** 1214-1217.
82. Mawn VB, Fleischer ABJ (1993) A survey of attitudes, beliefs, and behavior regarding tanning bed use, sunbathing, and sunscreen use. *J Am Acad Dermatol* **29:** 959-962.

Chapter 13

What can be done to reduce personal ultraviolet radiation exposure?

Brian L. Diffey, D.Sc., Ph.D.
Regional Medical Physics Department, Newcastle General Hospital, Newcastle upon Tyne, UK

Key words   sun avoidance, shade, clothing, sunscreens, risk management

INTRODUCTION

There is adequate evidence that exposure to solar ultraviolet (UV) radiation is a major etiological factor in human skin cancer [1]. Managing the risk of skin cancer does not necessarily mean reducing or avoiding the hazard, i.e., exposure to the sun's ultraviolet rays. For example, a walker who spends the day hiking across the hills on a summer's day is choosing not to minimize personal risk of skin cancer, but rather to face it and embrace it as part of an attempt to maximize their enjoyment and quality of life. A pragmatic approach, therefore, is to adopt strategies that control the hazard commensurate with the need or desire to be outdoors.

The approach here is to adopt a risk management model [2] to explore the feasibility of various strategies in controlling exposure to solar ultraviolet radiation, termed the "hazard" in the remainder of the chapter.

D. Hill et al. (eds.), Prevention of Skin Cancer, 241-258.
© 2004 *Kluwer Academic Publishers. Printed in the Netherlands.*

1.   PREVENT THE CREATION OF THE HAZARD

UV radiation is an integral component of terrestrial sunlight, which in addition comprises infrared and visible radiation (see Chapter 3). Solar radiation is responsible for the development and continued existence of life on Earth. Besides serving as the ultimate source of our food and energy, sunlight also acts on us to alter our chemical composition, control the rate of our maturation and drive our biological rhythms.

2.   REDUCE THE AMOUNT OF HAZARD BROUGHT INTO BEING

Rather than a reduction in ambient UV radiation, there is concern that depletion of the stratospheric ozone layer may result in increased levels of UV at ground level. Whilst there is unequivocal evidence concerning stratospheric ozone depletion, we cannot be sure, as yet, whether this depletion is accompanied by increases in terrestrial UV radiation. This does not mean that no systematic trend exists, simply that the 95% confidence intervals on estimated trends are likely to encompass zero [3].

3.   MODIFY THE RATE AND DISTRIBUTION OF THE RELEASE OF THE HAZARD

Both the *quality* (spectrum) and *quantity* (intensity) of terrestrial ultraviolet radiation varies with the elevation of the sun above the horizon, or *solar altitude*. The solar altitude depends on the time of day, day of year, and geographical location. On a summer's day, UVB (when taken as 290-320 nm) comprises approximately 6 per cent of terrestrial UV, and UVA (when taken as 320-400 nm) the remaining 94 per cent. But since UVB is much more effective than UVA at causing biological damage, solar UVB contributes about 80% towards most of the harmful effects we associate with sun exposure, with solar UVA contributing the remaining 20%.

The quality and quantity of solar UV are modified on its passage through the atmosphere. The principal interactions in the stratosphere (~10 to 50 km above sea level) are absorption by ozone and scattering by molecules such as N_2 and O_2. In the troposphere (0 to ~10 km asl) absorption by pollutants such as ozone, NO_2 and SO_2, and scattering by particulates (e.g., soot) and clouds are the main attenuating processes.

Clouds reduce UV intensity, although not to the same extent as infrared (heat) intensity. This is because water in clouds attenuates solar infrared much more than ultraviolet, and so the risk of overexposure is increased because the warning sensation of heat is diminished. Roughly speaking, the ambient annual UV radiation is about two thirds that estimated for clear skies in temperate latitudes, rising to about 75% for the tropics [4]. Light clouds scattered over a blue sky make little difference to UV intensity unless directly covering the sun, whilst complete light cloud cover reduces terrestrial UV to about one half of that from a clear sky. Even with heavy cloud cover, the scattered ultraviolet component of sunlight (often called skylight) is seldom less than 10% of that under clear sky [5]. However, very heavy storm clouds can virtually eliminate terrestrial UV even in summertime.

Reflection of solar UV radiation from most ground surfaces is normally less than 10% [6]. The main exceptions are gypsum sand, which reflects about 15-30%, and snow, which can reflect up to 90%. Contrary to popular belief, calm water reflects only about 5% of incident UV radiation, although up to 20% is reflected from choppy water. Since UV rays pass easily through water, swimming in either the sea or open-air pools offers little protection against sunburn.

In people with white skins living in the tropics (30°N to 30°S), sun protection is necessary all year, whereas for those living in temperate latitudes (40° to 60°) sun awareness is generally limited to the 6-month period encompassing the summer solstice.

4.   SEPARATE THE HAZARD FROM HUMANS

The sun's UV rays are strongest in the four-hour period around local noon when 50-60% of a summer's day UV is received. Figure 13.1 illustrates that avoiding summer sun for 2 hours around solar noon in the tropics (latitude ~20°) results in a similar sun exposure to all-day exposure at more temperate latitudes (~50°). Table 13.1 summarizes the percentage of ambient UV radiation present at different times during a summer's day. The data are applicable to all latitudes between tropical and temperate, i.e., 20° to 60°, and assume that solar noon occurs at 1:00pm. So someone going in the sun between 10:30 am to 11:30 am and again from 4:30 pm until the end of the day avoids 100-(12+4+2+1) = 81% of the ambient UV available. Hence simply keeping out of the sun by staying indoors, particularly around the middle of the day in tropical latitudes, is a powerful way of controlling personal exposure to solar UV radiation.

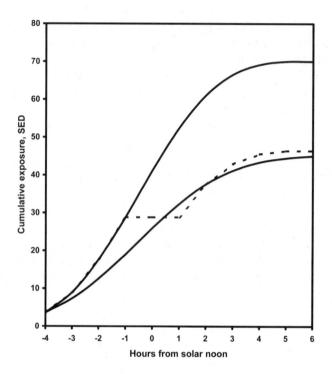

Figure 13.1 The effect of sun avoidance around noon on UV exposure during a summer's day. The upper and lower solid curves show the cumulative ambient exposures throughout a day at 20°N (e.g., Honolulu) and 50°N (e.g., London), respectively; the broken curve shows how the cumulative exposure at 20°N is modified by seeking shade for 2 hours around noon.

Table 13.1 Approximate percentage of ambient UV received during a clear summer's day from tropical (20°) to temperate (60°) latitudes. Solar noon is assumed to occur at 1:00 pm.

Hourly interval	% daily UV
Before 9:30 am	6
9:30 am to 10:30 am	8
10:30 am to 11:30 am	12
11:30 am to 12:30 pm	15
12:30 pm to 1:30 pm	17
1:30 pm to 2:30 pm	15
2:30 pm to 3:30 pm	12
3:30 pm to 4:30 pm	8
4:30 pm to 5:30 pm	4
5:30 pm to 6:30 pm	2
After 6:30 pm	1

5.   SEPARATE THE HAZARD FROM HUMANS BY A BARRIER

5.1   Shade

Shade can be provided naturally by trees, by utilizing canopies and semi-permanent structures, or by constructed shade in areas where large numbers of people may gather. In addition to protecting against UV exposure, shade can also provide wind and rain protection, improve acoustics, and enhance the environment.

It is important that any shade structure blocks the line-of-sight path from most of the sky, as well as that from the sun. A substantial proportion of solar UV radiation is received from the sky, as a result of scattering in the atmosphere. At temperate latitudes, a minimum of around 50% of solar UV radiation is received from the sky. This minimum occurs under clear skies around noon in summer, i.e., when the solar elevation is at a maximum. Under cloudy conditions or when the sun is lower in the sky, the proportion of total UV radiation received from the sky is greater. At lower latitudes, the contribution from the sky is smaller than that directly from the sun, but is never insignificant. This effect is more pronounced for UV radiation than visible radiation, so that observing the amount of shade provided by a structure by looking at its shadow may provide an over-estimate of its UV protective properties.

Small shade structures, such as parasols, can leave large amounts of sky visible to the occupant and may provide only low UV protection, typically equivalent to protection factors of 3 to 10. For these reasons, it is not valid to determine the protection provided by a shade structure from the protection factor of its fabric, in an analogous way to the evaluation of protection factors for clothing [7].

Trees provide a natural means of shade, but the diversity of genus and tree canopy dimensions can make it difficult to generalize the degree of protection afforded. Protection factors for single trees can range from around 4 to greater than 50, depending on foliage and proximity to the periphery of the shadow cast by the tree. Venturing into even a small wooded area can essentially eliminate all UV exposure with protection factors of 100 and greater [8]. British trees commonly found in recreational areas, such as beech and sycamore, generally provide better protection [8] than common Australian trees, such as eucalypts and Norfolk Island pines [9].

5.2   Clothing and hats

One consequence of the increasing concern about sun exposure has resulted in methods to determine the ultraviolet (UV) protection afforded by clothing fabrics [10] and the introduction of the so-called *Ultraviolet Protection Factor (UPF)*, which is analogous to the ubiquitous *Sun Protection Factor (SPF)* associated with sunscreens. The common method of determining the UPF is to use an *in vitro* method. Briefly, this method utilizes a source of UV radiation and a photodetector to measure the UV intensity, before and after passing through the fabric sample. The ratio of these two measurements is numerically equal to the UPF.

Clothing does not suffer from the uncertainties of sunscreen application (see Section 5.4), and a fabric whose UPF is 15, say, really does provide this level of sun protection. National radiation laboratories in Australia and the UK have determined UPFs on several thousand summer-weight clothing fabrics with the following results [11,12]:

- Almost 90% of summer clothing has UPFs >10 and, in practice, provides equivalent protection to sunscreens of SPF 30 or higher (see Section 5.4.1);
- 80% of summer clothing has UPFs >15 and under normal exposure patterns will offer virtually complete protection.

A number of factors affect the protection offered by fabrics against solar UV radiation; these include weave, color, weight, stretch and wetness [10,13].

Clothing is an effective and reliable source of protection against solar UV radiation, provided the garment exhibits good coverage of the skin and the fabric prevents most of the incident UV radiation from reaching the skin beneath it. There are a number of commercial companies who market sun protective clothing claiming high UPFs (30+). Whilst these claims are perfectly justified, it should be borne in mind that such high photoprotection may not be necessary except for highly sun-sensitive individuals or for all day exposure in harsh solar environments. What is perhaps more useful to people who may be concerned about limiting unnecessary sun exposure are some of the items marketed by Australian cancer organizations. These include fingerless and palmless gloves to protect the backs of the hands of gardeners, and a sleeve to be worn on the offside arm by drivers with short-sleeved shirts who like to keep their side window open.

Wide-brimmed hats provide protection equivalent to a factor 5 or so over much of the face. A baseball-style hat provides good protection to the nose but leaves the cheeks and neck unprotected [14]. Legionnaire style hats, with a flap of fabric covering the neck and ears, are particularly effective.

5.3   Optical filters

Materials that are visibly clear will absorb UV radiation to varying extents. For example window glass transmits radiation down to 310 nm (within the UVB), whereas plastics such as perspex® and polycarbonate do not transmit below 370 nm. In general, windscreens on cars transmit some UVA but block UVB, unlike cockpit windscreens on airplanes, which block UVB and UVA.

5.4   Topical sunscreens

Topical sunscreens act by absorbing or scattering UV radiation and are widely available for general public use as a consumer product. Behavioral aspects of sunscreen use are discussed in detail in Chapter 12.

By far the most common reason for using sunscreens, cited by 80% of people in one survey [15], was to protect against sunburn. Other reasons that people use sunscreens include:

- Know dangers of sun exposure
- Perceive themselves at risk of skin cancer
- Know people who had skin cancer
- Protect against ageing and wrinkling
- Extend time in the sun

The protection provided by a sunscreen is expressed by its *Sun Protection Factor* (SPF). This is popularly interpreted as how much longer skin covered with sunscreen takes to burn compared with unprotected skin [15]. A more appropriate definition of the SPF is that it is the ratio of the least amount of ultraviolet energy required to produce a minimal erythema on sunscreen protected skin to the amount of energy required to produce the same erythema on unprotected skin [16]. At the start of the 1990s most commercially available sunscreen products had SPFs less than 10, but by 2000 most manufacturers produced products with factors of 15 to 30 and it is not uncommon to find products claiming a factor of 50 or higher.

It goes without saying that the primary purpose of sunscreens is to reduce the occurrence of sunburn, and so it is somewhat disturbing to see data which showed [17] that whilst this expectation was realized for natural measures of sun protection (clothing and shade), people who usually or always wore SPF 15+ sunscreen reported a higher incidence of sunburn than people who rarely or never used sunscreen.

The mismatch between the expected protection achieved by sunscreens and that observed in practice depends upon a number of factors, as discussed below.

5.4.1   Application thickness

The protection offered by a sunscreen – defined by its Sun Protection Factor – is assessed after phototesting *in vivo* at an internationally agreed application thickness of 2 mg/cm^2. Yet a number of studies have shown that consumers apply much less than this [18-23], typically between 0.5 to 1.5 mg/cm^2. Application thickness has a significant effect on protection, with most users probably achieving a mean value of between 20-50% of that expected from the product label as a result of common application thickness [24,25]. A useful rule-of-thumb is that the protection most people get from a sunscreen is numerically equal to about one-third the SPF.

A simple method has been suggested that would allow users to apply a quantity of sunscreen that would result in closer agreement between the expected and delivered protection [26]. The "rule of nines" is used to assess the extent of a patient's burns as a percentage of the patient's body surface area [27]. The "fingertip unit" is used to measure the amount of cream or ointment to be used in dermatology: it is a strip of product squeezed on to the index finger, from the distal crease to the fingertip [28].

With the rule of nines, the body's surface area is divided into 11 areas, each representing roughly 9% of the total according to:

Body areas by "rule of nines" for extent of burns:
1   Head, neck, and face
2   Left arm
3   Right arm
4   Upper back
5   Lower back
6   Upper front torso
7   Lower front torso
8   Left upper leg and thigh
9   Right upper leg and thigh
10   Left lower leg and foot
11   Right lower leg and foot

Sunscreen can be applied to each of these areas at a dose of 2 mg/cm^2 if two strips of sunscreen are squeezed out on to both the index and middle fingers from the palmar crease to the fingertips. The application of this "two fingers" of sunscreen will provide a dose of the product that approximates to that used during the laboratory determination of the Sun Protection Factor. Such a dosage guide is a means of ensuring that users are protected according to their expectations. Users are unlikely to be willing to cover themselves or their families with such a copious layer of sunscreen and would prefer to apply half this amount. A less daunting proposition, and the one actually suggested, is to apply one finger of sunscreen, with the corollary that the resultant protection would be only about half that stated on the product. Users should be encouraged to reapply one finger's worth within half an hour of the initial application in order to achieve optimal protection (see Section 5.4.5).

5.4.2.   Application technique

When sunscreens are tested in the laboratory to determine their SPF, great care is taken to achieve a uniform layer of sunscreen over the test area by spreading with a gloved finger. In practice, of course, nothing like this care is taken when consumers apply sunscreen to the skin. Quantitative estimates of the distribution of sunscreen surface density have been made using fluorescence spectroscopy [18,29,30]. In one study [29], volunteers were asked to apply sunscreen to one forearm "as if you were on the beach" using a quantity of sunscreen sufficient to produce an average thickness of 1 mg/cm^2 over the forearm. The same quantity of sunscreen was then placed in the other palm and the subjects were instructed to apply the cream "as evenly as possible" to the remaining forearm.

Whilst no significant difference was found between the median thickness following crude and careful application, there was, however, a statistically significant difference in the distribution of surface densities between the two methods of application, with careful application showing much less variability in thickness than crude application. Moreover, following crude, but not careful, application most subjects were shown to have some sites where no sunscreen had been applied.

Not only is sunscreen not applied uniformly to exposed sites, but also users choose not to apply it to all exposed sites. This is illustrated in Figure 13.2, which summarizes the results of the author asking 100 British adults (age range 19-61 years; 51 male) the following question: *"If you decide to use a sunscreen, do you always apply it to each of these sites if they are uncovered?"* It is clear from Figure 13.2 that less than half the people questioned always apply sunscreen to all uncovered sites, even if they decide to use sunscreen. An American study examining the use of summertime sun protection by children reported similar findings [31], where the areas most likely to be missed during sunscreen application were the ears, neck, feet and legs.

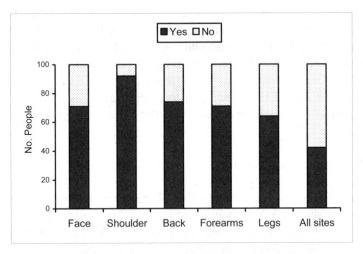

Figure 13.2 100 people were asked *"If you decide to use a sunscreen, do you always apply it to each of these sites if they are uncovered?"*. 71 people said they always applied sunscreen to their face, whilst 29 people said they didn't always do this, and so on.

5.4.3   Sunscreen type

In general, sunscreens containing inorganic chemicals, such as titanium dioxide, as the sole active ingredient are less cosmetically acceptable than products incorporating organic filters and, as a consequence, users may compensate for this by applying less quantity and so reduce the photoprotection achieved. This is unfortunate because inorganic sunscreens are often marketed as *total sunblocks* and will tend to be used by sun-sensitive individuals, including those with photosensitive disorders.

In a blind, within-subject study [21], it was shown that a SPF 25 sunscreen containing only inorganic filters (ZnO and TiO_2) was more difficult to spread on the skin than a product with the same SPF but containing only organic filters (Parsol MCX, Parsol 1789 and oxybenzone). As a consequence, subjects applied less of the inorganic sunscreen than the organic sunscreen (median thickness 0.94 mg/cm^2 and 1.48 mg/cm^2, respectively). This reduction in amount applied is likely to lead in practice to the inorganic sunscreen providing a SPF of about one-half of that achieved with the organic sunscreen [24].

5.4.4   Substantivity

Topical sunscreens are designed to be substantive so that they remain on the skin under stressful conditions. Indeed, most commercially available sunscreens are water resistant, while a few also claim to be rub resistant and/or sand resistant.

Typical results using excised human epidermis as a substrate to evaluate water resistance [32,33] are shown in Figure 13.3. Products that claimed to be waterproof or water-resistant exhibited a gradual decrease in protection over four immersions, whilst day-care products and sunscreens that made no claims concerning water resistance were readily washed-off.

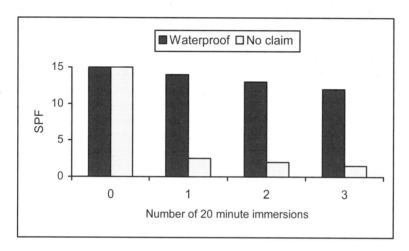

Figure 13.3 The change in SPF with water immersion for an SPF 15 product that claimed to be waterproof and an SPF 15 product that made no claim concerning water resistance [33]

Similar *ex* vivo techniques [34] have been developed to evaluate sand-resistance of sunscreens. The results on all products tested were largely consistent. The SPFs increased significantly immediately after sand agitation, because sand adhered to the skin surface as a result of moisture in the epidermis itself and the sticky nature of the sunscreens, but after removal of excess sand by gentle rubbing with a tissue, the SPFs were significantly lower (typically half to two-thirds) than those prior to sand agitation.

5.4.5   Re-application

The reasons for reapplying sunscreen during sun exposure are to compensate for initial under-application so as to achieve a SPF more in line with the rated value, and to replace sunscreen that may have been removed by water, vigorous toweling, or friction with clothing or sand. Inadequate application is the primary purpose for reapplication since modern waterproof or water-resistant sunscreens exhibit good substantivity [35] even after immersion in water [31].

Guidance on sunscreen packs about reapplication is generally to "reapply frequently" or "reapply regularly." Given considerations of cost, convenience and human nature, it is unlikely many users will reapply sunscreens frequently or regularly. Also, general guidance to reapply sunscreens frequently or regularly is vague and non-specific, and there are few published data on how well consumers comply with this advice. A common recommendation by many public health agencies [36] is to reapply sunscreen every 2-3 hours.

A mathematical analysis [37] has shown that using a sunscreen that is readily removed from the skin achieves little in the way of sun protection, no matter when it is reapplied. For sunscreens that bind moderately or well to skin, typical of modern waterproof or water-resistant products, the lowest skin exposure results from early reapplication into the sun exposure period, and not at 2-3 hours, after initial application. Typically, reapplication of sunscreen at 20 minutes into a 4-hour exposure to strong summer sunshine results in 60-85% of the UV exposure that would be received if sunscreen were reapplied at 2 hours.

Further calculations showed that a single reapplication of a substantive SPF 15 sunscreen at 20 minutes into a 6-hour exposure period resulted in a lower skin UV dose at the end of this period than either an initial application only or reapplication at 2 and 4 hours (Table 13.2). This finding reinforces the need to apply an adequate quantity of sunscreen early into the sun exposure period; a conclusion that is independent of the sunscreen rated SPF or the solar UV intensity. Clearly, the magnitude of skin exposure decreases with increasing SPF and decreasing UV intensity. The data in Table 13.2 indicate that reapplication of sunscreen results in a skin exposure that is 2-3 times less than achieved with a single application of sunscreen. The same increase in protection from sunburn with sunscreen reapplication was found in an experimental study using 104 adult Caucasian volunteers [38].

Table 13.2 Skin exposure following an application of a highly substantive SPF 15 sunscreen at 1 mg/cm^2 on each occasion during a 6-hour exposure period of mean skin irradiance 6 SED/h [37].

No. sunscreen applications	Time(s) of application	Skin exposure after 6-h, SED
1	0	8.9
2	0 & 20-min	3.7
3	0, 2-h & 4-h	4.0

Consumers are advised to apply sunscreen liberally or generously. However, many studies have shown that users feel uncomfortable with application at 2 mg/cm^2, and prefer to apply quantities averaging at around one half this thickness. It is likely, therefore, that campaigns to encourage people to apply a greater quantity of sunscreen at a single application will fail. An important factor in sunscreen performance is the uneven nature of the skin surface. If an opaque sunscreen is applied to the skin, particularly at low surface densities typical of actual usage, the epidermal markings become visible as the surface grooves, or sulci, are filled [39]. With further application, the intervening ridges are also covered and the surface becomes more featureless. The situation is analogous to painting a wall with a textured surface when two coats of paint are almost always required for satisfactory coverage. In the same way, two "coats of sunscreen" may be required for adequate protection.

Advising people to reapply sunscreen early into their sun exposure period may well be more successful than the common public health recommendation [36] to reapply at 2-3 hours when the reasons they have for being in the sun are more likely to make them forget to reapply sunscreen. The advice given to sunscreen users should be as follows [37]:

- Apply sunscreen liberally to exposed sites 15 to 30 minutes before going out into the sun.
- Reapply sunscreen to exposed sites 15 to 30 minutes after sun exposure begins.
- Further reapplication of sunscreen is necessary after vigorous activity that could remove sunscreen, such as swimming, toweling or excessive sweating and rubbing.

When photoprotective measures are used in combination, it is possible to reduce exposure to solar UV radiation to within acceptable levels without seriously limiting the range of outdoor activities that can be safely pursued. So applying an SPF 15 to the face at typical thickness achieves a 5-fold reduction in skin exposure. Much the same is achieved by wearing a broad-brim hat. But applying sunscreen *and* wearing a hat results in an approximate 25-fold reduction in exposure.

6. MAKE HUMANS MORE RESISTANT TO THE HAZARD

6.1 Tanning

Delayed tanning, or melanogenesis, becomes noticeable about a few days after sun exposure, gradually increases for several days and may persist for weeks or months. Following solar UV radiation exposure there is an increase in the number of functioning melanocytes and activity of the enzyme tyrosinase is enhanced [40]. This leads to the formation of new melanin and hence an increase in the number of melanin granules throughout the epidermis.

6.2 Epidermal hyperplasia

Thickening (hyperplasia) of the epidermis is a significant component of a mild sunburn reaction. In the first 48 hours after exposure there is some thickening due to inter- and intracellular edema, but by 72 hours there is an increased mitotic rate of the cells in the basal layer leading to hyperplasia. When the acute inflammatory stage has subsided, all layers of the epidermis appear thickened. In the absence of further stimulation, the epidermis returns to normal after about 2 months [41].

6.3 Photoadaptation

Although a tanned skin does confer a degree of photoprotection, such protection seems to be no more than moderate, a factor of only two to three being achieved by repeated sub-erythemal exposure to solar-simulated radiation in subjects who tan poorly or moderately (skin types II and III) [42]. In Caucasians skin thickening is probably more important than tanning in providing endogenous photoprotection [43], although in darkly pigmented races it is likely that skin pigmentation is the most important means of protection against solar UV radiation.

7. IMMEDIATELY COUNTER THE DAMAGE DONE

Conventional photoprotection by sunscreens is entirely prophylactic and of no value once DNA damage has occurred. An intriguing development, which has yet to be exploited commercially, is to incorporate the DNA-repair enzyme photolyase into sunscreens [44]. On exposure to photoreactivating light, this enzyme converts cyclobutane dimers into their original DNA structure. It is suggested that this enzyme could be combined as an after-sun strategy with conventional sunscreens to provide photoprotection and repair at the same time. The bacterial enzyme, T4 endonuclease, when incorporated into a liposome lotion may also be a practical way to remove lesions in DNA and slow the progression of skin cancer [45].

8. REPAIR AND REHABILITATE

Despite the fact that people are exposed to potentially harmful levels of solar UV radiation, mechanisms have evolved to protect cells and to repair damaged molecules. The cell component most vulnerable to injury is nuclear DNA, but, in general, damage can be repaired by one of three mechanisms [46]:

1. Photoreactivation, or photoenzymatic, repair in which an enzyme (photolyase) binds to specific photolesions such as cyclobutanne pyrimidine dimmers, and after absorption of visible light reverses the damage *in situ*;
2. Excision repair, which involves a variety of proteins that recognize damaged nucleotides, incise surrounding DNA and remove the DNA fragment containing the photodamage;
3. Postreplication, or recombinational, repair in which UV-damaged DNA can replicate in such a way that gaps are left in the daughter strand opposite the damaged sites, with subsequent filling of the gaps by DNA synthesis.

CONCLUSION

The feasibility of various strategies for reducing personal ultraviolet radiation exposure has been described using a risk management model. The most effective strategy is to avoid outdoor exposure at those times of the day and year when solar UV levels are high. When this is neither practicable nor desirable, clothing and shade provide more effective and visible means of protection than applying topical sunscreens, since use of the latter is problematic.

SUMMARY POINTS

- Topical approaches using sunscreens can be problematic and vagaries of human behavior are such that the protection achieved in practice is frequently no greater than 10-fold of that using no protection.
- Clothing is generally more effective with almost 90% of summer clothing offering more than 10-fold protection and providing equivalent protection to sunscreens of SPF 30 or higher.
- Seeking shade can be an effective way of reducing exposure to solar UV radiation, provided that, as well as direct sunlight, a significant part of the sky is blocked, in order to attenuate both direct and scattered UV radiation. Effective shade structures, either trees or canopies, are capable of providing a 20-fold or more reduction in exposure.
- Avoiding sunlight by staying indoors especially around the middle of the day in tropical latitudes should be encouraged.

IMPLICATIONS FOR PUBLIC HEALTH

There is strong evidence that exposure to solar ultraviolet radiation can have adverse effects on health, notably an increased risk of potentially fatal cancers of the skin. There is equally convincing evidence that limiting outdoor exposure, especially intense, intermittent exposures when solar UV levels are high, can reduce this risk. This can be achieved, without seriously compromising outdoor pursuits, by avoiding direct exposure to sunlight around noon in summer, seeking shade, wearing clothing, and by applying sunscreen to unprotected parts of the body. However, protection by sunscreens is less certain than that provided by other means and, in particular, sunscreens should not be used to intentionally prolong exposure.

REFERENCES

1. International Agency for Research on Cancer Expert Group (1992) *Solar and Ultraviolet Radiation.* IARC Monographs on the Evaluation of Carcinogenic Risks to Humans, Vol. 55. Lyon, France: IARC Press.
2. Haddon W Jr (1980) Advances in the epidemiology of injuries as a basis for public policy. *Public Health Rep* **95**: 411-420.
3. Diffey BL (2000) Sunlight, skin cancer and ozone depletion. In: Hester RE, Harrison RM, eds. *Causes and environmental implications of increased UV-B radiation.* Issues in Environmental Science and Technology, Vol 14. London: Royal Society of Chemistry, pp107-119.

4. Frederick JE, Alberts AD (1992) The natural UV-A radiation environment. In: Urbach F, ed. *Biological responses to ultraviolet A radiation*. Overland Park: Valdenmar Publishing Company, pp. 7-18.

5. Paltridge GW, Barton IJ (1978) Erythemal ultraviolet radiation distribution over Australia - the calculations, detailed results and input data. *Division of Atmospheric Physics Technical Paper 33*, Australia: Commonwealth Scientific and Industrial Research Organisation.

6. Madronich S (1993) The atmosphere and UV-B radiation at ground level. In: Young AR, Björn LO, Moan J, Nultsch W, eds. *Environmental UV Photobiology*. New York: Plenum, pp. 1-39.

7. Wong, C F (1994) Scattered ultraviolet radiation underneath a shade-cloth. *Photodermatol Photoimmuno. Photomed* **10**: 221-224.

8. Diffey B, Diffey J (2002). Sun protection with trees. *Br J Dermatol* **147**: 397-399.

9. Parsons PG, Neale R, Wolski P, Green A (1998). The shady side of solar protection. *Med J Aus* **168** 327-330.

10. Gies HP, Roy CR, Elliott G, Zongli W (1994) Ultraviolet radiation protection factors for clothing. *Health Phys* **67**: 131-139.

11. Gies HP, Roy CR, McLennan A (1996) Textiles and sun protection. In: Volkmer B, Heller H, eds. *Environmental UV-radiation, risk of skin cancer and primary prevention*. Stuttgart: Gustav Fischer, pp. 213-234.

12. Driscoll CMH (2000) Clothing protection factors. *Radiological Protection Bulletin*, Chilton: National Radiological Protection Board, No 222.

13. Clark IES, Grainger KJL, Agnew JL, Driscoll CMH (2000) Clothing protection measurements. *Rad Prot Dosim* **91** 279-281.

14. Diffey BL, Cheeseman J (1992) Sun protection with hats. *Br J Dermatol* **127**: 10-12.

15. Sunscreens and the Consumer (1996) London: Health Education Authority

16. Department of Health and Human Services FDA, USA (1978) Sunscreen drug products for over the counter use: proposed safety, effectiveness and labelling conditions. *Federal Register* 43 (166): pp. 38206-38269.

17. Dixon H, Shatten R, Borland R. (1997) Reaction to the 1995/1996 SunSmart Campaign: results from a representative household survey of Victorians. In: *SunSmart Evaluation Studies No 5*. Melbourne: Anti-Cancer Council of Victoria, pp. 70-96.

18. Azurdia RM, Pagliaro JA, Diffey BL, Rhodes LE (1999) Sunscreen application by photosensitive patients is inadequate for protection. *Br J Dermatol* **140**: 255-258.

19. Bech-Thomsen N, Wulf HC (1993) Sunbathers' application of sunscreen is probably inadequate to obtain the Sun Protection Factor assigned to the preparation. *Photodermatol Photoimmunol Photomed* **9**: 242-244.

20. Hart GC, Wright AL, Cameron RG (2000) An assessment of the adequacy of sunscreen usage. *Rad Prot Dosim* **91**: 275-278.

21. Diffey BL, Grice J (1997) The influence of sunscreen type on photoprotection. *Br J Dermatol* **137**: 103-105.

22. Gottlieb A, Bourget TD, Lowe NJ (1997) Sunscreens: effects of amounts of application of Sun Protection Factors. In: Lowe NJ, Shaath NA, Pathak MA, eds. *Sunscreens: development, evaluation, and regulatory aspects*. New York: Marcel Dekker Inc, pp. 583-588.

23. Stenberg C, Larkö O (1985) Sunscreen application and its importance for the Sun Protection Factor. *Arch Dermatol* **121**:1400-1402.

24. Stokes RP, Diffey BL (1997) How well are sunscreen users protected? *Photodermatol Photoimmunol Photomed* **13**:186-188.

25. Brown S, Diffey BL (1986) The effect of applied thickness on sunscreen protection: in vivo and in vitro studies. *Photochem Photobiol* **44**: 509-514.
26. Taylor S, Diffey B (2002) Simple dosage guide for suncreams will help users. *Br Med J* **324**:1526.
27. Lund CC, Browder NC (1944) The estimation of the areas of burns. *Surg Gyn Obs* **79**: 352-358.
28. Long CC, Finlay AY (1991) The fingertip unit…a new practical measure. *Clin Exp Dermatol* **16**: 444-447.
29. Rhodes LE, Diffey BL (1996) Quantitative assessment of sunscreen application technique by *in vivo* fluorescence spectroscopy. *J Soc Cosmet Chem* **47**:109-115.
30. Rhodes LE, Diffey BL (1997) Fluorescence spectroscopy: a rapid, non-invasive method for measurement of skin surface thickness of topical agents. *Br J Dermatol* **136**: 12-17.
31. Robinson JK, Rigel DS, Amonette RA (2000) Summertime sun protection used by adults for their children. *J Am Acad Dermatol* **42**: 746-753.
32. Stokes RP, Diffey BL, Dawson LC, Barton SP (1998) A novel *in vitro* technique for measuring the water resistance of sunscreens. *Int J Cosmet Sci* **20**: 235-240.
33. Stokes RP, Diffey BL (1999) Water resistance of sunscreen and day-care products. *Br J Dermatol* **140**: 259-263.
34. Stokes RP, Diffey BL (2000) A novel *ex vivo* technique to assess the sand/rub resistance of sunscreen products. *Int J Cosmet Sci* **22**: 329-334.
35. Agin PP, Levine DJ (1992) Sunscreens retain their efficacy on human skin for up to 8h after application. *J Photochem Photobol B* **15**: 371-374.
36. Mackie RM (1996) *Skin Cancer*. 2nd edition. London: Martin Dunitz, p.331.
37. Diffey BL (2001) When should sunscreen be reapplied? *J Am Acad Dermatol* **45**: 882-885.
38. Pruim B, Green A (1999) Photobiological aspects of sunscreen re-application. *Aus J Dermatol* **40**: 14-18.
39. Farr PM, Diffey BL (1985) How reliable are sunscreen protection factors? *Br J Dermatol* **112**: 113-118.
40. Fitzpatrick TB, Szabo G, Wick MW (1983) Biochemistry and physiology of melanin pigmentation. In: Goldsmith LA, ed. *Biochemistry and Physiology of the Skin*. Oxford: Oxford University Press, pp.687-712.
41. Johnson BE (1984) Natural and artificial radiation of the skin. In: Jarrett A, ed. *The physiology and pathophysiology of the skin*. Vol. 8. London: Academic Press, pp.2434.
42. Sheehan JM, Potten CS, Young AR (1998) Tanning in human skin types II and III offers modest photoprotection against erythema. *Photochem Photobiol* **68**: 588-592.
43. Gniadecka M, Wulf HC, Mortensen NN, Poulsen T (1996) Photoprotection in vitiligo and normal skin. A quantitative assessment of the role of stratum corneum, viable epidermis and pigmentation. *Acta Dermato-Venereol* **76**: 429-432.
44. Stege H, Roza L, Vink AA, *et al.* (2000) Enzyme plus light therapy to repair DNA damage in ultraviolet-B-irradiated human skin. *Proc Natl Acad Sci* **97**: 1790-1795.
45. Yarosh DB (2001) Liposomes in investigative dermatology. *Photodermatol Photoimmunol Photomed* **17**: 203-212.
46. Eller MS (1995) Repair of DNA photodamage in human skin. In: Gilchrest BA, ed. *Photodamage*. Oxford: Blackwell Science Inc, pp.26-51.

Chapter 14

Impact of intervention strategies to reduce UVR exposure

Karen Glanz[1], Ph.D., M.P.H.; Mona Saraiya[2], M.P.H., M.D.; Peter Briss[3], M.D.
[1]Cancer Research Center of Hawaii, University of Hawaii; [2]Division of Cancer Prevention and Control, U.S. Centers for Disease Control and Prevention; [3]Epidemiology Program Office, U.S. Centers for Disease Control and Prevention

Key words: interventions, health promotion, melanoma, sun exposure

INTRODUCTION

It has been well documented in this book and elsewhere that skin cancer is a significant and, in many parts of the world, growing health problem (see Chapters 1 and 5) [1]. While skin cancer is among the most common cancers, it is also one of the most preventable. Behavioral recommendations for primary prevention of skin cancer aim to reduce exposure to ultraviolet radiation (UVR). The most often recommended behavioral strategies for reducing UVR exposure include: limit time spent in the sun, avoid the sun during peak hours, use a broad spectrum sunscreen when outside, wear protective clothing (hats, shirts, pants) and sunglasses, seek shade when outdoors, and avoid sunburn (Chapter 13).

Although awareness about skin cancer is growing, the practice of preventive behaviors remains variable, and is relatively low in many populations (Chapter 12). Thus, a variety of intervention strategies have been proposed for changing behaviors related to UVR exposure and their

D. Hill et al. (eds.), Prevention of Skin Cancer, 259-293.

determinants, including media campaigns, educational programs, and changes in sun-protective environments and policies. Because UVR exposure during childhood is believed to account for a significant proportion of total lifetime exposure and thus to play a causative role in skin cancer (see Chapters 6 and 12) [2], children and their caregivers are the main audiences for many of these interventions.

This chapter provides a review of the efficacy of health promotion intervention strategies for reducing UVR exposure in specific populations and settings. It is based on a recently completed comprehensive evidence review (see Section 1 for details) [3]. The key question addressed is: What interventions, or combination of interventions, are most effective for increasing sun protection behaviors (SPBs) [using sunscreen, hat use, shirt use, sunglasses, shade seeking, and sun avoidance]? In addition to summarizing what is known about how to reduce UVR exposure, the chapter will identify issues that influence interpretation of the literature, gaps in knowledge, and some key issues related to putting the evidence about preventive interventions into practice. Because the literature includes both controlled efficacy trials and effectiveness studies in real-world settings, this chapter reflects a mix of both.

1.   METHODS

This chapter is based on an evidence review of interventions to prevent skin cancer that is being coordinated by the authors for the *Guide to Community Preventive Services* ("the *Guide*"). The *Guide* is a comprehensive effort being undertaken in the United States to synthesize research results and translate them into evidence-based recommendations for public health interventions [4].

1.1   Search strategies and inclusion criteria

This evidence review follows the established procedure for systematic evidence reviews for the *Guide*. Studies are first identified for inclusion in the review, and then a detailed abstracting procedure is used to summarize the design, intervention, analysis, execution, and limitations of the research [5]. The skin cancer prevention review relied principally on articles in journals, supplemented with key published reports and new studies. An extensive list of key words relevant to skin cancer prevention was used for the search. To be included, the reference must be a primary study related to primary prevention of skin cancer, provide information on the efficacy or effectiveness of one or more intervention strategies in changing one or more outcomes of interest, and report on research conducted in a developed country (United States or other). Exclusion criteria include: publication before 1966, published in a language other than English, or set in a developing country. Also excluded are studies focusing solely on early detection, and etiologic trials, because the relationship between UV exposure and skin cancer is covered in other chapters (Chapters 3, 4, 5, 6), and we took this to be established as a starting point for our review.

Thus far, the review has identified 1,332 citations, of which 457 were considered for possible inclusion based on their titles and abstracts. After more detailed review of the papers, 79 studies have been formally abstracted in detail. Several of the studies are reported in multiple publications. The studies reviewed here may still be incomplete as the larger review is still in progress. Studies that use experimental designs have traditionally been considered the most informative because of their ability to minimize the effects of confounding variables. Non-experimental research is also included in this review where there are not significant limitations to interpretation. Studies using pre-experimental design are reported in limited detail when they suggest creative strategies and promising avenues to pursue. By including a range of designs, it is possible to take advantage of the strengths and minimize the weaknesses of each type of design. Recent review papers were used to supplement the primary sources [6,7].

1.2   Review and analysis

The studies reported here were reviewed and abstracted in detail. For most of the categories of studies, the main points are summarized in tables describing the intervention, evaluation methods, and main results. Following these summaries, a semi-quantitative analysis of significant findings examined the results for various behavioral endpoints, designs, measurement methods, and types of strategies.

2.   TYPES OF INTERVENTIONS, AUDIENCES, AND SETTINGS

There is no single, clear-cut way to classify interventions to reduce UVR exposure. While some studies can be easily identified within a single category (e.g., education for school-age children), many more involve multiple methods or communication strategies. Further, intervention studies often target multiple audiences, for example both parents and children, or physicians and patients. The nature of intervention strategies is also often influenced by their organizational context, or setting. Bearing in mind these complexities, it is useful to provide a broad typology of four types of interventions that readers may use to group various strategies and studies: 1) individual-directed strategies; 2) environmental, policy, and structural interventions; 3) media campaigns; and 4) community-wide multi-component interventions. Each type of intervention is briefly characterized here.

2.1   Individual-directed strategies

Individual-directed strategies include informational and behavioral interventions aimed primarily at individuals or groups. These interventions usually occur within an organizational context, such as a school, recreation program, or health care setting. They typically aim to teach and motivate individuals by providing knowledge, attitudes, and behavioral skills for skin cancer prevention. They include the use of small media (brochures, pamphlets, printed materials, etc.), didactic programs (e.g., classroom lessons, lectures), interactive activities (games, multimedia programs), and skill development (role-play, teaching sunscreen application, etc.). These strategies can be directed toward any age, occupational, or risk group and are often combined with other strategies.

2.2   Environmental, policy, and structural interventions

Environmental, policy, and structural interventions aim to provide and/or maintain a physical, social, and/or information environment that supports sun protection and sun safety practices. These interventions aim to improve the sun protective conditions for *all* people in a defined population (school, community setting, etc.), and not just for those who are most motivated. They reach populations by passively reducing UV radiation exposure, providing sun protection resources, and broadening the accessibility and reach of skin cancer prevention information. Examples include increasing shade areas, supplying sunscreen, providing environmental sources of information and/or prompts, and many other possible strategies. *Policies* establish formal rules or standards, for organizational actions or legal requirements or restrictions related to skin cancer prevention measures. Policies may be developed by a school, school board, or community organization, or by other legal entities such as municipal, state, and federal governments. *Environmental* strategies involve providing supportive resources for skin cancer prevention in the physical, social, and/or information environment. They may be based on, and restricted or assisted by, policies. However, environmental supports can also be undertaken in the absence of a formal policy.

2.3   Media campaigns

Media campaigns use mass media channels such as print (newspaper, magazines) and broadcast media (radio, television), and the Internet to disseminate information and behavioral guidance to a wide audience. They may be aimed at specific types of target audiences but are typically characterized by broad distribution channels. Media campaigns have some of the characteristics of individual-directed interventions but without the face-to-face interpersonal interaction and "captive audience" in a defined organizational setting. Media campaigns tend to have a public health orientation and often seek to raise levels of awareness or concern, and to help shape the policy agenda that drives other interventions.

2.4   Community-wide multi-component interventions

Community-wide multi-component interventions often called population-wide programs or campaigns, seek to combine elements of the three other types of strategies into an integrated effort in a defined geographic area (city, state/province, or country). They often include individual-directed strategies, environmental and policy changes, media campaigns, and a variety of setting-specific strategies delivered with a defined theme, name/logo, and set of messages [8,9].

Table 14.1 further illustrates the range of target audiences, settings, and types of applicable interventions to reduce UVR exposure. It is important to remember that most efforts cut across categories and can be informative about more than a single audience, setting, and/or strategy. For ease of presentation, the next section will use primarily a setting-specific approach to reviewing the evidence, recognizing that setting specific programs can be individual-directed with or without environmental/policy changes. In addition, we report on four types of interventions that do not readily fit into single setting categories: mass media, parent/caregiver, and community-wide interventions, as well as providing information on message testing studies.

Table 14.1 Audiences, settings, and examples of skin cancer prevention strategies[1].

Target population	Setting	Examples of strategies
Infants and toddlers	Pre-school Health care	Training for staff Adding shade structures
School-age children and adolescents	Primary or secondary school Outdoor recreation Home	Education in classrooms Peer education Providing sunscreen, hats
Adults	Occupational Outdoor recreation Home	Protective clothing, hats Information posters, shade Mailed or posted information
Health care providers	Health care setting Professional education or in-service training	Training for prevention counseling Systems changes: prompts, incentives, supports
Caregivers	Home Pre-School School Outdoor recreation Community-wide	Training and education Supportive resources (sunscreen, hats, etc.) Guidance on structural change
High-risk groups Patients	Home Health care settings	Phone or mail information and counseling Physician/nurse/group education of patients, families
Any audience or combination of audiences	Community-wide (may include various settings)	Mass media Small media (brochures, etc.) Policy and environmental strategies Combinations of strategies

[1] These are examples only, and are not exhaustive.

3.   REVIEW OF FINDINGS: IMPACT OF INTERVENTIONS TO REDUCE UVR EXPOSURE

This section reviews the impact of interventions in nine categories. The first five categories are defined by setting: child care centers/pre-schools; primary and secondary schools; outdoor recreation settings; workplace settings; and health care settings. Additional categories include mass media, interventions for parents and caregivers, community-wide interventions, and message testing studies. The placement of a given study into a particular category was done on the basis of its main emphasis and the type and/or context of outcomes reported. A few studies report outcomes on more than one type of audience and therefore may be reported in a secondary category as well, particularly for studies of children that also studied an intervention's impact on parents and caregivers.

3.1   Setting-specific interventions

3.1.1   Child care centers/pre-schools

UV radiation exposure during childhood contributes to the development of skin cancer, and most UV exposure occurs during childhood and adolescence. Further, many young children are cared for in childcare centers or pre-schools where they play outside for part of the day. Therefore, these settings are well suited to efforts to reduce UVR exposure. Table 14.2 summarizes five studies that reported on strategies to promote UVR reduction in childcare or pre-school settings. Four of the five studies addressed training or education for teachers and staff, and four included parent education materials and lectures. Three studies were randomized trials with a fourth being embedded within a community-randomized study of a comprehensive program. The findings showed improvements in knowledge in two studies, and changes in policy and/or structural factors in three studies; however, none of these studies reported improved sun protection behaviors (SPBs) in parents, teachers/staff, or children.

Table 14.2 Interventions in pre-schools and day care centers

Citation & location	Intervention	Evaluation[1,2]	Results[3]
Boldeman et al., 1991 Sweden [69]	Context: community wide sun safety. Sun awareness lecture (45 min.) + discussion session (1-2 hours) for nursery school managers	Exposed community (high v. low participation) vs. unexposed control community - post-program only. n = 574 matrons (managers) of nursery schools. 6 months intervention to assessment	High participation more likely to disseminate to staff & parents (87% v. 45-70% other gps). Higher knowledge in high-participation group. No change found in sunbathing habits
Loescher et al., 1995 Arizona (USA) [98]	Curriculum for 4-5 year olds plus take home activities. Focus on cover up, find shade, and ask for sun-safe things (e.g., sunscreen)	RCT by class (n = 12), Intervention v. Control n = 150, 142. Measured knowledge, comprehension and application using a self-report pictorial instrument	Improvements in knowledge, comprehension in Intervention classes. No improvement in application of concepts; children may be too young for processing application concepts
Crane et al., 1999b Colorado (USA) [87]	3-hour workshop for staff, working session to develop protection plans for centers, activity packets for parents. Aimed at both individual and structural factors. Continued across 2 summers	RCT by preschool/center (n = 27), Intervention v. wait-list Control. Measures: interviews, observations, review of policies. Parent survey n = 201	Trend in increased knowledge of directors. Increased proportion of centers with sun-screen (SS) policy, decrease in SS available at centers. No improvements in observed SPBs at centers. No difference in parent knowledge, SPBs. Trend to reduced sunburns in Intvn. children
Wolf et al. 1999 Arizona (USA) [103]	Statewide prevention, education, and sun safety policy program in day care. Training for staff members. Parent education kits	RCT: Training sites v. Controls n = 245 day care centers. Knowledge assessments, on-site policy and practices review	Training outcomes not reported. State-level policy changes achieved: sun safety mandates added to licensing regulations
Grant-Petersson et al., 1999 New Hampshire (USA) [92]	Policy discussions, curriculum materials. Take-home print materials. Teacher training. Group meetings, sunscreen. Based on social cognitive theory	Director policy survey. Teacher curriculum evaluation. n=31 child care settings. Context: 5 intervention, 5 control communities	Process evaluation data only. 44-91% taught curriculum (various parts). Increased policies to recommend/require hat & sunblock for children and teachers

[1] RCT = Randomized controlled trial
[2] Sample description = combined "n" given as pre, post for baseline and final assessment
[3] SPB = sun protection behavior

3.1.2   Primary and secondary schools

Formal educational settings have been the most-often reported sites for sun safety program evaluations. School settings allow for integrating skin cancer education into existing learning situations as well as for supportive policy and environmental interventions. The literature reports on such programs and accompanying evaluations that have been conducted in Australia, the United States, Canada, Scotland, England, and France. Because recent review articles include detailed descriptions and tables reporting the methods of many of these studies [5,10], a detailed summary table is not included in this chapter. Twenty-four studies were reviewed, including 20 in primary schools, 3 in secondary schools, and one that included both.

A wide range of strategies has been used for *short duration presentations*, including: didactic classroom teaching [11-14], health fairs [15], a toolkit and measurement of the UV Index [16], an educational picture book [17], Sun Awareness Week [18], teaching by medical students [19], interactive CD-ROM multimedia programs [20-22], and peer education [23-24]. The majority of these programs improved sun safety knowledge, but few of them led to improvements in behavioral intentions and/or sun protection behaviors (SPBs).

Multi-unit presentations included multiple curricular sessions [25-28], games and educational packages [29], peer education supplemented with problem-based learning [21], and two programs that continued across more than one year [30-31]. Like the short duration presentations, the majority of these efforts led to improvements in knowledge. Most of the multi-unit programs also contributed to changes in attitudes about sun protection. Some evaluations also found behavioral change through short-term follow-up periods. The Kidskin intervention in Western Australia compared a control condition with moderate and high intensity interventions [32] and has recently reported two-year results [33]. The findings showed that the children receiving the intervention had less sun exposure but did not change their sunscreen or hat use behaviors relative to the controls. The only randomized study that continued across three years, and was directed at adolescents, resulted in improved knowledge but no significant behavior changes [31].

One study specifically reported on an intervention to increase adoption of comprehensive skin protection policies in primary and secondary schools in Australia [34]. Intervention strategies included either a mail-only intervention, or mail plus a staff development module. The intervention led to increased adoption of comprehensive policies in elementary schools, with the mail and staff support condition proving more effective than mail alone

(+10.7% vs. +6.0%). However, there were no significant differences in policy adoption by secondary schools, and no significant effects on adoption of SPBs in either level of school.

3.1.3   Outdoor recreation settings

Recreation settings provide unique opportunities to promote appropriate sun protection practices because recreation and sports programs involve supervised activities and are conducted mostly or entirely outdoors. Parents and recreation leaders are in an excellent position to introduce children to the importance of sun protection habits, and to facilitate their adoption by providing necessary resources (e.g., sunscreen, hats). Further, parents and recreation leaders can serve as role models for sun safety and can influence, develop, and implement supportive policies, so their actions should also be the focus of prevention efforts (see Section 3.2.2).

Table 14.3 summarizes six studies of skin cancer prevention programs conducted in swimming pools, outdoor recreation programs, zoos, and for tourists. Four of the studies were group-randomized trials, one used a non-equivalent control group design, and the other used a time-based design. Two studies found significant increases in hat use [35,36]; one found increases in several SPBs [37]; and the others found improvements in SPBs, sunscreen, and shade use [38,39]. An evaluation of a brochure for tourists traveling to a sunny region of Australia led to significantly greater sun avoidance, but no difference in other SPBs or sunburn [40]. While some behaviors improved significantly in these studies, effect sizes were fairly small, except for the time series study reported by Lombard [37] which could have overestimated effects due to lack of a concurrent comparison. Larger effects were found in policies and environmental supports, particularly sunscreen and shade availability, in Glanz's studies in outdoor recreation [38] and swimming pool settings [39]. However, a comparison study revealed that education plus environmental/policy change was no more effective than education alone in promoting desirable sun protection behaviors (SPBs) among children [38].

Table 14.3 Interventions in outdoor recreation settings.

Citation & location	Intervention	Evaluation[1,2]	Results[3]
Lombard et al., 1991 Virginia (USA) [37]	**Swimming pools** Posted prompting and feedback, goal setting, commitment, lifeguard training, behavioral modeling, free sunscreen, information posters	Baseline followed by intervention phase (A-B). Two pools, intervention 3-6 weeks. Outcomes measured by observations of behavior: shirt, shade, hats, sunglasses, zinc oxide, sunscreen bottles, use of free sunscreen (pool users & lifeguards)	Children increased SPBs 6 to 27%. Adult SPBs increased 22 to 38%. Lifeguards increased SPBs 17 to 64%
Mayer et al., 1997 California (USA) [35]	**Swimming pools** Project SunWise – 4 poolside UVR lessons for swim classes, home-based activities for children & parents	RCT, group randomized. 48 YMCA aquatics classes. 6 week intervention. N=169 (92% follow-up), age 7 years. Outcomes: SPBs reported by parents, tanness measured by colorimeter	76% exposed to at least 3 lessons. 72% did most of the family activities. Significant increase in hat use in Intervention. No significant increase in SPB, sunscreen use, or tanness
Glanz et al., 1998 Glanz et al., 2000 Glanz et al., 2001 Hawaii (USA) [38,100,104]	**Outdoor recreation** Hawaii SunSmart program – Educational: staff training, on-site activities, take-home family booklets, behavior monitoring scoreboards, incentives. Environmental: free sunscreen, posters, shade tents, policy consultation	Field test (1998) – pre-post test, 5 sites, 6 wks n=156,113 parents/children, 45,41 staff. RCT (2000,2001) – control [C] v. education [E] v. education + environment [E+E] 14 sites; baseline, 6 weeks, 3 mo follow-up. Measured SPBs, knowledge, sun protection policies, norms – by surveys. N=756,383 (cohort),285 – children/parents. N=176,144,66 – staff	Field test (1998): increased SPB, knowledge norms, reported policies: 3-20% improvement. RCT (2000,2001): children increased SPB and sunscreen use with intervention, increase in E+E no greater than E; changes partly maintained at follow-up. Staff: increased knowledge, SPBs, norms, SP policies with intervention. E+E no greater than E
Mayer et al., 1999 Mayer et al., 2001 California (USA) [36,105]	**Zoos** SunWise Stampede – tipsheets for parents, children's activities, prompts/reminders, coupons, discount prices for sunscreen and hats	Non-equivalent control group design; baseline and intervention phase (A-B). Intervention vs. Evaluation only zoo. Summer and winter studies, 4 weeks observation + intervention	Increased sales of sunscreen & hats in summer; sunscreen only in winter. Increased "ideal hat" use in winter (+0.8%), no increase in summer study. High exposure to and satisfaction with intervention
Segan et al., 1999 Australia [40]	**Tourism** Six-page color brochure "The SunSmart Holiday Guide"; emphasis on reducing sun exposure, avoiding sunburn; harm minimization during holiday experience	RCT, randomized across 21 flights. Pre- and post-holiday surveys. n=449 baseline, 373 follow-up (84%). Adults, mean age 33.4 years	Intervention group avoided sun more. No difference in other SPBs. No difference between groups in sunburn. Those receiving brochure read it & liked it
Glanz et al., 2002 Geller et al., 2001 Hawaii & Massachusetts (USA) [39,68]	**Swimming pools** Pool Cool – staff training, 8 sun safety lessons, interactive poolside activities; providing sunscreen, shade, signage, promoting sun safe environments. 6 weeks intervention	RCT, 28 pools: sun protection (15 pools) v. Injury Prevention control (13 pools). Repeated cross-sectional surveys, pre & post. n=1,010, 842 (parents/children). n=220, 194 lifeguards/aquatic instructors. Measured knowledge, SPB, norms, reported SP policies, sunburns, observations of pool environments (baseline, mid, end)	Children increased SPBs, sunscreen, shade use, reported SP policies. Parents increased SPBs, hat use, reported SP policies. Observations – increased sunscreen availability, signage, lifeguard shirt use; no change in shade

[1] RCT = Randomized controlled trial
[2] Sample description = combined "n" given as pre, post for baseline and final assessment
[3] SPB = sun protection behavior

3.1.4   Workplaces

Outdoor workers receive intense and prolonged exposure to the sun, and thus interventions that are educational and environmental are well suited to the workplace. For adults who work indoors, the workplace may also be a viable setting for educational programming. We reviewed six evaluations of workplace solar exposure prevention strategies (see Table 14.4). Most of the participants in these studies were male. Three of the studies reported improvements in knowledge, sun exposure, and some sun protection behaviors [41-43]. One case-control comparison of an occupational cancer prevention program for water company workers in Israel suggested that regulations were more effective among employees who had already received an educational program [44].

3.1.5   Health care settings

Health care settings provide opportunities for both patient-directed interventions and provider- or system-directed interventions. Thirteen studies were reviewed, including five that were patient-directed, six provider-directed, and two pharmacy interventions (see Table 14.5). Among the *patient-directed interventions*, two programs for newborns used the hospital environment as an opportunity to educate and support sun safety practices for infants [45,46]. Mothers who received the interventions reported low levels of sun exposure. Another study compared message sources and various types of messages to activate members of a Health Maintenance Organization (HMO) to call-in for educational materials. While only 7% of participants called in, they were more likely to do so if the letter came from their physician or health care organization [47]. One study for patients at high-risk led to increased knowledge and intentions for SPBs, but only led to increased SPBs in those with higher perceived risk [48]. Another novel investigation used feedback and instruction on adequate sunscreen application for photosensitive patients, and successfully improved thickness of sunscreen at 2 week and 6 month follow-ups [49]. Interestingly, two of the studies found that patient behavior changes were associated with higher perceived skin cancer risk [47,48].

Provider-directed interventions that have been evaluated are mainly health professional curricula or continuing education to improve knowledge, skin cancer detection skills, and skin cancer prevention counseling practices. Several interventions reported improvements in knowledge and/or clinical skills in lesion identification and management [50-53]. Others found improved attitudes and increased physician-reported and patient-reported clinician sun protection advice [54-55].

Table 14.4 Interventions in workplaces.

Citation & location	Intervention	Evaluation[1,2]	Results[3]
Borland et al., 1991 Australia [41]	Worksite campaign, marketing approach: posters, video (man dying of melanoma), lapel buttons, brochures; group and individual activities	RCT by work team (3 Int. v. 3 control sites) Outdoor telecom workers n = 599, 627 observations Observations of hat, shirt, shade, overall SPB	Increased hat wearing Shirt wearing interaction effect (control group decreased shirt use) No significant difference in shade Intervention group overall higher SPB
Girgis et al., 1994 Australia [42]	Skin screening and risk feedback plus lecture (one-time intervention)	RCT Intervention v. Control Outdoor electrical workers n = 142, 98% male Measured by diary: weather, clothing, sunscreen; validated by observation @ pre-test	Increased SPB post-test in Intervention group Increased knowledge No change in attitudes
Friedman et al., 1995 Texas [106]	Video presentation, physician skin exam, SSE pamphlet and written materials	Pre-, post-, follow-up; non-experimental n = 324 hospital employees in cohort at high/moderate risk for skin cancer Surveys of psychosocial factors 7 months after baseline	Inconclusive for impact of intervention Intentions to practice SPBs and Skin Self-Examination (SSE) not significantly correlated
Hanrahan et al., 1995 Australia [108]	2 educational brochures about melanoma	RCT Intervention v. Control Male workers in an industrial complex n = 204, age 45 +	Increased knowledge of melanoma (+19.8%) No increased ability to recognize or count pigmented or malignant lesions
Azizi et al., 2000 Israel [43]	Local safety officer training 90 minute didactic health education Skin and eye examination Supply of protective gear & sunscreen	RCT Group Randomized trial (4 sites) Minimal [M] vs. Partial [P] vs. Complete [C] Outdoor water company workers, males n = 213 baseline, 144 cohort (all surveys) 3 surveys; results based on final Measured % exposed skin and UVR based on surveys & solar UV ratings to get MED Collected blood samples for serum Vitamin D but results not reported	Protocol deviation made P more Complete Increased sunscreen use in C and P groups Reduced sun-exposed skin in C and P groups Increased SSE with intervention
Shani et al., 2001 Israel [44]	Health education & sun-protection regulations (free supply & required use of sun protection gear)	Opportunistic case-control comparison of those in former program or non-participating Outdoor water company workers, males n = 101; 50 former involved, 51 non-involved	Higher SPBs among program-involved, i.e. "educated" employees Lower melanin presence scores among program-involved employees

[1] RCT = Randomized controlled trial
[2] Sample description = combined "n" given as pre, post for baseline and final assessment
[3] SPB = sun protection behavior

Table 14.5. Interventions in health care settings.

Citation & location	Intervention	Evaluation[1,2]	Results[3]
Patient-directed interventions			
Bolognia *et al.*, 1991 Connecticut (USA) [45]	**Education for mothers of newborns** "Low level" = printed guidelines and printed postcard reminder to limit sun "High level" = guidelines, pamphlets, sunscreen samples, baby sun hat, sun umbrella	RCT: control v. low level v. high level Baseline, follow-up surveys of sun exposure and SPBs n = 275 mothers of newborns, 90% white	Both intervention groups decreased sun exposure Intervention groups spent less unprotected time in sun No difference Low v. High level
Geller *et al.*, 1999 Massachusetts (USA) [46]	Education in newborn nurseries Behavioral package, educational kits, tip sheets, pamphlets, bibs, hats, magnets, sand pails Health provider advice (nurses)	Post-test surveys n = 187 (136 surveyed) mothers Measured recall, satisfaction, sunburn, changes in sun exposure, knowledge SPB Survey one year after intervention	88% recalled the information and reported it was timely Two-thirds of mothers said it was the only sun protection information they received from a health provider 89% reported child always wears hat outside 90% reported child spends < 3 hrs/week in sun 13% reported child had sunburn in past year
Gerbert *et al.*, 1997 California (USA) [47]	Education for HMO members Mailed materials from one of 3 sources: their physician, their HMO, junk mailer **Messages** emphasized effects of UVR on either: skin cancer risk, aging and wrinkling, or both	RCT: source and message varied Baseline survey, outcome measured by call-in for more information n = 933 HMO members	Over-all call-in rate low at 7% More calls if letter from MD or HMO Message emphasis had no effect Skin cancer risk predicted patient activation
Robinson *et al.*, 1995 Illinois (USA) [48]	Education for **NMSC patients and helpers** Delivered by physicians and nurses	Pre-post design n = 200 pairs of patients (P) and relative/friend (R/F) Measured risk, SPBs, attitudes, knowledge Post-test survey 1 year after intervention	Increased knowledge in P and R/F Increased intention to practice more SPBs SPBs increased only in those with higher perceived risk
Azurdia *et al.*, 2000 United Kingdom [49]	Education for **photosensitive patients** Feedback and instruction on adequate sunscreen application	Pre-post with follow-up: baseline, 2 weeks, six months n = 6 patients with photosensitive conditions Measure was fluorescence spectroscopy to assess adequacy and thickness of sunscreen application	Education improved sunscreen application Baseline thickness 0.11 mg/cm^2 to 0.82 at 2 weeks and 1.13 at 6 months
Provider-directed interventions			
Gooderham *et al.*, 1999a Canada [50]	**Medical school curriculum** Week-long dermatology curriculum during Sun Awareness Week: didactic + case study + teaching primary school students	Pre-post design, 2 month interval n = 98 first-year medical students Survey of knowledge, attitudes, behaviors	Improved knowledge, attitudes Increased intentions for SPB Couldn't assess actual behavior in short time, not during summer
Mikkilineni *et al.*, 2001 Rhode Island (USA) [55]	**Continuing medical education** 2 hour multicomponent educational curriculum on skin cancer triage, prevention, and counseling	Pre-post test Surveys of MD's, patient exit interviews HMO primary care providers n = 28,22	Improved attitudes to total body skin exam and skin cancer prevention Increase in reported MD skin cancer counseling Patient exit interviews corroborated MD reports

Reference	Intervention	Methods/Sample	Results
McCormick et al., 1999 Texas (USA) [51]	**Nurse training module** 1 week didactic + clinical skin cancer prevention training module 20 hours clinical included triage for skin lesions, skin exam practice	Quasi-experiment, intervention v. comparison Baseline, post-intervention, 3 months n = 32 intervention, 87 comparison nurses Measured knowledge, screening ability, attitudes, self-efficacy, organizational factors	Increased knowledge, screening ability, self-efficacy; but no change in organizational barriers
Dolan et al., 1997 Illinois (USA) [53]	**Continuing medical education** 2 1-hour seminars on skin cancer conducted by general internist with a dermatologist	RCT, intervention v. control n = 82 housestaff and attending MD's Measures: knowledge, attitudes, beliefs, treatment decision ability Exit interviews of moderate & high risk patients before & after (n = 82, 113)	Incomplete attendance (22% attended none) Increased self-efficacy, risk factor identification No increase I vs. C in lesion identification and management Greater increase in patient reported SC counseling by intervention MDs (+19% v. −8%)
Harris et al., 2001 Arizona (USA) [52]	**Continuing medical education** Internet-based CME; interactive, self-paced Focus on guidelines for recognizing malignant melanoma	Pre-post test n = 354 physicians Online survey of knowledge, clinical skills, MD confidence	Significant improvements in knowledge (85% vs. 52% pre-test) Increased MD confidence, clinical skills scores (90% vs. 81% pre-test) High user satisfaction
Dietrich et al., 2000 New Hampshire (USA) [54]	**Continuing education + office visits** Meeting + 2 visits to assist with office system set-up to promote SC prev. to children and parents: practice routine, handouts, waiting room ed materials, sunscreen samples	Context of SunSafe community intervention with 5 intervention + 5 control towns Self-report, observation, parent interviews n = 41 cooperating MD's at follow-up (family practice + pediatrics) N = 837 parents surveyed	MD's receiving intervention used more handouts, education materials, sunscreen samples Parents in intervention towns reported more clinician sun protection advice (34% vs. 27%)

Pharmacy Interventions

Reference	Intervention	Methods/Sample	Results
Leinweber et al., 1995 Alberta (Canada) [56]	**Pharmacy campaign** One-month campaign to increase knowledge, awareness by pharmacists, staff, customers. Education materials:posters, mobiles, point-of-purchase signs, buttons for staff Bag stuffer, pamphlets and cards for customers	Pre-post surveys of pharmacists n = 409, 349 retail pharmacists Measures of knowledge, attitudes, pharmacy practice, and barriers	Increased knowledge in selected areas Majority (63%) gave favorable feedback Pamphlets and posters rated most useful 34% said the campaign increased contact with customers
Mayer et al., 1998a Mayer et al., 1998b California (USA) [57,58]	**Pharmacy training and materials** Training, video + print materials, feedback on SC counseling performance, incentives, environmental prompts	RCT, n = 54 pharmacies n = 113,105 pharmacists (80 cohort) Primary measure of counseling: use of confederates Pharmacist survey of knowledge, self-efficacy, attitudes, reported counseling Counts of brochures & sunscreen samples used	Increased counseling by intervention pharmacists (relative increase + 70%) Knowledge, self-rated skills, self-reported counseling increased No change in favorable attitudes to counseling

[1] RCT = Randomized controlled trial
[2] Sample description = combined "n" given as pre, post for baseline and final assessment
[3] SPB = sun protection behavior

Two additional health care interventions took place in *pharmacies*, and combined provider-directed and system-directed strategies. A one-month campaign in pharmacies in Canada led to increased knowledge, pharmacist satisfaction, and reported increases in contact with customers [56]. A longer-term program with training, videos and print materials, feedback on skin cancer counseling performance, incentives, and environmental prompts in California was found to increase objectively assessed counseling (using study confederates) by intervention pharmacists, as well as knowledge, self-rated skills, and self-reported counseling [57,58].

3.2   Other types of interventions

3.2.1   Mass media

Mass media are a recognized vehicle for reaching wide audiences, particularly for the purpose of raising awareness and/or concern about an issue. Specific interventions that include mass media as part of a prevention strategy have been reported recently in the United States, Sweden, and New Zealand (see Table 14.6). A principal goal of evaluations of these campaigns has been to assess awareness of the campaigns and their messages. Generally, studies have reported increased awareness and/or substantial recall of the media information [59-65]. In Australia, Theobald and others evaluated a three-segment television program that emphasized early detection and the dangers of sun exposure and sunburn. Viewers reported significantly greater awareness and personal concern about sun protection than did non-viewers, but there were no differences between groups in attitudes toward tanning, perceived barriers to protection, and the seriousness of too much UVR exposure [66]. Some studies found that respondents reported changes in the use of sunscreen and/or sun avoidance [60,62,63], though others did not [61,62,65,67]. Three of the studies have specifically examined the consequences of media reporting of skin cancer advisories in the form of UV Index and/or "burn time" [62,63,65]. On balance, those types of strategies appear to lead to sun avoidance in about half of the respondents who say they are aware of the information and messages.

Table 14.6 Mass media interventions.

Citation & location	Intervention	Evaluation [1,2]	Results [3]
King et al., 1983 & Putnam et al., 1985 Hawaii (USA) [59,60]	Mailed educational comic book and TV and radio PSA's 6-8 month period	Pre-post surveys Statewide & Caucasian target areas n = 1616, 1403 for state surveys n = 318, 304 for target area	45% recalled comic book and 90% of those read, understood, & enjoyed it Increased awareness of peak sun hours Increased sunscreen, protective clothing among readers
McGee & Williams, 1992 New Zealand [61]	SunSmart media campaign aimed at teens 2 years duration	Post-campaign survey n = 345 adolescents (13-15 years) Reference made to pre-campaign survey, but no details given	High awareness of campaign Positive attitudes toward tanning common High exposure without protection Associations between exposure, awareness, and SPBs
Boutwell et al., 1995 Gelb et al., 1991 Texas (USA) [62,107]	Skin cancer advisories and behavioral messages via mass media Telephone call-in line to request print materials 3 months	Pre- and post- campaign surveys Beginning and end of summer n = 250, 250	Improvement since pre-campaign survey Awareness increase (12.4% to 62.4%) No significant change in use of sunscreen, hats, clothing Increase in sun avoidance (15.8% to 27.5%)
Geller et al., 1997 MMWR, 1997 USA [63,64]	Broadcast of UV Index on TV and newspaper weather reports, with behavioral messages	Telephone survey of weather forecasters (n=185) and newspaper review (n=58) Survey of white adults in 12 "high exposure" and 12 "low exposure" cities; n = 700	71% of TV stations broadcast UVI 61% of newspapers reported UVI 64% public awareness, 90% able to describe 38% reported behavior change; most common was sun avoidance No difference, high vs. low exposure cities
Kiekbusch et al., 2000 Sweden [67]	Multimedia campaign on malignant melanoma 3 years	Mail survey in campaign town and non-campaign comparison n = 782, 793	Campaign town – no major change in SPB but negative change in comparison In men, trend of increased knowledge and SPB
Bulliard & Reeder, 2001 New Zealand [65]	Media weather reporting of burn time and UV Index	Telephone survey over 4 weeks of summer n = 396	Greater awareness of "burn time" than UVI UVI better understood, recalled, but less used to guide SPB General perceived understanding greater than comprehension (96% vs. 65%)

[1] Respondents are adults unless indicated
[2] Sample description = combined 'n' given as pre, post for baseline and final assessment
[3] SPB = sun protection behavior

3.2.2   Interventions for parents and caregivers

Because of the importance of reducing UVR exposure in children, educational and behavioral strategies aimed at parents and caregivers (such as sports coaches, lifeguards, teachers, and so on) have been the focus of some efforts. Some studies that seek to improve children's sun protection behaviors have also evaluated the impact on parents and caregivers, who may be persuaded to improve their own sun safety so they can act as role models [38,68].

Seven studies were identified with emphases on parents and caregiver outcomes (see Table 14.7). Two studies were educational programs for preschool staff and parents of young children. One, in Sweden, found that lectures as a supplement to mailed information increased the effectiveness of the sun safety message [69]. Another found that using a combined didactic-experiential prevention program improved, not only knowledge, but also attitudes, beliefs, and SPBs [70]. A third study used computer-altered visual stimuli (photos) to influence adolescent female day camp staff. Those receiving the altered stimuli (showing aging with or without disfigurement from skin cancer lesions) increased their sunscreen use at the time of a six-week follow-up [71].

Training programs for sports and outdoor recreation were conducted and evaluated in several locations in the United States. The SunSmart Hawaii program achieved increases in knowledge, SPBs, and norms [38]; a Georgia program for soccer coaches and parents led to greater knowledge and more promotion of sun safety among youth [72]; and the "Pool Cool" aquatics sun safety program led to reduced sunburning and improvements in sun protection policies, but not to significant differences in SPBs between experimental and control groups [68].

In Australia, Dobbinson and others [73] evaluated a ten-year sponsorship program for beach lifeguards (known as "lifesavers" in Australia) that aimed to promote sun protection and role model behavior with training, education, informational prompts, policy implementation, and structural changes. Evaluation data included surveys of lifeguards and beach-goers in the state with the sponsorship program and a comparison state without the program. Lifeguards in the state with the sponsorship program reported higher rates of SPBs, less sunburn, and more favorable views of themselves as role models, but no differences in their attitudes toward intentional tanning.

Table 14.7 Interventions for parents and caregivers.

Citation & location	Intervention	Evaluation[1,2]	Results[3]
Boldeman et al., 1991 Sweden [69]	Lectures for participating preschool staff and mailed information nationally	Post-program survey to preschools in lecture area and a remote reference area. Total sample = 674 with varying programs	Lectures more effective to improve sun awareness than mailed information alone. SPB message twice as effective in areas that received lectures
Rodrigue, 1996 Florida (USA) [70]	Comprehensive Prevention Program (CPP) and Information Only Condition (IOC). CPP = didactic + experiential (discussion, role play, survivor speaker, risk assessment)	RCT: CPP vs. IOC vs. no-intervention control. n = 55 Caucasian mothers w/ children < 10 yrs. Post-test 3 months after pre-test	CPP and IOC showed increased knowledge. CPP increased SPB, attitudes, beliefs
Novick, 1997 New York (USA) [71]	Computer-altered visual stimuli: photos to show aging and skin cancer lesions. One-time intervention, 6 week assessment	RCT, no alterations v. aging v. aging + disfigurement. n = 30 white females, 13-18 yrs; day camp staff	No change in sun exposure. Increased sunscreen use with visual stimuli
Parrott et al., 1999 Georgia (USA) [72]	Training program for soccer coaches and parents: didactic, role plays, strategies for sun-safe soccer teams	Outcomes measured by sunscreen logs and sun exposure. Pilot study; pre-post surveys of kids & adults. n = 12 coaches, 50 parents, 61 youths	Coaches & parents increased knowledge and trend to increased self-efficacy and intentions to promote sun-safety. Youth reported an increase in parents and coaches telling them to use sunscreen. Pilot study: Improved SPB parents, trends for staff
Glanz et al., 1998 Glanz et al., 2000 Hawaii (USA) [38,104]	Educational program for staff, children; and education/environmental program in outdoor recreation settings. Program included interactive take-home activity guides for children & parents	Pilot study pre-post test all components. Main trial group RCT by site, 14 rec sites in 3 conditions: Control, Education, Ed + Envir. Pilot study, parents n=156, 113 (cohort = 94); and staff n=45, 41 (cohort = 30). Main trial, staff n = 176, 144 (n=66 @ 3 mo FU). Outcomes knowledge, SPB, sunscreen, norms, program sun protection policies	Main trial: increases in knowledge, SPBs, norms, sun protection policies. Education + Environment not superior to Education alone
Dobbinson et al., 1999 Australia [73]	Lifesaver (lifeguard) sponsorship program aimed at changing norms, role modeling. Education, sunscreen provision, policies. Sponsorship contracts requiring hats and shirts, funding for shade and clothing. Training, education, informational prompts	After 10 years of program: survey to compare with pre-program, & comparison with another state without a program. Surveys of beach-goers in state with program and another state with no program. n = 128, 134 lifesavers (with/without program). n = 228, 153 beachgoers (with/without program)	Higher rates of SPBs - lifesavers with program. Less sunburn among those with the program. Significant improvements over pre-program. More favorable views of selves as role models with the program. No differences in attitudes toward tanning
Geller et al., 2001 Hawaii & Massachusetts (USA) [68]	Sun protection program at swimming pools. Staff training + leading lessons	RCT: Sun protection v. injury prevention control. Randomized swimming pools (n = 28 pools). n = 220, 194 lifeguards/aquatic staff	No significant differences in SPB by groups. Reduced sunburning at Sun Protection pools. Increased sun protection policies at SP pools

[1] RCT = Randomized controlled trial
[2] Sample description = combined "n" given as "n" given as pre, post for baseline and final assessment
[3] SPB = sun protection behavior

3.2.3   Community-wide interventions

Community-wide sun safety programs aim to achieve broad changes in defined geographic areas through multi-component and multi-sectoral interventions in various settings that can include entire communities, schools, workplaces, health care, recreation, media, and other organizations. These efforts include not only education, but also significant efforts to institute policy and structural supports to sun safety. Such programs have been in place for two decades in Australia, with the longest-standing and best evaluated one being the Slip! Slap! Slop! and SunSmart campaigns in Victoria, in the south of the country [9]. Two American programs, the SafeSun Project in New Hampshire [8,74] and the Falmouth Safe Skin Project in Massachusetts [75], have used similar strategies on a smaller scale (see Table 14.8).

The efficacy of community-wide interventions has been established through a series of evaluation studies conducted for the Australian programs in Victoria [9,76,77] and related publications on specific program components and surveys. Since the start of the program, there have been major decreases in pro-tanning attitudes and positive changes in SPBs including sunscreen, hat and shirt use, sun avoidance, and shade seeking, as well as reduction in sunburns [9,76]. The program has further been effective for improving accessibility, availability, and prices of sun protection items. While these programs' successes have been remarkable among public health interventions [78], important areas of resistance persist. These include changing adolescents' behaviors and use of wide-brimmed hats. An important question regarding the wide applicability of these results is whether these strategies would be viable in geographic areas where rates of skin cancer are lower.

The SafeSun Project was evaluated in a group-randomized controlled trial with 10 small towns in the state of New Hampshire. The main outcomes were assessed by observing children at beaches. After one and two years, increased body covering and sunscreen use were found in the intervention communities [8,74]. However, no differences were found in use of protective clothing or shade at either time point.

The Falmouth Safe Skin Project evaluation showed increases in sunscreen use by 6 to 13-year-olds, greater knowledge, and fewer sunburns among very young children. However, there was less hat use and shirt use among 6 to 13-year-olds after the three-year intervention [75]. The evaluation involved two cross-sectional surveys without a comparison community.

Table 14.8 Community-wide interventions.

Citation & location	Intervention	Evaluation[1,2]	Results[3]
Miller et al., 1999 Massachusetts (USA) [75]	**Falmouth Safe Skin Project** Community-wide intervention, 1 town of about 2,000 families Hospital maternity unit, child care centers, schools, summer camps, local media, community activism & participation w/ volunteer assistance (social networks) 3 year component	Repeated cross-sectional surveys, pre-post 3 years between surveys Parents with children ages 0-13 (analyzed 0-5, 6-13) n = 401, 404 Measured sun exposure, SPBs, knowledge, role modeling, self-efficacy, sunburns	Significant decrease in sunburns 0-5 year olds Increase in usual sunscreen 6-13 year olds Significant decrease in shirt use, 6-13 years Trend toward less hat use, 6-13 year olds Increased knowledge
Dietrich et al., 1998 Dietrich et al., 2000a New Hampshire (USA) [8,74]	**SafeSun Project** Multi-sectoral intervention: schools, day care centers, primary care practices, Beach areas Used organizational vehicles to get consistent messages out 2 year intervention	RCT, n = 10 towns, Intervention v. Control Main evaluation = observation of children at the beach (age 2-9) and parent interviews, Measured SPBs and covering up n = 865, 1065 children observed	At one year: a) significantly more children had at least some body covering by sunscreen or clothes (+9% vs. −5%) b) more sunscreen use in intervention towns c) no difference in use of protective clothing or shade At two years: same, approximately the same I vs. C difference in at least some body covering (+17% vs. +3%)
Montague et al., 2001 Hill et al., 1993 (Australia) [9,76]	**Slip! Slap! Slop! and SunSmart** Multi-component, long term programs from 1980 to 2000 in Victoria, AUS Public education + mass media SunSmart schools: curriculum, training, accreditation Community support: workplace, sporting groups, government, policy/structural supports Training for health professionals	Repeated cross-sectional population surveys Surveys of individuals in target groups - adults, children, organizations Specific project evaluations	Decrease in pro-tanning attitudes (61% to 35%) Positive changes in SPB: shade seeking, hat, sunscreen, covering up, sun avoidance Reduction in sunburns Structural changes, including policies/facilities Improved accessibility, availability, price of sun protection items Continued room for improvement, especially in some difficult audiences, e.g., adolescents

[1] RCT = Randomized controlled trial
[2] Sample description = combined "n" given as pre, post for baseline and final assessment
[3] SPB = sun protection behavior

### 3.2.4	Message testing studies

An important area of inquiry in the arena of behavioral research to reduce UVR exposure concerns the relative effectiveness of various messages. Eight studies have examined various types of persuasive strategies, including fear arousal or emotional appeals; various types of "message framing" approaches, or relative emphases in persuasive messages; humor; and inductive versus deductive styles of communication. Buller, Burgoon *et al.* [79,80] studied language intensity and logical style in printed sun safety messages for parents of children aged 5 to 11 years. They found that high-intensity messages, formatted in deductive style, were most persuasive at achieving intentions to practice sun safety [80] and that deductive messages were most effective for parents with mixed intentions [79].

Prentice-Dunn and others [81] compared the effectiveness of appearance-based messages focusing on the benefits of tanning and the efficacy of prevention on students' sun protection intentions. They found that students who were less concerned about appearance expressed greater intentions to take precautions, and that conveying "low benefits" of tanning also encouraged protective behaviors.

Several studies tested various types of message framing, including "gain vs. loss" and "high efficacy vs. low efficacy" conditions. Block and Keller [82] found that for low efficacy messages, negative framing was more effective; and Rothman *et al.* [83] found that positively framed pamphlets were more likely to lead to requests for sun protection while negatively framed messages influenced intentions for skin examination. Detweiler *et al.* [84] conducted a study at the beach, and found that gain-framed messages led to more requests for sunscreen and greater intentions to use varieties that were SPF 15 or higher.

Richard and others [85] compared humorous and alarmist (high-fear) pamphlets with neutral versions and a no-pamphlet control. Those who received the humorous pamphlet were more likely to read it, but those receiving the alarmist version had greater increases in knowledge. One concern raised in the conclusions was that alarmism might interfere with reading while humor might decrease the impact of the message. Stephenson and Witte's experiment [86] is consistent with these findings, but extends them to suggest that a fear appeal combined with a strong efficacy message emphasizing the effectiveness of recommended behaviors promoted more sun protective behaviors.

These studies, while for the most part not conducted as widely distributed interventions, are very useful in helping to guide the content of messages used in setting-specific, community-wide, or mass media interventions to reduce UVR exposure.

4. DISCUSSION

4.1 What success can be achieved?

The ideal intervention strategies to reduce UVR exposure are coordinated, sustained, community-wide approaches that combine education, mass media, and environmental and structural changes. The longest-established and most-studied of these programs, SunSmart in the state of Victoria in Australia, has reduced several skin cancer risk behaviors by roughly one-half, although some sub-groups and behaviors present continuing challenges [9]. Because SunSmart (with its predecessor Slip! Slap! Slop!) appears to have achieved society-wide normative changes, it has good prospects for continuing to build on this success. What is less clear is whether this type of effect can be accomplished in areas with lower skin cancer rates, larger populations, or more ethnically mixed populations. The results of the SunSafe Project in New Hampshire, in the United States [8,74], at least suggest that movement in the same direction is possible in another culture and location.

4.2 What can we conclude about settings?

As described in this chapter, many studies have reported interventions located within specific organizational settings. These venues provide useful ways to reach important audiences like children and high-risk patients. They can also increase the relevance of the intervention, as with programs in outdoor recreation, outdoor workplaces, and health care settings. Organizational settings also provide clear opportunities for policy and structural supports to complement educational efforts.

With regard to specific settings for which larger numbers of studies are reported, we can draw additional conclusions. Schools appear to provide a good foundation for sun safety education, but have been limited in their success at influencing long term behavioral changes. Most likely, they should link with other community organizations and with families, to achieve transfer to those occasions when children are selecting sun protective products and spending time outdoors. Health care settings appear to be appropriate and feasible places to teach health care providers (including pharmacists) better skin cancer diagnostic and counseling skills. The salience of prevention messages in health care settings is likely to be high. However, attendance at provider education programs has been a limitation, and skin cancer prevention is likely to compete with other priorities for the attention of doctors and nurses. Also, while the promise of system changes to bring skin cancer prevention into health care is strong, much less is known about whether this will lead patients or populations to increase their solar protection behaviors.

4.3   What is known about environmental, policy, and structural interventions?

It is generally agreed that environmental and structural changes are necessary components of successful skin cancer prevention efforts. An analysis of the studies reviewed here reveals that environmental supports, policy changes, and/or structural interventions have been part of carefully evaluated prevention programs in virtually all types of settings, although their impact has not been specifically studied in school programs. In pre-school settings, policies regarding hats and sunscreen have been most prominent. Outdoor recreation settings have used free or discounted sunscreen, shade supports, environmental prompts (signs, posters), and free or reduced-price hats. Supply of protective gear and sunscreen, as well as regulations, have been used in workplace settings. A broad range of structural changes has been used in comprehensive community-wide programs [9,54].

Despite the wide inclusion of environmental, policy and structural changes in health promotion efforts, the research reveals some limitations to their efficacy. Adoption of sun protection policies is often a strategy for change *and* an outcome in itself. Several studies found that changes in the adoption of policies are not necessarily accompanied by changes in the "clients" – children, patients, and/or workers [44,68,87]. Other studies have not measured changes in the intended beneficiaries of prevention strategies [56]. Another complication is the increasing public demand for supportive sun safety items, which can make it difficult to separate their influence from educational programs [39,43].

When do environmental and structural supports make a difference? They may take longer than individual-directed strategies to make a difference. They may need to be stronger or more intense than they have been in reported programs. And finally, some supports (e.g., free sunscreen, hats) may be effective mainly by reducing obstacles to action for already motivated people, rather than changing behaviors of those who are unmotivated.

4.4   What type of messages work best?

The only type of message for which there are enough studies to analyze their impact are the general category of fear-arousing messages, emotional appeals, and risk information. These have been variously tested in the form of "high intensity messages" [80], alarmism [85], fear appeals [86], negatively framed messages [82], risk feedback [42], and experiential programming with survivors or patients dying of melanoma [41,62]. Most of these strategies have shown some effect on behavior or behavioral intentions, though their specific impact cannot be separated in multi-component interventions. In the SunSmart media campaign, a fear-arousing television spot showing a graphic depiction of skin cancer removal was tested and found to generate very high awareness and recall [77].

Another issue regarding the type of message has not been discussed in detail in reports of interventions. That is: is it more effective to give a "strict" message of total sun protection (wide brim hat, long sleeves, long pants, routine sun avoidance, etc.) or to encourage gradual behavior change? Theories of human behavior suggest that gradual change may be more successful for achieving both individual [88] and social change [89]. One formative study supported this notion that small changes would be considered more acceptable and would not cause the audience to "tune out" to the intervention [90].

4.5   What outcomes are most influenced?

Of all outcomes measured, increases in knowledge are the most-often reported. Among behavioral outcomes, the use of sunscreen is the main outcome for which success is reported. Increased sunscreen use also seems to account for much of the increase in "composite sun protection behaviors" (SPBs) in many reports. Some studies have found increases in hat use or general covering-up, but this has been less common. Some media interventions, especially those emphasizing the UV Index and weather conditions, have succeeded in promoting sun avoidance.

4.6   Design and analysis considerations

Of the studies reviewed, about half used experimental designs and many involved group-randomized trials. Most of the randomized controlled trials are studies of individuals or setting-specific strategies, while the majority of evaluations of mass media and community-wide interventions used other designs. Some studies have used repeat cross-sectional or time series designs. The remaining studies have used various non-experimental designs.

These designs make causal inference more difficult, but can reduce problems with internal validity, like contamination. The importance of experimental designs is illustrated by some studies that found improvements in the control groups as well as experimental groups. Others found negative trends in control groups [39,42,67], again underscoring the importance of studying appropriate controls.

Duration of interventions and length of follow-up are other limitations to our knowledge of strategies for reducing UVR exposure. About two-thirds of the interventions had a duration of less than 6 weeks, and more than half the evaluations followed subjects for less than 3 months. The trend toward multi-year interventions and longer follow-up periods is an important advance, though the commitment of research resources may constrain longer-term programs and evaluations.

One of the most vexing and difficult to assess factors in reported intervention studies is the *quality of the intervention* [91]. An encouraging trend can be seen in the conduct of formative research and pre-testing of interventions before they are implemented [36,41,90]. More studies are reporting process evaluation data to assist in interpretation [35,51,92]. A related consideration is testing whether the hypothesized "active ingredients" or mediating factors changed, and whether changes in these factors are associated with behavior change. Few studies in the solar protection area have reported on mediators' analysis up to now. There is also substantial variability in the rigor of *data analytic methods*, and many studies do not control for relevant confounders such as risk levels and weather conditions.

4.7   Measurement of outcomes

This area of research faces important challenges in both conceptualizing and operationalizing the main behavioral outcomes of interest. UVR exposure behaviors are both habitual and contingent, multi-dimensional, and not necessarily additive (for example, staying indoors may make wearing sunscreen or a hat unnecessary). The complex interactions among different sun protection behaviors have seldom been studied. Also, the distinction between intentional and incidental sun exposure has not been well studied. The adequacy of the items used, or of how they are used, is also usually not accounted for in self-report measures although new tools may enable us to improve on these measures [49].

Most studies rely on self-report of behaviors and their presumed determinants. Intervention studies in schools rely almost exclusively on self-reports. Self-report is particularly vulnerable to social desirability bias. A few studies have used multiple measures, for example both surveys and diaries, and examined their relative merits for assessing behavior [93].

Studies in non-school settings have more often used observations and, occasionally, physical measures [94]. Observations may not reflect adoption of a "habit" but only a moment in time [36]. Physical measures such as colorimeters [95] and poplysulphone dosimeters [96] are useful, but may be impractical in large trials, and measures of tanness (skin darkening as measured by a colorimeter), may not be valid in non-white populations. There is also a need for further development of measures of environmental and policy change strategies for sun safety.

5.   THEORY AND EVIDENCE FOR PLANNING INTERVENTIONS

Like other types of health promotion efforts, skin cancer prevention programs are most likely to succeed when they are based on a clear understanding of the targeted health behaviors and their environmental context. Theories about why people do or do not engage in sun protection behaviors (SPBs), and data about a given target audience, are often helpful in guiding the search for promising and suitable interventions [97]. Population-wide surveys such as those described in Chapter 12 have been used to examine the distribution of behaviors and their determinants, and contribute to the design of strategies to increase SPBs. Other formative research methods such as focus groups have also been used to develop targeted skin cancer prevention programs, especially when working with understudied audiences in new locations such as multiethnic Hawaii [90].

Although some evaluation reports do not describe the theoretical bases of skin cancer prevention interventions, many of the more recent publications specify one or more theories that have guided their programs. These include learning theories [98], theories of message framing and fear arousal [79-85], applied behavioral analysis [37], stages of change [99], social cognitive theory [38,100] and ecological approaches [9]. Theories that suggest both individual-directed and environmental strategies are most compatible with multi-component and community-wide interventions. Persons who engage in the planning of skin cancer prevention programs – whether for community health improvement or for scientific evaluation – should identify and examine their assumptions and, in turn, build on the theories underlying their approaches to improve sun protection in their communities and audiences.

6.   RESEARCH NEEDS AND WORK IN PROGRESS

The field of behavior change for skin cancer prevention has progressed significantly in the past decade, but there are important areas for further advancement. As outlined above, these include design, measurement, communicating about interventions, developing a better understanding of how environmental and policy interventions work, and studies in multi-ethnic populations. The use of new communication technology and international collaborations can make significant contributions to these advances.

Currently, there are several other large-scale sun protection intervention studies in progress, some of which have been completed but not yet reported in published form. These include interventions at beaches [99], and in pre-school settings [101], pediatric health care settings [102], and schools [16]. In addition, innovative studies are examining personalized counseling for siblings of melanoma patients, tailored print materials for people at high-risk for skin cancer, and preventive interventions for workers in the ski industry and postal workers. The results of these studies will further advance our understanding of what changes can be achieved through educational, motivational and environmental interventions.

CONCLUSIONS

There is good evidence from evaluations in Australia that, in a country with high skin cancer rates, a sustained comprehensive community-wide program can substantially increase solar protection behaviors. It is less clear whether such efforts can be successfully transferred to locations where skin cancer is a less prominent public health concern and the population includes a higher proportion of dark-skinned individuals.

Prevention programs in specific settings can, by themselves, achieve significant improvements in reducing UVR exposure and contribute to wider efforts in the community. Media programs are effective for increasing awareness and possibly for promoting sun avoidance during high UV periods. School programs have thus far proven effective mainly for increasing knowledge and in some cases, short-term behavioral improvements. Other settings such as outdoor recreation settings, health services, and outdoor workplaces may have high salience and thus be valuable venues for prevention.

Methodological issues such as design and measurement continue to present challenges to behavioral researchers and health promotion experts. Also, little attention has been devoted to the efficiency, or cost to achieve improvements in health behavior, in the available intervention literature (see Chapter 15). Advancements in these domains should complement further action and evaluation, with the prospect of stemming the tide of skin cancer internationally.

SUMMARY POINTS

- Comprehensive, community-wide programs can increase solar protection behaviors and reduce UVR exposure
- Prevention programs in specific settings, such as recreation settings and outdoor workplaces, can also achieve significant improvements in behavior
- Media programs can increase awareness about skin cancer and UVR exposure, and school programs have been shown most effective for improving knowledge and attitudes, and in some cases for improving short-term behaviors

IMPLICATIONS FOR PUBLIC HEALTH

- Skin cancer rates are increasing and more attention should be devoted to designing and evaluating programs to effectively reduce exposure to ultraviolet radiation, especially in high risk populations
- There is a need to develop programs that are effective in countries where skin cancer is not of as high a priority as in Australia, and the experiences in Australia provide an excellent starting point
- Intervention studies need to attend to the issues of study design, measurement, and cost-effectiveness. There is also a need for studies of diffusion of successful program strategies.

REFERENCES

1. Howe HL, Wingo PA, Thun MJ *et al.* (2001) Annual report to the nation on the status of cancer (1973 through 1998), featuring cancers with recent increasing trends. *J Natl Cancer Inst* **93:** 824-842.
2. Whiteman DC, Whiteman CA, Green AC (2001) Childhood sun exposure as a risk factor for melanoma: a systematic review of epidemiologic studies. *Cancer Causes Cont* **12:** 69-82.
3. Saraiya M, Briss P, Nichols P, White C, Das D, Glanz K. Preventing skin cancer by reducing exposure to ultraviolet light: A report on the recommendations of the Task Force on Community Preventive Services. *Morbidity and Mortality Weekly Reports.* (in press).

4. Briss PA, Zaza S, Pappaioanou M *et al.* (2000) Developing an evidence-based Guide to Community Preventive Services – Methods. *Am J Prev Med* **18(1S):** 35-43.
5. Zaza S, Wright-DeAguero L, Briss PA et al. (2000) Task Force on Community Preventive Services: Data collection instrument and procedure for systematic reviews in the Guide to Community Preventive Services—Methods. *Am J Prev Med* **18:** 44-74.
6. Buller DB, Borland R (1999) Skin cancer prevention for children: A critical review. *Health Educ Behav* **26:** 317-343.
7. Stanton W (Ed.) (1996) *Primary Prevention of Skin Cancer in Australia.* Report of the Sun Protection Programs Working Party. Canberra: NHMRC
8. Dietrich AJ, Olson AL, Sox CH *et al.* (1998) A community-based randomized trial encouraging sun protection for children. *Pediatrics* **102:** e64.
9. Montague M, Borland R, Sinclair C (2001) Slip! Slap! Slop! and SunSmart, 1980-2000: Skin cancer control and 20 years of population-based campaigning. *Health Educ Behav* **28:** 290-305.
10. Buller DB, Borland R (1998) Public education projects in skin cancer prevention: Child care, school, and college-based. *Clin Dermatol* **16:** 1-13.
11. Vitols P, Oates RK (1997) Teaching children about skin cancer prevention: why wait for adolescence? *Aust NZ J Public Health* **21:** 602-605.
12. Labat KL, DeLong MR, Gahring S (1996) Evaluation of a skin cancer intervention program for youth. *J Family Consumer Sci* **88:** 3-10.
13. Mermelstein RJ, Riesenberg LA (1992) Changing knowledge and attitudes about skin cancer risk factors in adolescents. *Health Psychol* **11:** 371-376.
14. McWhirter JM, Collins M, Bryant I, Wetton NM, Bishop JN (2000) Evaluating 'Safe in the Sun', a curriculum programme for primary schools. *Health Educ Res* **15:** 203-217.
15. Buller MK, Goldberg G, Buller DB (1997) SunSmart Day: A Pilot Program for photoprotection education. *Pediatric Dermatol* **14:** 257-263.
16. Cantor M, Rosseel K, Rutsch L (1999) The United States Environmental Protection Agency SunWise School Program. *Health Educ Behav* **26:** 303-304.
17. Thornton C, Piacquadio DJ (1996) Promoting Sun Awareness: Evaluation of an Educational Children's Book. *Pediatrics* **98:** 52-55.
18. Fleming C, Newell J, Turner S, Mackie R (1997) A study of the impact of Sun Awareness Week 1995. *Br J Dermatol* **136:** 719-724.
19. Gooderham MJ, Guenther L (1999b) Sun and the skin: evaluation of a sun awareness program for elementary school students. *J Cutan Med Surg* **3:** 230-235.
20. Hornung RL, Lennon PA, Garrett JM, DeVellis RF, Weinberg PD, Strecher VJ (2000) Interactive Computer Technology for Skin Cancer Prevention Targeting Children. *Am J Prev Med* **18:** 69-76.
21. Fork HE, Wagner RFJ, Wagner KD (1992) The Texas peer education sun awareness project for children: primary prevention of malignant melanoma and nonmelanocytic skin cancers. *Cutis* **50:** 363-364.
22. Buller DB, Hall JR, Powers PJ *et al* (1999) Evaluation of the "Sunny Days, Healthy Ways" sun safety CD-ROM program for children in grades 4 and 5. *Cancer Prev Control* **3:** 188-195.
23. Reding DJ, Fischer V, Lappe K, Gunderson P (1994) Health education delivery by Wisconsin veterinarians. *Wisconsin Med J* **93:** 627-629.
24. Reding DJ, Fischer V, Gunderson P, Lappe K, Anderson H, Calvert G (1996) Teens teach skin cancer prevention. *J Rural Health* **12**(4 suppl S): 265-272.
25. Buller DB, Buller MK, Beach B, Ertl G (1996) Sunny days, healthy ways: evaluation of a skin cancer prevention curriculum for elementary school-aged children. J *Am Acad Dermatol* **35:** 911-922.

26. Buller MK, Loescher LJ, Buller DB (1994) "Sunshine and skin health": a curriculum for skin cancer prevention education. J *Cancer Educ* **9**: 155-162.

27. Hughes BR, Altman DG, Newton JA (1993) Melanoma and skin cancer: evaluation of a health education programme for secondary schools. *Br J Dermatol* **128**: 412-417.

28. Ramstack JL, White SE, Hazelkorn KS, Meyskens FL (1986) Sunshine and skin cancer: a school-based skin cancer prevention project. *J Cancer Educ* **1**: 169-176.

29. Bastuji-Garin S, Grob JJ, Grognard C, Grosjean F (1999) Melanoma prevention: evaluation of a Health Education Campaign for Primary Schools. *Arch Dermatol* **135**: 936-940.

30. Girgis A, Sanson-Fisher RW, Tripodi DA, Golding T(1993) Evaluation of interventions to improve solar protection in primary schools. *Health Educ Qtly* **20**: 275-287.

31. Lowe JB, Balanda KP, Stanton WR, Gillespie AM (1999) Evaluation of a Three -Year School-Based Intervention to Increase Adolescent Sun Protection. *Health Educ Behav* **26**: 396-408.

32. Milne E, English DR, Cross D, Corti B, Costa C, Johnston R (1999) Evaluation of an intervention to reduce sun exposure in children: design and baseline results. *Am J Epidemiol* **150**: 164-173.

33. Milne E, English DR, Johnston R *et al.* (2000) Improved sun protection behaviour in children after two years of the Kidskin intervention. *Aust N Z J Public Health* **24**: 481-487.

34. Schofield MJ, Edwards K, Pearce R (1997) Effectiveness of two strategies for dissemination of sun-protection policy in New South Wales primary and secondary schools. *Aust N Z J Public Health* **21**: 743-750.

35. Mayer JA, Slymen DJ, Eckhardt L *et al.* (1997) Reducing ultraviolet radiation exposure in children. *Prev Med* **26**: 516-522.

36. Mayer JA, Lewis EC, Eckhardt L *et al.* (2001) Promoting sun safety among zoo visitors. *Prev Med* **33**: 162-169.

37. Lombard D, Neubauer TE, Canfield D, Winett RA (1991) Behavioral community intervention to reduce the risk of skin cancer. *J Appl Behav Anal* **24**: 677-686.

38. Glanz K, Lew RA, Song V, Murakami-Akatsuka L (2000) Effects of skin cancer prevention in outdoor recreation settings: the Hawaii SunSmart Program. *Eff Clin Pract* **3**: 1-5.

39. Glanz K, Geller AC, Shigaki D, Isnec MR, Maddock JE (2002) A randomized trial of skin cancer prevention in aquatics settings: The *Pool Cool* program. *Health Psychology*: In press.

40. Segan CJ, Borland R, Hill D (1999) Development and evaluation of a brochure on sun protection and sun exposure for tourists. *Health Educ J* **58**: 177-191.

41. Borland RM, Hocking B, Godking GA, Gibbs AF, Hill DJ (1991) The impact of a skin cancer educational package for outdoor workers. *Med J Aust* **154**: 686-688.

42. Girgis A, Sanson-Fisher RW, Watson A (1994) A workplace intervention for increasing outdoor workers' use of solar protection. *Am J Public Health* **84**: 77-81.

43. Azizi E, Flint P, Sadetzki S *et al.* (2000) A graded work site intervention program to improve sun protection and skin cancer awareness in outdoor workers in Israel. *Cancer Causes Control* **11**: 513-521.

44. Shani E, Rachkovsky E, Bahar-Fuchs A, Rosenberg L (2001) The role of health education versus safety regulations in generating skin cancer preventive behavior among outdoor workers in Israel: an exploratory photosurvey. *Health Promot Internation* **15**: 333-339.

45. Bolognia JL, Berwick M, Fine JA, Simpson P, Jasmin M (1991) Sun protection in newborns. A comparison of educational methods. *Am J Dis Child* **145**: 1125-1129.

46. Geller AC, Sayers L, Koh HK, Miller DR, Steinberg BL, Crosier-Wood M (1999) The New Moms Project: educating mothers about sun protection in newborn nurseries. *Pediatr Dermatol* **16:** 198-200.

47. Gerbert B, Wolff M, Tschann JM *et al.* (1997) Activating patients to practice skin cancer prevention: response to mailed materials from physicians versus HMOs. *Am J Prev Med* **13:** 214-220.

48. Robinson JK, Rademaker AW (1995) Skin cancer risk and sun protection learning by helpers of patients with nonmelanoma skin cancer. *Prev Med* **24:** 333-341.

49. Azurdia RM, Pagliaro JA, Rhodes LE (2000) Sunscreen application technique in photosensitivepatients: a quantitative assessment of the effect of education. *Photodermatol Photoimmunol Photomed* **16:** 53-56.

50. Gooderham MJ, Guenther L (1999a) Impact of a sun awareness curriculum on medical students' knowledge, attitudes, and behavior. *J Cutan Med Surg* **3:** 182-187.

51. McCormick LK, Masse L, Cummings SS, Burke C (1999) Evaluation of skin cancer prevention module for nurses: Change in knowledge, self-efficacy, and attitudes. *Am J Health Promot* **13:** 282-289.

52. Harris JM, Salasche SJ, Harris RB (2001) Can Internet-based continuing medical education improve physicians' skin cancer knowledge and skills? *J Gen Intern Med* **16:** 50-56.

53. Dolan NC, Ng JS, Martin GJ, Robinson JK, Rademaker AW (1997) Effectiveness of a skin cancer control educational intervention for internal medicine housestaff and attending physicians. *J Gen Intern Med* **12:** 531-536.

54. Dietrich AJ, Olson AL, Sox CH, Winchell CW, Grant-Petersson J, Collison DW (2000b) Sun protection counseling for children: primary care practice patterns and effect of an intervention on clinicians. *Arch Fam Med* **9:** 155-159.

55. Mikkilineni R, Weinstock MA, Goldstein MG, Dube CE, Rossi JS (2001) The impact of the basic skin cancer triage curriculum on provider's skin cancer control practices. *J Gen Intern Med* **16:** 302-307.

56. Leinweber CE, Campbell HS, Trottier DL (1995) Is a health promotion campaign successful in retail pharmacies? *Can J Pub Health* **86:** 380-383.

57. Mayer JA, Slymen DJ, Eckhardt L, Rosenberg C, Stepanski BM, Creech L *et al.* (1998a) Skin cancer prevention counseling by pharmacists: specific outcomes of an intervention trial. *Cancer Detect Prev* **22:** 367-375.

58. Mayer JA, Eckhardt L, Stepanski BM, Sallis JF, Elder JP, Slymen DJ *et al.* (1998b) Promoting skin cancer prevention counseling by pharmacists. *Am J Public Health* **88:** 1096-1099.

59. King PH, Murfin GD, Yanagisako KL, Wagstaff DA, Putnam GL, Hajas FL *et al.* (1982) Skin cancer/melanoma knowledge and behavior in Hawaii: changes during a community-based cancer control program. *Prog Clin Biol Res* **130:** 135-144.

60. Putnam GL, Yanagisako KL (1985) Skin cancer comic book: evaluation of a public educational vehicle. *J Audiov Media Med* **8:** 22-25.

61. McGee R, Williams S (1992) Adolescence and sun protection. *NZ Med J* **105:** 401-403.

62. Boutwell WB (1995) The Under Cover Skin Cancer Prevention Project. A community-based program in four Texas cities. *Cancer* **75:** 657-660.

63. Geller AC, Hufford D, Miller DR, Sun T, Wyatt SW, Reilley B *et al.* (1997) Evaluation of the Ultraviolet Index: media reactions and public response. *J Am Acad Dermatol* **37:** 935-941.

64. MMWR (1997) Media dissemination of and public response to the Ultraviolet Index-- United States, 1994-1995. *Morbidity & Mortality Weekly Report* **46:** 370-373.

65. Bulliard JL, Reeder A (2001) Getting the message across: Sun protection information in media weather reports in New Zealand. *N Z Med J* **114:** 67-70.
66. Theobald T, Marks R, Hill D, Dorevitch A (1991) "Goodbye Sunshine": Effects of a television program about melanoma on beliefs, behavior, and melanoma thickness. *J Am Acad Dermatol* **25:** 7171-723.
67. Kiekbusch S, Hannich HJ, Isacsson A, Johannisson A, Lindholm LH, Sager E *et al.* (2000) Impact of a cancer education multimedia device on public knowledge, attitudes, and behaviors: a controlled intervention study in Southern Sweden. *J Cancer Educ* **15:** 232-236.
68. Geller A, Glanz K, Shigaki D, Isnec MR, Sun T, Maddock J (2001) Impact of skin cancer prevention on outdoor aquatics staff: The *Pool Cool* program in Hawaii and Massachusetts. *Prev Med* **33:** 155-161.
69. Boldeman C, Jansson B, Holm LE (1991) Primary prevention of malignant melanoma in a Swedish urban preschool sector. *Cancer Educ* **6:** 247-253.
70. Rodrigue JR (1996) Promoting healthier behaviors, attitudes, and beliefs toward sun exposure in parents of young children. *J Consult Clin Psychol* **64:** 1431-1436.
71. Novick M (1997) To burn or not to burn: use of computer-enhanced stimuli to encourage application of sunscreens. *Cutis* **60:** 105-108.
72. Parrott R, Duggan A, Cremo J, Eckles A, Jones K, Steiner C (1999) Communicating about youth's sun exposure risk to soccer coaches and parents: a pilot study in Georgia. *Health Educ Behav* **26:** 385-95.
73. Dobbinson S, Borland R, Anderson M (1999) Sponsorship and sun protection practices in lifesavers. *Health Promot Internation* **14:** 167-175.
74. Dietrich AJ, Olson AL, Sox CH, Tosteson TD, Grant-Petersson J (2000a) Persistent Increase in Children's Sun Protection in a Randomized Controlled Community Trial. *Prev Med* **31:** 569-574.
75. Miller DR, Geller AC, Wood MC, Lew RA, Koh HK (1999) the Falmouth safe skin project: evaluation of a community program to promote sun protection in youth. *Health Educ Behav* **26:** 369-384.
76. Hill D, White V, Marks R, Borland R (1993) Changes in sun-related attitudes and behaviours, and reduced sunburn prevalence in a population at high risk of melanoma. *Eur J Cancer Prev* **2:** 447-456.
77. Anti-Cancer Council of Victoria (1999) *SunSmart Evaluation Studies, No. 6.* Melbourne Victoria: Anti-Cancer Council of Victoria.
78. Carter R, Marks R, Hill D (1999) Could a national skin cancer primary prevention campaign in Australia be worthwhile?: an economic perspective. *Health Promot Internation* **14:** 73-82.
79. Buller DB, Borland R, Burgoon M(1998) Impact of behavioral intention on effectiveness of message features: Evidence from the family sun safety project. *Hum Communication Res* **24:** 433-453.
80. Buller DB, Burgoon M, Hall JR, Levine N, Taylor AM, Beach BH *et al.* (2000) Using language intensity to increase the success of a family intervention to protect children from ultraviolet radiation: predictions from language expectancy theory. *Prev Med* **30:** 103-113.
81. Prentice-Dunn S, Jones JL, Floyd DL (1997) Persuasive appeals and the reduction of skin cancer risk: The roles of appearance concern, perceived benefits of a tan, and efficacy information. *J Appl Soc Psychol* **27:** 1041-1047.
82. Block LG, Keller PA (1995) When to accentuate the negative: The effects of perceived efficacy and message framing on intentions to perform a health-related behavior. *J Marketing Res* **32:** 192-203.

83. Rothman AJ, Salovey P, Antone C, Keough K, Martin CD (1993) The influence of message framing on intentions to perform health behaviors. *J Exp Soc Psychol* **29:** 408-433.

84. Detweiler JB, Bedell BT, Salovey P, Pronin E, Rothman AJ (1999) Message framing and sunscreen use: Gain-framed messages motivate beach-goers. *Health Psychol* **18:** 189-196.

85. Richard MA, Martin S, Gouvernet J, Folchetti G, Bonerandi JJ, Grob JJ (1999) Humour and alarmism in melanoma prevention: a randomized controlled study of 3 types of information leaflet. *Br J Dermatol* **140:** 909-914.

86. Stephenson MT, Witte K (1998) Fear, threat, and perceptions of efficacy from frightening skin cancer messages. *Public Health Rev* **26:** 147-174.

87. Crane LA, Schneider LS, Yohn JJ, Morelli JG, Plomer KD (1999b) "Block the Sun, Not the Fun": Evaluation of a Skin Cancer Prevention Program for Child Care Centers. *Am J Prev Med* **17:** 31-37.

88. Prochaska, JO, DiClemente, CC, Norcross, JC (1992) In search of how people change: Applications to the addictive behaviors. *Am Psychol* **47:** 1102-1114.

89. Rogers EM (1995) *Diffusion of innovations.* 4th Edition. New York: The Free Press.

90. Glanz K, Carbone E, Song V (1999) Formative research for developing targeted skin cancer prevention programs for children in multiethnic Hawaii. *Health Educ Res* **14:** 155-166.

91. Rimer BK, Glanz K, Rasband G (2001) Searching for evidence about health behavior and health education interventions. *Health Educ Behav* **28:** 231-248.

92. Grant-Petersson J, Dietrich AJ, Sox CH, Winchell CW, Stevens MM (1999) Promoting sun protection in elementary schools and child care settings: the SunSafe Project. *J School Health* **69:** 100-106.

93. Glanz K, Silverio R, Farmer A (1996) Diary reveals sun protective practices. *Skin Ca Fdn J* **14:** 27-28.

94. Creech LL, Mayer JA (1998) Ultraviolet radiation exposure in children: a review of measurement strategies. *Annals Behav Med* **19:** 399-407.

95. Eckhardt L, Mayer JA, Creech L, Johnston MR, Lui KJ, Sallis JF, Elder JP (1996) Assessing children's ultraviolet radiation exposure: the potential usefulness of a colorimeter. *Am J Public Health* **86:** 1802-1804.

96. Diffey BL, Gibson CJ, Haylock R, McKinlay AF (1996) Outdoor ultraviolet exposure of children and adolescents. *Br J Dermatol* **134:** 1030-1034.

97. Glanz K, Lewis FM, Rimer BK (Eds.) (1997) *Health Behavior and Health Education: Theory, Research and Practice (2nd Edition).* San Francisco: Jossey-Bass Inc.

98. Loescher LJ, Emerson J, Taylor A, Christensen DH, McKinney M (1995) Educating preschoolers about Sun Safety. *Am J Public Health* **85:** 939-943.

99. Weinstock MA, Rossi JS, Redding CA, Maddock JE, Cottrill SD (2000) Sun protection behaviors and stages of change for the primary prevention of skin cancers among beachgoers in southeastern New England. *Annals Behav Med* **22:** 286-293.

100. Glanz K, Maddock JE, Lew RA, Murakami-Akatsuka L (2001) A randomized trial of the Hawaii SunSmart program's impact on outdoor recreation staff. *J Am Acad Dermatol* **44:** 973-978.

101. Tripp MK, Herrmann NB, Parcel GS, Chamberlain RM, Gritz ER (2000) Sun Protection is Fun! A skin cancer prevention program for preschools. *J School Health* **70:** 395-401.

102. Crane LA, Ehrsam G, Mokrohisky S *et al.* (1999a) Skin cancer prevention in a pediatric population: The Kaiser Kids Sun Care program. *Health Educ Behav* **26:** 302-303.

103. Wolf S, Swanson LA, Manning R (1999) Projects SPF (Sun Safety, Protection, and Fun): Arizona Department of Health Services Early Childhood Skin Cancer Prevention Education Program. *Health Educ Behav* **26:** 301-302.

104. Glanz K, Chang L, Song V, Silverio R, Muneoka L (1998) Skin cancer prevention for children, parents, and caregivers: a field test of Hawaii's SunSmart program. *J Am Acad Dermatol* **38:** 413-417.

105. Mayer JA, Eckhardt L, Lewis EC (1999) Sunwise Stampede – A sun safety program for zoo visitors. *Health Educ Behav* **26:** 304-305.

106. Friedman LC, Webb JA, Bruce S, Weinberg AD, Cooper HP (1995) Skin cancer prevention and early detection intentions and behavior. *Am J Prev Med* **11:** 59-65.

107. Gelb BD, Boutwell WB, Cummings S (1994) Using Mass Media Communication for Health Promotion: Results from a Cancer Center Effort. *Hosp Health Serv Adm* **39(3):** 283-293.

108. Hanrahan PF, Hersey P, Watson AB, Callaghan TM (1995) The effect of an educational brochure on knowledge and early detection of melanoma. *Aust J Public Health* **19:** 270-274.

Chapter 15

Skin cancer prevention: an economic perspective

Rob Carter, Grad.Dip.Pop.Health, B.A.(Hons), M.A.S., Ph.D.
Centre for Health Program Evaluation, Melbourne, Victoria, Australia

Key words: cost-effectiveness, economic efficiency, cost of illness (COI),
burden of disease (BOD)

INTRODUCTION

The purpose of this chapter is to explore the economics of skin cancer, particularly the economics of skin cancer prevention. The chapter starts with a discussion of the contribution that the discipline of economics can offer to an understanding of skin cancer, explaining the separate but related tasks of description, prediction and evaluation. The discussion covers the important distinction between "positive" and "normative" economics and its significance for policy prescriptions about what constitutes "value" and the rationale for government intervention. Using these concepts of description, prediction and evaluation, the chapter then explores what is known about the economics of skin cancer and skin cancer prevention, using the situation in Australia as a case study. Readers already familiar with economic theory may choose to skip to Section 2 of this chapter for its particular applications to skin cancer prevention.

D. Hill et al. (eds.), Prevention of Skin Cancer, 295-317.
© 2004 *Kluwer Academic Publishers. Printed in the Netherlands.*

1.   ECONOMICS DISCIPLINE AND UNDERSTANDING SKIN CANCER

1.1   How can the economics discipline contribute?

The starting point for understanding the contribution that health economics can offer, is to appreciate that the discipline carries out three separate but related tasks, viz: "description," "prediction," and "evaluation."

With "description," the task is to measure and report on current activities, health status, resource use, behavior, or system effects. There is naturally a heavy emphasis on empirical data collection and analysis. While economics brings its own techniques to empirical studies, it is often heavily dependent on other disciplines for data input and analysis. Those disciplines include, for example, epidemiology for disease incidence/prevalence data; demography for population trends; clinical medicine for treatment pathways; biostatistics for data analysis; and accounting for cost records. Importantly, description often involves the construction of particular concepts and this process of construction may involve particular assumptions or definitions. In estimating the cost of illness (COI), for example, assumptions are required concerning the elements of illness that represent a "cost." All COI studies will estimate the cost of disease management and care, while many will try to estimate lost production due to illness in the broader economy and some will also try to impute a cost to pain and suffering. COI studies, along with epidemiological assessments of incidence/prevalence and disease burden provide different pictures of the impact of disease on society.

With "prediction", the task is to estimate future trends in health status, resource use, risk factors, or system effects. As the research question moves from describing the status quo, to predicting future trends, it becomes increasingly important for assumptions to be clearly specified. Those arguing for the importance of particular diseases, for example, will quite often use disease models based on current practice to predict future "needs." Sometimes this is done without clearly specifying that their predictions are based on assumptions that current practice is acceptable (i.e., efficacious, efficient, affordable, etc.) or that technology and/or societal expectations will not change. Further, the task of prediction requires that the concept of evidence be supported by measures of uncertainty associated with the predictions.

While the tasks of description and prediction have their contentious aspects, it is the third task of "evaluation" – with its central role of judging "value" – that is the most debated and often the most misunderstood contribution of economics. Evaluation in economics has distinctive characteristics that separate it from evaluation as practiced by other disciplines. Evaluation in economics involves both a comparison of alternatives (one of which is often the status quo and the other an option for change) and importantly, has regard to both their costs and benefits. A prime task in economic evaluation is to address the question: "What difference will the proposed intervention make compared to current practice?" Evaluation often involves both description (e.g., describing current practice and the current health burden) and prediction (e.g., estimating cost and benefit streams through time), but importantly, involves a judgment (implied or explicit) about the "appropriate" use of resources. The issue of appropriateness is guided by decision rules that relate incremental benefit achieved by the proposed intervention to its incremental cost. These decision rules in turn raise an important issue about how "benefit" is defined – is it just health gain or are there broader dimensions involving acceptability, equity and social justice? The task of economic evaluation is thus intimately linked to the contribution economics can make to health service planning and priority setting.

The discipline distinguishes between "positive economics" and "normative economics", with the former covering "what is", and the latter "what ought to be." Positive economics is meant to be as value free as possible and is dominated by the task of description. There is an unavoidable normative judgment that data is worthwhile collecting and that particular definitions are appropriate. Beyond this, positive economics strives to be value free. Normative economics on the other hand is quite consciously based on value judgments that underlie suggested change. The failure of some economists to make these values transparent can lead to confusion as to whether pronouncements for change are based upon economic theory, empirical work, or ideology. Nowhere is this confusion more apparent than in debates about whether governments ought to intervene in the market; and if so, how. Clarity about ethical values goes to the heart of what is meant by the term "economic evidence" and what is meant by the term "efficient."

1.2   What is meant by the term "efficiency" in economics?

Economics generally distinguishes three concepts of efficiency. The first two address the supply side and are sometimes rolled into one in introductory textbooks. "Technical efficiency" is achieved when production is organized so that maximum output is produced with the resource inputs available (i.e., land, labor, capital and enterprise). It is an engineering-based notion of efficiency that depends on the physical production function. "Productive efficiency" (sometimes called "cost-effectiveness efficiency") is achieved when production is organized to minimize the cost of producing a given output. It thus takes into account both the production function and prevailing factor input prices (i.e., rent, wages, interest and profit). The third and arguably the most important concept of efficiency, particularly for strategic planning and priority setting, is "allocative efficiency." Allocative efficiency incorporates the demand side and is achieved when resources are allocated so as to produce the "optimal" level of each output in line with the "value" consumers place on them.

It is important to appreciate three aspects of these efficiency concepts. First, that efficiency is a purely instrumental concept – it has meaning only if an explicit objective has been articulated against which efficiency can be assessed. Second, there exists a hierarchical relationship between these concepts – technical efficiency is required to achieve productive efficiency and productive efficiency is in turn required to achieve allocative efficiency. Third, and arguably the most important, there exist alternative ways to define "optimal" and to define "value" within the key concept of allocative efficiency. The assessment of these alternative ways to define and measure allocative efficiency is at the heart of a paradigm clash that has emerged in the normative economics of health, a clash between the orthodox tradition of what is termed "welfare economics" and newer theoretical frameworks that might be termed "non-welfarism." It is worth the effort to understand the essence of this debate, for the matters discussed underlie the difference between pronouncements from economic rationalists (who advocate market-based solutions) and many health economists (but not all) who see a far greater role for government in the health sector.

The orthodox "welfare economics" framework rests squarely on notions of individual utility or preference as the foundation of analysis. This tradition is very much in accord with political values that hold individual autonomy to be paramount. Social welfare (an increase in which is at the heart of economics) is a function only of individual welfare (or utility) and judgments about the superiority of one policy option over another are made by reference to the sum of these individual utilities. Moreover, the individual utilities are essentially a function of goods and services consumed (there are caveats made to this generalization in the literature, but the focus on goods and services remains). It is assumed that individuals are the best judges of their own welfare (the "consumer sovereignty" assumption) – a view that with a few added conditions gives substance to the neoclassical faith in free markets.

"Non-welfarism" refers to frameworks for normative economic analysis that reject the exclusive focus of welfare economics on the utilities of individuals. This approach relaxes this assumption to enable other aspects of policy change to be included in the assessment of efficiency. Since in the welfarist approach the focus of social welfare is utility received from the consumption of goods and services, an important theme of non-welfarism are characteristics that may have value in and of themselves, and not simply as a means of obtaining utility. The appropriate characteristics involved are subject to debate and ongoing research, but obvious candidates include individual health status, together with notions of equity and social justice.

The most important non-welfarist strand from a historical perspective was undoubtedly the notion of "merit goods." Musgrave [1] raised this term in his *Theory of Public Finance* in 1959, describing them as goods whose consumption is considered so meritorious (by government) that they are made available on terms that are more generous than in the market place. The concept of merit goods was a watershed because it plainly involved the possibility of governments overruling the judgments of individuals about what was of value to them. It raised the fundamental issues of what arguments should be included in the social welfare function and what weight should be attached to each argument. The health sector has been particularly responsive to these non-welfarist ideas; in part because of features of health care that raise doubts about the appropriateness of the free market approach; and in part because the role of health care in the health production function provides greater scope for third-party judgment than for many other goods [2].

1.3   Role of the free market approach in the health sector?

In orthodox welfare economics the free market is relied upon to answer the three fundamental economic questions that all societies must answer – i.e. what should be produced? ("allocative efficiency"), how should it be produced? ("technical" & "production efficiency"), and who should receive it? ("distributive equity"). Economists often argue, therefore, that if there is no impediment to the free operation of markets, the market mechanism will ensure that resources are allocated to minimize cost and maximize community welfare. In recent years, for example, there has been a surge of interest in reforming the organization and delivery of health care systems by replacing government regulation with a greater reliance on market forces.

This has led several health economists [3-7], particularly Thomas Rice, to provide authoritative reviews of the traditional market model, its underlying assumptions and applicability to health. These authors argue that because the free market cannot be relied upon to allocate health care resources efficiently, there is an efficiency rationale for governments to intervene in the funding and provision of health care. They have challenged in particular the implicit assumption behind the resurgence of interest in market competition that "economic theory" demonstrates that competition in health care will lead to superior social outcomes. They argue persuasively that the belief in the superiority of market-based systems stems from a misunderstanding of economic theory as it applies to health. Rice summarizes the position thus:

> "As will be shown, such conclusions are based on a large set of assumptions that are not met, and cannot be met in the health sector. This is not to say that competitive approaches in this sector of the economy are inappropriate; rather, their efficacy depends on the particular circumstances of the policy being considered and the environment in which it is to be implemented. There is, however, no a priori reason to believe that such a system will operate more efficiently, or provide a higher level of social welfare, than alternative systems that are based instead on government financing and regulation. This argument is further bolstered by the fact that so many other developed countries have chosen to deviate from market-based health systems." [7, p.3]

It is important to acknowledge, however, that in responding to market failure, governments often create impediments to the free operation of markets (such as licensing requirements that impact on freedom of entry and/or funding arrangements that distort choice). The possibility of "government failure" clearly exists as the mirror image of market failure. It is quite possible that government intervention may further aggravate rather than ameliorate problems associated with market failure and/or that governments may carry out their priority setting tasks inefficiently. Thus, while the presence of market failure is a necessary pre-condition to justify government intervention on an efficiency rationale, it is not a sufficient condition unless any government failure involved is less distorting than the market failure it is trying to address. In this context it is opportune that economists and policy-makers in a number of countries are addressing the issue of priority setting with renewed interest.

It also important to recognize that while "market failure" may provide an efficiency rationale for government intervention in the health sector, it is by and large not the main reason why governments become involved. Rather than pursuing efficiency, most governments intervene for reasons associated with equity and social justice. Market-based systems ration access to health care on the basis of ability-to-pay and/or people's ability to acquire health insurance. Under this system individuals are required to set and fund their own priorities. Societies generally choose not to use this system of allocation for health care – among various reasons, chief is the widespread concern that citizens have access to health care in accordance with their needs, not in accordance with their ability-to-pay. Thus, in all developed countries a form of health care insurance is made available, and in most countries there is also government intervention, albeit to varying extents, to regulate the production and distribution of health care. Having intervened initially for largely equity-based reasons, most governments would still seek to avoid and/or minimize the possibility of government failure.

2.   DESCRIPTION: WHAT IS THE SIZE OF THE SKIN CANCER PROBLEM AND HOW MUCH IS SPENT ON IT?

2.1   Overview

Governments, health authorities, research departments and a range of other bodies often seek reliable information on the burden of disease (BOD), both in terms of health status and its resource implications. The uses to which such descriptive information on the BOD can be put vary widely. BOD information is often utilized, for example, in developing measures of public health significance and/or monitoring trends through time. It can be employed to examine the performance of the health care system and its various components, in planning health service provision, in measuring the potential for health status gains and/or cost offsets and as an input into economic evaluation and priority setting.

Over and above its mortality and morbidity impacts, disease has important second-order effects on income and production patterns throughout the economy, as well as on resource utilization within the health care system. Cost-of-illness (COI) or disease costing studies are one type of BOD study that describe the relationship between current disease incidence and/or prevalence and the consequent resource implications, particularly for the structure and utilization of health services. It is important to recognize that they are descriptive studies (i.e., describing the status quo), not evaluation studies that compare the status quo with options for change. Nonetheless, being able to examine how health resources are currently funded and allocated among different users, different health services and different diseases can be useful in considering a variety of equity, access and utilization issues. Of particular interest to those in the health promotion field, for example, is the use of limited resources in the diagnosis, treatment and management of preventable illness. Planners may wish to have this information to identify what potential changes in service utilization may follow the achievement of population goals and targets, or to develop broad order estimates of the potential health care offsets to the cost of prevention activities.

Economists make a distinction in COI studies between the "direct costs" of providing health care services, "indirect costs", and "intangibles" (such as pain and suffering). Direct costs (such as hospitals, medical and allied health services, pharmaceuticals, etc.) are the least contentious, but there is an important issue related to study perspective. Studies are often dominated by the perspective of third-party funders, and while including some cost impacts on patients (such as insurance co-payments), other cost impacts on patients will be ignored (such as the value of carer time; travel and waiting time; home modifications, etc.). Intangibles are not often costed in COI studies and (arguably) are best measured through health status indicators such as the quality adjusted life year (QALY) or disability adjusted life year (DALY). Apart from measurement difficulties in placing dollar values on pain and suffering, there is also a danger in studies that focus only on costs, to lose sight of the central role of community welfare in economic thinking.

Indirect costs focus on lost production in the economy attributable to illness and premature death, but may also include costs impacting outside the health care sector (such as police and court costs for drug abuse; vehicle damage for alcohol abuse; etc.). The estimation of production effects has been a contentious issue in the COI literature. In part this reflects the variety of measurement techniques available, in part it reflects the difficult ethical and equity issues involved, and in part it reflects the fact that when measurement is attempted, the resulting estimates often swamp direct costs. While the direct costs of disease have a clear meaning and usefulness, they do not provide a comprehensive "costing" of the impact of disease in the absence of the more contentious indirect costs and intangibles.

2.2   Case study: BOD/COI of skin cancer in Australia

The Australian Institute of Health and Welfare (AIHW) commenced a research program in 1992 to provide COI estimates for key diseases in the ICD-9 framework [8]. Titled the "The Disease Costs and Impact Study (DCIS)", the research has produced a number of reports (including *Health System Costs of Cancer in Australia 1993-94* [9]) that have proved to be of considerable interest to policy makers, evaluators and industry. Table 15.1 sets out direct cost and utilization estimates available for skin cancer in Australia (for the reference year 1994) that have been utilized for the various purposes described above. Estimates for indirect costs and intangibles are not included in the cost estimates available from the AIHW.

Table 15.1 Burden of disease (BOD) data for skin cancer[1] in Australia.

Data item	Number per annum	Cost per annum (Aust $m)
Mortality for Australia, 1996 (malignant neoplasms)		
Deaths	1,376	
Melanoma	978	
NMSC	398	
Deaths as a % of deaths due to cancer, 1996 (34,526)	4.0%	
Deaths as a % of all deaths, 1996 (128,711)	1.0%	
Years of Life Lost (YLL)	16,672	
Melanoma	13,114	
NMSC	3,558	
YLL as a % of YLL due to cancer, 1996 (399,863)	4.2%	
YLL as a % of all YLL, 1996 (1,348,233)	1.2%	
Years Lived With Disability, Australia 1996 (YLD)	7,898	
Melanoma	6,896	
NMSC	1,002	
YLD as a % of YLD due to cancer, 1996 (78,716)	10.0%	
YLD as a % of all YLD, 1996 (1,162,041)	0.7%	
Disability Adjusted Life Years (DALY)	24,570	
Melanoma	20,010	
NMSC	4,560	
DALY as % of DALY due to cancer, 1996 (478,579)	5.1%	
DALY as a % of all DALY, 1996 (2,510,274)	1.0%	
Incidence cases, 1996	290,622	
Melanoma	7,797	
NMSC	282,825	
Utilisation & direct costs, 1994 (malignant neoplasms)		
Hospital admissions	54,700	100.3
Hospital bed days	118,100	
Non inpatient occasions of service	225,500	14.9
Medical consultations	1,892,200	63.7
GPs	834,700	28.3
Specialists	1,057,500	35.4
Prescriptions written	65,200	3.3
Referrals to Allied Health Professionals	130,600	2.3
Nursing home residents	161	5.9
Other		9.0
Total direct cost, 1994 (malignant neoplasms only)		**199.4**
Melanoma		16.7
NMSC		182.7
Costs as a % of cancer costs (malignant only) ($1,310m)		15.2%
Total direct costs, 1994 (all neoplasms)		**297.9**
Melanoma		65.6
NMSC		232.3
Costs as % of costs of all neoplasms ($1,904m)		15.6%
Costs as a % total direct health system costs ($31,397m)		0.95%

[1] Skin cancer is defined as either "all neoplasms" or "malignant neoplasms." "All neoplasms" is defined to include malignant neoplasms, benign neoplasms, in-situ neoplasms and neoplasms of uncertain behaviour. Malignant neoplasms include "melanoma" (ICD9: 172) and NMSC (ICD9: 173).

Sources:

1. The cancer incidence cases, YLL, YLD and DALY are for 1996 and are based on (Mathers *et al.*, 1999) [10].
2. The health service utilisation and cost data are for 1994 and are based on the AIHW DCIS publication for cancer (Mathers, 1998b) [9].

Also shown in Table 15.1 are DALY estimates taken from the Australian BOD study [10]. DALYs are calculated for a disease or health condition as the sum of years of life lost due to premature mortality (YLL) and the equivalent "healthy" years lost due to disability (YLD) for incident cases of the condition. The DALY, like the QALY, is an outcome measure that combines both the morbidity and mortality effects of disease into a single measure. The DALY was developed for the Global Burden of Disease Study (GBD) [11], undertaken in the first half of the 1990s by researchers at the Harvard School of Public Health and the World Health Organization (WHO). The GBD has generated considerable interest among health policy makers and researchers and an increasing number of national BOD studies are now underway.

The use of BOD/COI data to establish public health significance is illustrated in Table 15.1 by those data entries that show the mortality, morbidity and cost estimates associated with skin cancer as a percentage of all cancers and as a percentage of all disease. Recognition of the public health significance of skin cancer in Australia has led to its listing as one of seven priority cancers (along with lung cancer, cervical cancer, breast cancer, colorectal cancer, prostate cancer and non-Hodgkin's lymphoma). While NMSC is the most common cancer diagnosed, affecting a large number of individuals, the burden of disease is less than one quarter that due to melanoma. Australia has rates for these tumors at least three times those in other countries that consider that they have a public health problem with skin cancer [12-13].

The DALY and cost data have also been utilized to develop broad order estimates of the potential health benefit and cost offsets of introducing a national skin cancer prevention program in Australia [14]. This work suggested that the introduction of a national SunSmart program would yield a reduction in the disease burden by approximately 10,000 DALYs over a 10-year period (Melanoma: 8,135 DALYs; NMSC: 1,830 DALYs) while achieving cost offsets that resulted in net savings of approximately $A40 million. [Both cost and DALY estimates were discounted at 3% per annum to present value.] Further detail on this application is provided in Section 3.

2.3   Use and interpretation of descriptive data on direct costs of disease

While such direct cost estimates can certainly be useful to planners and researchers for the variety of purposes mentioned above, it is important that they are not over-interpreted. Disease costing analysis, like any analytical tool, can be misused and it is important that their uses and limitations be understood. From an economic perspective, the most important points to note are:

- Existing expenditure on a disease, no matter how large, is not sufficient in itself to justify further expenditure (i.e., description is not evaluation, but may input into evaluation). In other words, it is not so much the size of the disease burden per se that should guide resource allocation, but rather the efficiency of specific interventions designed to reduce the disease burden.

- Care should be taken in interpreting direct costs associated with disease treatment as an estimate of financial savings that would result from prevention of disease. Such "cost offsets" are not estimates of immediately realizable savings, but rather "opportunity cost" estimates measuring resources devoted to the treatment of preventable disease that could be available for other purposes. Conversion of opportunity cost savings into financial savings involves a number of practical issues (such as workforce restructuring, professional interests, management policies, public reaction, etc.) as well as theoretical issues (such as the mix between "fixed" and "variable" costs and "lumpiness" in the expansion/contraction of capital equipment and assets).

- Underlying COI studies are several conceptual and methodological issues that impact on the estimates produced. Examples include the study perspective mentioned above, which has an important impact on inclusion/exclusion criteria for cost categories. Data sources are also important, particularly whether a "top-down" approach (using broad aggregate data sets that are apportioned to individual diseases using various attribution formulae) or a "bottom-up" approach (care pathways based on patient level data) is being used. Similarly, it is important to appreciate whether a "prevalence-based" or "incidence-based" approach to costing is being employed. Prevalence-based costs measure the value of resources used in a specified period (usually one year) for *all existing cases* of the disease (regardless of the time of onset). Incidence-based costs measure the *lifetime costs* of *new cases* occurring in the specified period. The preferred approach depends on the purpose of the study and data availability. If the results are to be used for cost control or financial planning, then prevalence-based costs are preferable. If the estimates are to input into evaluation of prevention measures (as a description of current practice) then the incidence-based approach is preferable (as only new cases can be prevented).

Used sensibly and carefully, disease cost estimates (and burden of disease information in general) can have a role that goes beyond simple description and monitoring. Such information can also be a useful input into evaluation and the priority setting process. Carter [15] has argued, for example, that priorities for illness prevention and health promotion should be guided by information that includes the public health significance of health problems; their preventability (efficacy/effectiveness); and the relative cost-effectiveness (efficiency) of specific measures aimed at achieving the potential reductions in the disease burden.

3.   PREDICTION: WHAT FUTURE TRENDS ARE LIKELY IN REGARD TO SKIN CANCER?

With prediction, the task is to estimate future trends in risk factors, disease incidence/prevalence, health status, and resource use. In this chapter prediction will be illustrated within an evaluation context to help ascertain whether the introduction of a national skin cancer prevention program is likely to represent value-for-money. Readers interested in other aspects of prediction associated with skin cancer are encouraged to visit other chapters of the book.

4.   EVALUATION: ASSESSING EFFICIENCY IN SKIN CANCER PREVENTION

A number of skin cancer prevention programs have been developed and delivered in various countries throughout the world [16-21]. Behavioral evaluations and/or economic evaluations of comprehensive primary prevention programs are rare, but some have been published [22-23]. The case study [14] overviewed here should therefore be of international interest, particularly since it was part of a broader priority setting exercise in cancer control that trialed an innovative approach involving macro evaluation across multiple interventions.

The SunSmart campaign on which the proposed national program is modeled has been running in the State of Victoria, Australia, since 1987. It is the most comprehensive population-based primary prevention program for skin cancer reported in any country in the world. It comprises three elements: (i) a comprehensive education strategy including mass media, teaching resources and a sunlight protection policy and practice code; (ii) structural changes including guidelines for workers' sun protection and downward pressure on the price of sunscreens; and (iii) a variety of sponsorships. SunSmart provides a useful model to appraise a national skin cancer health promotion campaign, not only because of its comprehensiveness, but because it was introduced over a base level program that had been running in Victoria for several years (i.e., the "Slip! Slap! Slop!" campaign), with a more modest budget characteristic of current activities in many parts of Australia and overseas. The effectiveness rates that SunSmart achieved, therefore, hold promise of what a coordinated and well-run national strategy could achieve, over and above current levels of activity.

4.1   Calculation of the health benefit

The DALYs associated with melanoma and NMSC (refer Table 15.1) and the change expected with a national prevention program in place were derived by adapting the methods from the Australian BOD study [10]. The DALY benefit is estimated by analysis linking predicted changes in sunburn due to the intervention to corresponding reductions in total lifetime Ultraviolet Radiation (UVR) exposure and hence to anticipated outcomes in terms of reduced incidence of melanoma and NMSC. The lag period before reduced incidence is experienced was set at ten years for both melanoma and NMSC (i.e., the benefits were experienced in 2006 by our reference population), but the impact of variations in the time lag was also explored. There is no human data to allow a precise indication of this lag period and ten years is a judgment reflecting tumor development and dose-response equations.

The calculation of the health benefit involved a number of steps:

- Establish the DALY burden for melanoma and NMSC in 1996 (as per Table 15.1 from the Australian BOD study [10]);
- Estimate the BOD for 2006 for melanoma with and without a SunSmart program operating in 1996 (i.e., using counterfactual scenario analysis [24]); and

- Estimate the health benefit for NMSC using the 1996 ratio of deaths, YLL and DALY due to melanoma compared to NMSC (a simplifying assumption made due to the short timelines available for the study).

4.1.1   Estimating the BOD in 2006 assuming *no* national SunSmart program

The BOD for melanoma in 2006 without the intervention was estimated by using the projected Australian population in 2006 (instead of the 1996 population) in the DALY worksheets, which are available from the authors of the Australian BOD study. The worksheets were also modified to include an increase in the incidence of melanoma equal to its current rate of increase (i.e., 2.2% p.a. in males and 1.7% p.a. in females [25]). The mortality rates were assumed to stay at their present levels (as at 1996). The disability weights assumed in the Australian BOD study were not altered. Under this scenario the disease burden increased from 24,570 DALYs in 1996 to 33,131 DALYs in 2006 (26,936 for melanoma and 6,195 for NMSC).

4.1.2   Estimating the BOD in 2006 *with* a national SunSmart program

The BOD for melanoma in 2006 with a national SunSmart program in place was estimated assuming a fall in melanoma incidence derived from the performance of the SunSmart campaign in Victoria. Extensive and thorough evaluation of this program demonstrated substantial attitudinal and behavioral shifts, including increased hat wearing and sunscreen use [22]. A reduction in the crude proportion of sunburn in the population of Victoria from 11% to 7% was demonstrated, with the adjusted odds ratio being as follows: year 2/year 1: 0.75 (CI 0.57–0.99) and year 3/year 1: 0.59 (CI 0.43–0.81) [22].

Given the demonstrated one-third reduction in the incidence of sunburn, it was assumed that a 20% reduction in UVR exposure was plausible and that this equated with a 30% fall in cancer incidence. The rationale for this assumption is summarized in Table 15.2, which is discussed more fully in an article by Carter and colleagues [23]. The assumed fall in cancer incidence is a critical assumption and implies substantial and sustained reductions in sunburn. It is impossible to say exactly what the real relationship will be, but more conservative assumptions of between 15% and 30% falls were tested in the sensitivity analysis.

Table 15.2 Anticipated benefits from % reduction in lifetime UVR exposure.

NMSC[1]			Melanoma[2]	
% decrease in lifetime UVR	% decrease in incidence rate[3]	Decrease in number of deaths p.a.[4]	% decrease in incidence rate[5]	Decrease in number of deaths p.a.[6]
1	1.8	4	1.8	13
5	8.9	17	8.6	71
10	17.0	34	16.5	136
15	24.4	46	23.7	196
20	31.1	59	30.2	249

[1] Assumes NMSC incidence rate of 1000/100,000/year and baseline level of UVR of 2000 units

[2] Assumes melanoma incidence rate of 30/100,000/year.

[3] The regression equation from which these results are calculated is: (rate) = (a + b [dose]) where "a" = 4.82 and "b" = 9.32×10^{-4}

[4] The mortality data assume there is no change in the present early detection rate; a ratio of basal cell carcinoma/squamous cell carcinoma of 4.1; and a case fatality rate for squamous cell carcinoma of 0.7%.

[5] The regression equation from which these results are calculated is: (rate) = (a + b [dose]); where "a" = 1.0333 and "b" = 9×10^{-4}.

[6] The mortality data assume there is no change in the present early detection rate and that there is a case fatality rate for melanoma of 20%.

Source: Carter *et al.* (1999) [23]

The 30% reduction in melanoma incidence is then modeled in the DALY worksheet to determine the BOD in 2006 after the national SunSmart campaign. This assumes that current disease etiology and prognosis are representative of marginal changes for the time period over which the benefit stream applies. This analysis results in a health benefit of 699 fewer deaths from melanoma, corresponding to 5,757 fewer years of life lost (YLL) and 8,135 fewer DALYs.

The rest of the health benefit from the extension of the SunSmart campaign to a national level is the reduction in the incidence of, and therefore the morbidity/ mortality from, NMSC. This is approximated by maintaining the same ratio of deaths, YLL and DALY due to NMSC to melanoma as shown in Table 15.3. The DALY gains presented in Table 15.3 have been discounted at 3% to express them in present value terms (PV).

Table 15.3 Summary of health benefit experienced in 2006 due to a reduction of melanoma and NMSC lesions attributed to national SunSmart program, 1996.

	YLD[1]	Mortality	YLL[1]	DALYs[1]
Melanoma	2,378	699	5,757	8,135
NMSC	292	280	1,538	1,830
TOTAL	2,670	979	7,295	9,965

[1] Health benefit expressed in present value terms for 1996 (discounting at 3%).

Source: Carter *et al.*, 2000 [14]

4.2   Calculation of the incremental cost

The cost considered in this evaluation was the estimated cost to government of funding a comprehensive national health promotion campaign, coordinating initiatives in education, structural changes and sponsorships, less any savings in health care costs that could be anticipated from a reduction in management costs for skin cancer.

The anticipated costs of a national campaign of approximately $A5 million per annum is based on the Victorian SunSmart average cost of 28 cents per person over the 1988/89 to 1990/91 period, applied to the Australian population of 18 million people in 1996. Adjustment using the health price index [26] to express this cost in 1996 values (our reference year) takes the estimate to $A5.8 million. While simplistic, this per capita costing is based on an actual statewide program provided to 4.5 million people in Victoria that embodied the proposed elements of a coordinated comprehensive program.

The incremental cost of the proposed new national program (i.e., vis-à-vis the status quo) was estimated by deducting an estimate of current expenditure at the State/Territory level. Current average expenditure across Australia in 1995/96 at the State/Territory level was estimated at 14 cents per person or approximately $A2.5 million. This estimate was based on a survey [23] undertaken of State/Territory anti-cancer bodies, yielding an additional cost of approximately $A3.3 million per annum. This costing assumes that existing resources would be subsumed within any nationally coordinated program. The extent to which federal-state coordination would involve additional costs and whether these might be offset by economies of scale is not known. No provision has been included for these offsetting factors in this indicative costing.

4.2.1 Calculation of the health care offset

Estimates of the total direct costs of health care for melanoma and NMSC in 1994 were presented in Table 15.1 and were inflated to 1996 values using the health price index [26]. The difficulty is to determine by how much these health care management costs might change after the introduction of the primary prevention program. The best-case scenario is that the costs change in the same proportion as cancer incidence – a reduction of approximately 30%. The costs for skin cancer developing from exposure in 1996 are not incurred, however, until after the 10-year lag phase. The future cost offsets were thus discounted by 3% per annum to present value (PV) for the reference year (1996), as for the DALY gains. This calculation gave a cost offset (i.e., "opportunity cost" saving) of approximately $A40 million (PV) and yields a net saving to the national program of approximately $A36 million per annum.

It should be noted that this calculation uses the estimate of the current average cost of care to compute future cost offsets. The validity of this assumption will depend on whether cost structures change through time; what percentage of costs is avoidable; and the extent to which average costs are representative of target client/patient groups. As Richardson comments, this assumption is generally not unreasonable and is common practice in economic evaluation [27].

4.3 The cost-effectiveness ratios

Table 15.4 summarizes the estimated health gain, cost and average cost-effectiveness ratios for the proposed national primary prevention campaign compared with the "status quo." The cost-effectiveness ratios are shown with the potential cost offsets included and excluded. Also shown in Table 15.4 are the results when the anticipated costs of complying with SunSmart recommendations that impact on individuals are included.

From the government's perspective the proposed national SunSmart program is highly cost-effective. With cost offsets included, the intervention is "dominant", i.e., it both saves money and reduces the disease burden. Dominant programs naturally have very strong economic credentials for funding. Conversion of opportunity cost savings into financial savings should not be taken for granted, however, as previously discussed. It is for this reason that incremental costs are reported both as gross and net cost estimates in Table 15.4. With the cost offsets excluded, the option still yields highly cost-effective ratios of $A452 per life year and $A331 per DALY. When the costs impacting on individuals are included in the analysis, however, the cost-effectiveness ratios increase to $A21,069 per life year and

$A15,423 per DALY (no offsets) and to $A15,599 per life year and $A11,420 per DALY (with offsets included).

Table 15.4 Incremental benefits, costs ($A) and cost-effectiveness of a proposed national SunSmart program in Australia.

	Program costs ($m)	Cost offsets ($m)	Net cost (savings) ($m)	YLL	DALY	$/YLL (No cost offsets)	$/DALY (No costs offsets)
Program compared with status quo (30% reduction cancer incidence)	3.3	39.9	(36.6)	7,295	9,965	Dominant ($452 per YLL)	Dominant ($331 per DALY)

	National SunSmart program compared with status quo from government perspective	Add costs to individuals[1]
Health benefits		
YLL	7,295	7,295
DALY	9,965	9,965
Costs		
Program costs	$3.3m	$153.7m
Cost offsets	$39.9m	$39.9m
Net costs (savings in brackets)	($36.6m)	$113.8m
CEA results		
$/YLL no offsets	$452	$21,069
$/DALY no offsets	$331	$15,423
$/YLL with offsets	Dominant	$15,599
$/DALY with offsets	Dominant	$11,420

[1] Costing based on consumption of sunscreen equivalent to one tube per year (@ $A10 per tube) for every third person; and the use of hats equivalent to one extra hat every three years ($A10 per hat) for every second person. No estimate was included for clothing on the assumption that use of existing clothing would comply with the SunSmart recommendations. The savings to individuals from reduced co-payments due to lower incidence of cancer was deducted from the additional costs.

Source: Based on Carter *et al.* 2000 [14]

4.3.1   Sensitivity analysis

A probabilistic sensitivity analysis was performed using the @Risk computer software [28] and a conservative approach to estimating the health gain. In the primary analysis reported above, the value with the strongest evidence from the literature for each of the variables was used. In the sensitivity analysis a probability distribution was put around the variables and they were put through 2000 iterations (refer Table 15.5). The results of the sensitivity analysis suggest that some confidence can be placed in the results from the primary analysis – that is, the initiative has strong economic credentials under a plausible range of assumptions.

Table 15.5 Sensitivity analysis.

	Primary analysis		Add costs to individuals	
	Lower 95% CI level	Upper 95% CI level	Lower 95% CI level	Upper 95% CI level
Health benefit[1]				
YLL	3,459	6,677	3,459	6,677
DALY	4,842	9,148	4,842	9,148
Costs[2]				
Program costs ($A million)	2.97	3.63	121.7	184.1
Cost offsets ($A million)	22.5	44.3	22.5	44.3
Net cost (savings) ($A million)	(19.53)	(40.67)	99.2	139.8
CEA results				
$/YLL no offsets	445	1,049	18,227	52,223
$/DALY no offsets	325	750	13,303	38,021
$/YLL including offsets	Dominant	Dominant	14,857	40,416
$/DALY including offsets	Dominant	Dominant	10,845	28,872

[1] In the sensitivity analysis a conservative approach was taken to testing the sensitivity of the health gain. Thus the range set for the YLL and DALY estimates was below the point estimate assumed in the primary analysis. The variables and distribution used in the sensitivity analysis of the health benefit were as follows:

- *Increase in cancer incidence*: primary analysis assumed 2.2% p.a. in males and 1.7% in females. Risk uniform sensitivity distributions were adopted (0, 0.022) for males and (0, 0.017) for females. It was assumed that the increase in incidence might taper off as the cohorts aged.
- *Survival rates*: primary analysis assumed no change. Risk uniform sensitivity distributions were assumed (-0.01, 0.02). It was assumed survival rates might improve.
- *Dissemination ratio*: primary analysis assumed no change. Risk uniform sensitivity distributions were assumed (-0.01, 0.02). Assumed no dissemination group is more likely to increase.
- *Lag time*: primary analysis 10 years. Risk uniform sensitivity distribution assumed (5,15). Variation between 5 and 15 years based on expert judgement.
- *Reduction in incidence of skin cancer due to intervention*: primary analysis assumed 30%. Risk triangulation sensitivity distribution assumed (0.151, 0.302, 0.302). Only reductions in health gain were considered, down to 15% incidence reduction.

[2] The costs of the intervention were varied by taking the net cost of $A3.3 million and varying it by plus and minus 10%. The possible costs impacting on individuals were also modeled as shown in Table 15.4. The variations in the cost offsets mirrored the health benefit assumptions shown under 1.

Source: Based on Carter *et al.* (2000) [14]

CONCLUSIONS

The discipline of economics can contribute to an understanding of skin cancer, and perhaps more importantly, to an understanding of skin cancer prevention. This contribution can take various forms:

- Through *describing* the current disease burden (BOD) and the associated resource utilization implications (COI);
- Through *predicting* the changes in the BOD/COI through time, both with and without public health interventions; and
- Through *evaluating* the efficiency of different interventions designed to reduce the disease burden.

It is important to appreciate that the economic concept of "efficiency" is a purely instrumental concept – that is, it has meaning only if an explicit objective(s) has been articulated against which efficiency can be assessed. Thus there exist within economic theory alternative ways to define "value" in the key notion of "value-for-money" (or allocative efficiency). Value can be defined in terms of individual utility, but it can also be defined to include merit goods (such as good health), together with broader goals of equity and social justice. This in turn has implications for whether, and if so how, governments might intervene in the marketplace.

Of particular interest to those in the health promotion field is the use of limited resources in the diagnosis and treatment of preventable disease. The use of BOD/COI information to inform decision-makers about the public health significance of skin cancer was illustrated in Table 15.1. While such descriptive data has important uses, it also has its limitations, particularly as the sole basis to guide resource allocation. For economists, it is not so much the size of the disease burden per se that should guide resource allocation, but rather the efficiency of specific interventions in reducing the disease burden. Economic evaluation includes a set of techniques that economists use to assess efficiency.

Economic evaluation of skin cancer prevention programs is rare, so the case study presented in Section 4 should be of international interest. The purpose of the study was to establish in a general sense whether economic grounds existed to warrant further work to develop a national skin cancer health promotion program in Australia. The economic analysis was preliminary and scene setting and focused on "allocative efficiency" – that is, whether a comprehensive skin cancer prevention program along the lines of the SunSmart program in the State of Victoria represented potential value-for-money vis-à-vis other uses for limited health funds. While notions of cost-effectiveness are inherently subjective and vary from country to country, results below $A30,000 per DALY would be regarded favorably in Australia, having regard to how resources are currently deployed in the health sector.

Note that no attempt was made to address technical/productive efficiency. To answer these aspects of efficiency detailed marginal analysis would be necessary of the design aspects of individual program components and the level of resourcing that each warranted. Note also that adopting the initial perspective of the government as third-party funder simplified the analysis and was adequate for such preliminary assessments. Interestingly, however, sensitivity analysis suggested inclusion of costs impacting on individuals would have an important effect on the cost-effectiveness results. The costs to individuals would be even greater, for example, if the cost of lycra full body swim suits ($A40) was included.

The potential importance of costs falling on individuals in complying with national health promotion programs is an important result. Australian skin cancer primary prevention programs have relegated sunscreen use to secondary priority now for over 10 years. This has been done for a variety of reasons, including costs and concerns about the ease and adequacy of sunscreen application. The substantial increase in costs per DALY created by sunscreens alone reinforces this policy. Natural protection in the use of shade, avoidance of sunlight in the middle of the day and clothing remain the first priorities in the Australian prevention program.

SUMMARY POINTS

- Economic evidence on the efficiency of primary skin cancer prevention is scarce. There is some evidence to suggest, however, that primary prevention along the lines of the SunSmart program in the State of Victoria in Australia has the potential to provide excellent "value-for-money."
- Descriptive COI and BOD information on skin cancer can be informative, but it is not sufficient in its own right to guide resource allocation decisions. Priorities for illness prevention and health promotion should be guided by information that includes the public health significance of health problems, their preventability (efficacy/effectiveness), and their relative cost-effectiveness (efficiency).
- The financial impact on individuals in complying with public health guidelines needs to be borne in mind in framing policy recommendations; as such costs can have a substantial impact on cost-effectiveness results.

IMPLICATIONS FOR PUBLIC HEALTH

Primary skin cancer prevention programs in countries with high or increasing incidence and mortality rates (such as Australia) are likely to have strong economic credentials. Further work is necessary, however, to explore in more detail the value of the relative components of these campaigns as a way of ensuring that they continue to be cost-effective in the long term. The role given sunscreens in such programs, for example, warrants careful attention, particularly given the cost impact on individuals and their families.

Economic evaluation can play an important role, along with other disciplines, in aiding planners to make optimal decisions about what type of skin cancer prevention interventions to undertake, for how long and at what level of investment. For this to occur, however, it is important for planners and decision-makers to become informed users of what the discipline of health economics has to offer. Much is said in the name of "economic theory" that is founded more on ideology than on economic theory or empirical evidence. Users need to be aware when economics is being used in "positive" or "normative" mode and need to be conscious of the important distinctions between the tasks of description, prediction and evaluation.

REFERENCES

1. Musgrave RA (1959) *The Theory of Public Finance.* New York: McGraw-Hill.
2. Evans D (1984) *Strained Mercy: The Economics of Canadian Health Care.* Toronto: Butterworth.
3. Hurley J (2000) An overview of the normative economics of the health sector. In: Culyer A, Newhouse J, eds. *Handbook of Health Economics.* Volume 1A. Amsterdam: Elsevier.
4. Reinhardt U (1998) Abstracting from distributional effects, this policy is efficient. In: Bearer M, Getzen T, Stoddart G, eds. *Health, Health Care and Health Economics: Perspectives on Distribution.* Chichester, UK: Wiley and Sons.
5. Evans D (1998) Towards a healthier economics: reflections on Ken Bassett's problem. In: Bearer M, Getzen T, Stoddart G, eds. *Health, Health Care and Health Economics: Perspectives on Distribution.* Chichester, UK: Wiley and Sons.
6. Fuchs V (1996) Economics, values and health care reform. *Am Econ Rev* **86:** 1-24.
7. Rice T (1998) *The Economics of Health Reconsidered.* Chicago: Health Administration Press.
8. Mathers C, Stevenson C, Carter R, Penm R (1998a) *Disease Costing Methodology Used in the Disease Costs and Impact Study 1993-94.* Canberra: Australian Institute of Health and Welfare (Health and Welfare Expenditure Series No. 3). AIHW Cat. No. HWE 7.
9. Mathers C, Penm R, Sanson-Fisher R, Carter R, Campbell E (1998b) *Health System Costs of Cancer in Australia 1993-94.* Canberra: Australian Institute of Health and Welfare and National Cancer Control Initiative (Health and Welfare Expenditure Series No. 4). AIHW Cat. No. HWE 4.

10. Mathers C, Vos T, Stevenson C (1999) *The Burden of Disease and Injury in Australia.* Canberra: Australian Institute of Health and Welfare. AIHW Cat. No. PHE 17.

11. Murray CJ, Lopez AD (1996) *The Global Burden of Disease: A Comprehensive Assessment of Mortality and Morbidity from Diseases, Injuries and Risk Factors in 1990 and Projected to 2000.* Volume 1, Global Burden of Disease Study and Injury Series. Harvard: Harvard School of Public Health.

12. Magnus K (1991) The Nordic profile of skin cancer incidence. A comparative epidemiological study on the three main types of skin cancer. *Int J Cancer* **47**: 12-19.

13. Ko CB, Walton S, Keczkes K, Bury HPR, Nicholson C (1994) The emerging epidemic of skin cancer. *Br J Dermatol* **130**: 269-272.

14. Carter R, Stone C, Vos T *et al.* (2000) *Trial of Program Budgeting and Marginal Analysis (PBMA) to Assist Cancer Control Planning in Australia.* Report to the Cancer Strategies Group of the National Health Priorities Action Committee of AHMAC, Research Report 19, Centre for Health Program Evaluation.

15. Carter R (1994) A macro approach to economic appraisal in the health sector. *Aust Econ Rev* **106**: 105-112.

16. Cameron IH, McGuire C (1990) Are you dying to get a suntan? The pre- and post campaign survey results. *Health Educ J* **49**: 166-170.

17. Cody R, Lee C (1990) Behaviours, beliefs and intentions in skin cancer prevention. *J Behav Med* **13**: 373.

18. Robinson JR (1990) Behaviour modification obtained by sun protection education coupled with removal of skin cancer. *Arch Dermatol* **126**: 477-481.

19. Borland R (1992) Public awareness and reported effects of the 1989-90 SunSmart campaign. In: *SunSmart Evaluation Studies No. 2*. Melbourne: Anti-Cancer Council of Victoria.

20. Borland R, Hocking B, Godkin G, Gibbs A, Hill D (1991) The impact of a skin cancer control education package for outdoor workers. *Med J Aust* **154**: 686-688.

21. Boldeman C, Jansson B, Holm LE (1991) Primary prevention of malignant melanoma in Swedish urban pre-school sector. *J Cancer Educ* **6**: 247-253.

22. Hill D, White V, Marks R (1993) Changes in suntan-related attitudes and reduced sunburn prevalence in a population at high risk of melanoma. *Eur J Cancer Prev* **2**: 447-456.

23. Carter R, Marks R, Hill D (1999) Could a national skin cancer primary prevention campaign in Australia be worthwhile? An economic perspective. *Health Promot Internat* **14**: 73-81.

24. Murray CJ, Lopez AD (1999) On the comparable quantification of health risks: lessons from the Global Burden of Disease Study. *Epidemiology* **10**: 594-605.

25. Australian Institute of Health and Welfare (AIHW) and Australasian Association of Cancer Registries (AACR) (1999) *Cancer in Australia 1996: Incidence and Mortality Data for 1996 and Selected Data for 1997 and 1998.* Canberra: Australian Institute of Health and Welfare. AIHW Cat. No. CAN 7 (Cancer Series).

26. Australian Institute of Health and Welfare (1999). *Health Expenditure Bulletin No. 15. Australia's Health Services Expenditure to 1997-98.* Canberra: Australian Institute of Health and Welfare (Health and Welfare Expenditure Series).

27. Richardson J (2001). *Economics and Communicable Diseases.* Discussion Paper. Melbourne: Centre for Health Program Evaluation.

28. @RISK [computer software program], Version 4.0 (2001). Newfield, New York: Palisade Corporation.

Chapter 16

Conclusions

David J. Hill[1], Ph.D.; J. Mark Elwood[2], M.D., D.Sc.; Dallas R. English[3], Ph.D.
[1]*Centre for Behavioural Research in Cancer, The Cancer Council Victoria, Melbourne, Victoria, Australia;* [2]*National Cancer Control Initiative, Melbourne, Victoria, Australia;* [3]*Cancer Epidemiology Centre, The Cancer Council Victoria, Melbourne, Victoria, Australia*

In this final chapter, we consider three fundamental questions, based upon the arguments and evidence presented in previous chapters. First, is enough known about the causal pathways leading to skin cancer to make prevention worth considering? Second (and assuming sufficient is known about causation), what techniques for preventive interventions are effective or at least show promise? Third, how much can we expect preventive interventions to achieve in terms of reduced mortality or other benefits?

IS ENOUGH KNOWN ABOUT THE CAUSAL PATHWAYS TO MAKE PREVENTION WORTH CONSIDERING?

The answer to this question is undoubtedly yes. Evidence from epidemiological studies indicates that exposure to sunlight is the predominant cause of skin cancer in populations of European origin. The risks are highest in people with skin that is the most susceptible to the effects of sunlight. Evidence from animal and molecular studies indicates that it is the UVB component of the sun's radiation that is largely responsible, although UVA may play some role in melanoma. Randomized trials have

D. Hill et al. (eds.), Prevention of Skin Cancer, 319-323.
© 2004 *Kluwer Academic Publishers. Printed in the Netherlands.*

demonstrated that reductions in sun exposure can reduce the incidence of squamous cell carcinoma, solar keratoses and nevi.

Exposure early in life appears to be particularly important for basal cell carcinoma and probably for melanoma. This has led to a focus on reducing exposure among children and adolescents. However, exposure later in life is also important for squamous cell carcinoma and probably for melanoma. Randomized trials in adults have shown that reductions in exposure lead rapidly to reduced incidence of squamous cell carcinoma.

The circumstances of exposure and not just the total time people are exposed to sunlight are relevant to skin cancer. The intensity of sunlight and especially its UVB component depends upon the angle of the sun in the sky. Thus, UVB levels are inversely associated with latitude and are highest in summer and in the middle of the day. This means that limiting exposure in the middle of the day during summer has the greatest potential for reducing skin cancer incidence. Uncertainty about the relative potency of UVA and UVB means that it is prudent to use physical barriers that minimize transmission of all UV radiation, such as deep shade, clothing and as a last resort, broad spectrum sunscreens.

The epidemiology of basal cell carcinoma and melanoma is complex. These skin cancers appear to be influenced by individual patterns of exposure to sunlight. More intermittent, recreational, patterns of sun exposure are implicated in basal cell carcinoma and melanoma. On the other hand, squamous cell carcinoma may be influenced only by total exposure. Another complicating feature is that risk is strongly influenced by an individual's sensitivity to sunlight. The complexity of the dose-response relationships, the wide variations in sensitivity to sunlight and the different patterns of exposure in populations of European origin mean that there is no single prevention strategy that will work equally well for all skin cancers in all subgroups. Instead, successful strategies will require tailoring interventions according to the patterns of exposure and possibly also to the underlying sensitivity to sunlight. The best approach will be to encourage sun protection policies and practices that reduce sun exposure in both occupational and recreational settings, with the emphasis being on providing opportunities to reduce exposure in all situations.

WHAT TECHNIQUES FOR PREVENTIVE INTERVENTIONS ARE KNOWN TO BE EFFECTIVE OR AT LEAST SHOW PROMISE?

There is evidence that in populations of European origin exposure to UVR reaches levels that put many individuals at risk of avoidable skin cancer. There is thus plenty of room to lower exposure with the consequent potential to reduce skin cancer rates. It seems likely that many individuals have acted upon health information obtained from media even where no formal health education/health promotion programs have been run. Often these "responsive" individuals will be those with susceptible skins who know full well the effects of intense sunlight on unprotected skin. This informal dissemination has probably done much, at little or no public expense, to contain skin cancer rates.

The next step to consider is a major one: should there be distinct health promotion/health education programs designed to change the sun exposure of targeted at-risk populations or sub-populations? It should be noted that modern definitions of health promotion include "the combination of educational and environmental supports for actions and conditions of living conducive to health" [1]. Hence interventions including policy initiatives and environmental modification should be included as possibilities. For instance, codes of practice relating to the qualities of sunscreen, the use of solaria, occupational exposure to UVR and shade provision in public places.

There is now quite a body of health promotion literature that covers sun-related behavior and strategies to change it. Much of this work has been done among infant and school age groups, for two reasons: accessibility of these groups for research, and the belief that early-life sun exposure might be particularly hazardous.

While it is relatively easy to show improvements in knowledge and attitudes, behavior change has been more difficult to demonstrate in school-based studies. Studies in outdoor recreation settings have been less disappointing, although long-term changes in habitual behavior could not be demonstrated in such studies. Similarly, outdoor workplace studies have shown behavior change effects, at least in the short term. Studies of interventions designed to protect children by changing the behavior of parents and caregivers have had mixed results.

Consistent with health promotion theory, the most promising results are to be found with multi-component, community or population-wide interventions. These attempt to maximize individual and environmental change strategies and include the use of mass-media communications. Unfortunately, such interventions are few in number, and usually do not use randomized prospective designs. Indeed, lack of randomized control groups may be an unavoidable feature of research to assess the effects of multi-component strategies of whole populations. Rather than decry this, it may be more useful to consider other evaluation designs that provide high levels of confidence in attributions of causality, such as well-designed time-series analyses. Only in Australia and parts of the USA can evidence be found of sustained change in sun-related behaviors that are associated with the introduction of multi-component population-wide programs.

HOW MUCH CAN WE EXPECT PREVENTIVE INTERVENTIONS TO ACHIEVE IN TERMS OF REDUCED MORTALITY OR OTHER BENEFITS?

How much can be achieved depends on the size of the problem. The common skin cancers, basal cell and squamous cell carcinoma and melanoma, are significant problems only in light skinned peoples. In more pigment-favored communities, the issues of skin cancer are very different both qualitatively and quantitatively, and this review does not set out to deal with them. Within susceptible populations, the impact of skin cancer varies dramatically depending mainly on the overall intensity of sun exposure. Melanoma is amongst the five most common cancers in terms of incidence in Australia and New Zealand, but falls much further down the ranking in much of North America and Europe. The importance of skin cancer prevention relative to other health needs therefore varies greatly between countries.

Even in high-risk countries, preventive programs have to be justified by showing that the benefits will balance or outweigh the costs. Skin cancers other than melanomas cause few deaths and may be ignored in priority setting exercises dependent on mortality or years of life lost. However, they account for very considerable morbidity and cost; in Australia they are the most expensive cancers in health care costs because of their very large numbers. The impact of preventive programs on costs may however be paradoxical; programs aimed at prevention through avoidance of sun exposure may also encourage, either deliberately or coincidentally, increased awareness of skin lesions which may lead to increased demands on medical care and increased costs.

The clearest justification for preventive programs is in regard to melanoma, because despite the relatively good prognosis this accounts for a considerable number of deaths. Moreover, these occur at younger ages than other cancer deaths, leading to a larger total of years of life lost and greater personal, family and social consequences. Prevention of deaths from melanoma will depend on both reducing incidence and achieving earlier diagnosis. Programs of sun exposure modification that successfully prevent the occurrence of melanoma should also lead to a reduction in other skin cancers.

It is difficult to predict what reduction in sun exposure will result in a useful decrease in skin cancer incidence; a precise quantitative model demands more than our current understanding of the etiology and natural history of skin cancers. We may never have the empiric data necessary to accurately predict changes in incidence from changes in behavior. Better knowledge may come from prospective observational studies comparing populations with different degrees of changing sun exposure, prospective trials of sun exposure behavior modification, or integrated multi-center case-control studies assessing exposure with more precision and detail than has been done before. In Chapter 15, an argument is presented that in an Australian population, community based programs could produce a 20% reduction in total ultraviolet exposure, and that this could result in a 30% reduction in acute sunburn. It is then assumed that this equates to a 30% reduction in skin cancer incidence, both of melanoma and other types, with a lag time of 10 years. Cost benefit analyses have been based on these estimates, plus a range of values around these estimates. These several assumptions are all open to debate, and this assessment takes no account of the varying relationships of different skin cancers to patterns of sun exposure. However, as a first approximation, the results seem generally compatible with recent trends seen in melanoma incidence and mortality in Australia and other countries. This analysis leads to the conclusion that primary prevention programs will produce lower incidence rates of skin cancer, and a reduction in deaths from melanoma. Further, it shows that in Australia costs of about $A5 million annually to carry out a program would lead to health care cost savings of some $A40 million annually after a 10-year interval. This suggests that, even in lower incidence areas, primary prevention programs could be both worthwhile in terms of morbidity and mortality savings, and cost-effective.

REFERENCES

1. Green LW, Kreuter MW (1991) *Health Promotion Planning: An Educational and Environmental Approach* (2nd edition). Mountain View, CA: Mayfield, p4.

Index